PARASITIC ZOONOSES

Clinical and Experimental Studies

ACADEMIC PRESS RAPID MANUSCRIPT REPRODUCTION

Proceedings of the Sixth International Conference of the World Association for the Advancement of Veterinary Parasitology held at the Tierärzliche Hochschule, Vienna, Austria, September 18th to 20th, 1973.

PARASITIC ZOONOSES
Clinical and Experimental Studies

Edited by

E. J. L. SOULSBY

Department of Pathobiology
School of Veterinary Medicine
University of Pennsylvania
Philadelphia, Pennsylvania

ACADEMIC PRESS, INC.

New York San Francisco London 1974
A Subsidiary of Harcourt Brace Jovanovich, Publishers

ACADEMIC PRESS, INC.
111 Fifth Avenue, New York, New York 10003

United Kingdom Edition published by
ACADEMIC PRESS, INC. (LONDON) LTD.
24/28 Oval Road, London NW1

LIBRARY OF CONGRESS CATALOG CARD NUMBER: 74-16429

PRINTED IN THE UNITED STATES OF AMERICA

Contents

*Invited Paper

CONTENTS

*Invited Paper

CONTENTS

*Invited Paper

CONTENTS

*Invited Paper

List of Contributors

Numbers in parentheses indicate the pages on which the authors' contributions begin.

J. ARMOUR, Glasgow University Veterinary School, Bearsden, Glasgow, Scotland, (249)

A. M. ASSMANN, Laboratoire de Parasitologie, Faculté de Medicine de Dijon, France, (27)

J. M. BAFORT, Department of Malariology, Institute of Tropical Medicine, Antwerpen, Belgium, (109)

W. N. BEESLEY, Department of Veterinary Parasitology, Liverpool School of Tropical Medicine, Liverpool, England, (349)

W. P. BERESFORD-JONES, Royal Veterinary College, London, England, (383)

V. K. BEREZHKO, The All-Union K. I. Skryabin Institute of Helminthology, Moscow, USSR, (343)

A. S. BESSONOV, The All-Union K. I. Skryabin Institute of Helminthology, Moscow, USSR, (179)

J. K. A. BEVERLEY, Division of Pathology, University of Sheffield, Sheffield, England, (1)

ERLING BINDSEIL, Department of Pathology, The Royal Veterinary and Agricultural University, Copenhagen, Denmark, (313)

R. S. BRAY, M.R.C. Laboratories, Fajara, Nr. Banjul, The Gambia, (65)

Y. CAMPANA-ROUGET, Laboratoire de Parasitologie, Faculté de Medicine de Dijon, France, (27)

LIST OF CONTRIBUTORS

WILLIE L. CHAPMAN, JR., Department of Medicine and Surgery, College of Veterinary Medicine, University of Georgia, Athens, Georgia 30602, (117)

JULIA J. CHIEN, Department of Parasitology, College of Veterinary Medicine, University of Georgia, Athens, Georgia 30602, (117)

J. D. DARGIE, Glasgow University Veterinary School, Bearsden, Glasgow, Scotland, (249)

H. K. DENNIG, Institut für vergleichende Tropenmedizin der Ludwig Maximillians–Universität, München, Federal Republic of Germany, (79)

W. P. H. DUFFUS, UNDP/FAO Special Fund Project (Ken 22), c/o Veterinary Research Laboratory, P. O. Kabete, Kenya, (85, 97)

N. DŽAKULA, Veterinary Faculty, University of Zagreb, Zagreb, Yugoslavia, (195)

V. S. ERSHOV, The All-Union K. I. Skryabin Institute of Helminthology, Moscow, USSR, (343)

JACQUE A. EUZEBY, École Nationale Veterinaire, Lyon, France, (151)

HENRI GALLIARD, Faculté de Medicine, 15 Rue de l'École de Medicine, Paris VI, France, (295)

G. J. GALLIE, Department of Tropical Animal Health, Royal (Dick) School of Veterinary Studies, Easter Bush, Roslin, Midlothian, Scotland, (187)

RAINER GOTHE, Institute of Parasitology and Parasitic Diseases of Animals, Justus Liebig University, Giessen, Federal Republic of Germany, (369)

WILLIAM L. HANSON, Department of Parasitology, College of Veterinary Medicine, University of Georgia, Athens, Georgia 30602, (117)

I. V. HERBERT, Department of Applied Zoology, University College of North Wales, Bangor, United Kingdom, (199)

G. HÖSL, Institut für vergleichende Tropenmedizin der Ludwig Maximilians–Universität, München, Federal Republic of Germany, (79)

TOSHIO ISHII, Nippon Institute for Biological Sciences, Tokyo, Japan, (35)

F. W. JENNINGS, Glasgow University Veterinary School, Bearsden, Glasgow, Scotland, (133)

P. KAGERUKA, Department of Veterinary Medicine, Institute of Tropical Medicine, Antwerpen, Belgium, (109)

LIST OF CONTRIBUTORS

A. D. KASHINSKY, The All-Union K. I. Skryabin Institute of Helminthology, Moscow, USSR, (343)

KLAUS KUNZE, Department of Clinical Neurophysiology, Center of Neurology, Justus Liebig University, Giessen, Federal Republic of Germany, (369)

J. LAMINA, Abtlg für Parasitologie und Zoologie der TU–München, Federal Republic of Germany, (305)

G. LÄMMLER, Institute for Parasitology and Parasitic Diseases of Animals, Justus Liebig University, Giessen, Federal Republic of Germany, (327)

F. LEVITTE, Laboratoire de Parasitologie, Faculté de Medicine de Dijon, France, (27)

SHEELAGH LLOYD, Department of Pathobiology, School of Veterinary Medicine, University of Pennsylvania, Philadelphia, Pennsylvania 19174, (231)

BARBARA MACHNICKA, Polish Academy of Sciences, Department of Parasitology, Warsaw, Poland, (213)

SUSUMU MAKIMURA, Department of Parasitology, Obihiro University, Hokkaido, Japan, (35)

B. MARAN, Veterinary Faculty, University of Zagreb, Zagreb, Yugoslavia, (195)

P. K. MURRAY, Glasgow University Veterinary School, Bearsden, Glasgow, Scotland, (133)

MAX MURRAY, Glasgow University Veterinary School, Bearsden, Glasgow, Scotland, (133, 249)

M. I. NAUMYTCHEVA, The All-Union K. I. Skryabin Institute of Helminthology, Moscow, USSR, (343)

G. S. NELSON, London School of Hygiene and Tropical Medicine, Keppel Street, London, England, (273)

KATHRYN H. NEPOTE, Department of Pathobiology, School of Veterinary Medicine, University of Pennsylvania, Philadelphia, Pennsylvania 19174, (241)

I. A. NISENBAUM, The All-Union K. I. Skryabin Institute of Helminthology, Moscow, USSR, (343)

CARLOS OBERG, Instituto de Patologia Animal, Facultad de Medicina Veterinaria, Universidad Austral de Chile, Valdivia, Chile, (199)

YOSHITAKA OMATA, Department of Parasitology, Obihiro University, Hokkaido, Japan, (35)

LIST OF CONTRIBUTORS

Z. S. PAWLOWSKI, Clinic of Parasitic Diseases, Medical Academy of Poznan, Poznan, Poland, (241)

JERZY PTASIŃSKI, Clinic of Neurosurgery, Medical Academy, Warsaw, Poland, (223)

MIODRAG RISTIC, College of Veterinary Medicine, University of Illinois, Urbana, Illinois 61801, (41)

EDWARD L. ROBERSON, Department of Parasitology, College of Veterinary Medicine, University of Georgia, Athens, Georgia 30602, (117)

R. RUDOLPH, Institute of Veterinary Pathology, Justus Liebig University, Giessen, Federal Republic of Germany, (327)

E. J. RUITENBERG, Rijks Instituut voor de Volksgezondheid, Bilthoven, Netherlands, (319)

B. RUSHTON, Glasgow University Veterinary School, Bearsden, Glasgow, Scotland, (249)

TJ. SCHILLHORN VAN VEEN, Department of Parasitology and Entomology, Faculty of Veterinary Medicine, Ahmadu Bello University, Zaria, Nigeria, (287)

M. M. H. SEWELL, Department of Tropical Animal Health, Royal (Dick) School of Veterinary Studies, Easter Bush, Roslin, Midlothian, Scotland, (187)

WIESLAW ŚLUSARSKI, Department of Parasitology, Polish Academy of Sciences, Warsaw, Poland, (223)

RONALD D. SMITH, College of Veterinary Medicine, University of Illinois, Urbana, Illinois 61801, (41)

E. J. L. SOULSBY, Department of Pathobiology, School of Veterinary Medicine, University of Pennsylvania, Philadelphia, Pennsylvania 19174, (231, 241)

P. A. STEERENBERG, Rijks Instituut voor de Volksgezondheid, Bilthoven, Netherlands, (319)

NAOYOSHI SUZUKI, Department of Parasitology, Obihiro University, Hokkaido, Japan, (35)

J. S. TEPPEMA, Rijks Instituut voor de Volksgezondheid, Bilthoven, Netherlands, (319)

ISAMU TOMODA, Department of Parasitology, Tokyo University, Tokyo, Japan, (35)

G. M. URQUHART, Glasgow University Veterinary School, Bearsden, Glasgow, Scotland, (133)

R. VOLLERTHUN, Institute of Veterinary Pathology, Justus Liebig University, Giessen, Federal Republic of Germany, (327)

LIST OF CONTRIBUTORS

G. G. WAGNER, U. S. Department of Agriculture, Co-operative Research Project, c/o East African Veterinary Research Organization, Muguga, P. O. Box 32, Kikuyu, Kenya, (85, 97)

T. WIKERHAUSER, Veterinary Faculty, University of Zagreb, Zagreb, Yugoslavia, (195)

H. ZAHNER, Institute for Parasitology and Parasitic Diseases, Justus Liebig University, Giessen, Federal Republic of Germany, (327)

WANDA ZAPART, Intestinal Diseases Consulting Unit, Medical Academy, Warsaw, Poland, (223)

M. ŽUKOVIC, Veterinary Faculty, University of Zagreb, Zagreb, Yugoslavia, (195)

Preface

The zoonoses, those diseases and infections naturally transmitted between animals and man, assume increasing importance in the modern world. In part, this is due to economic development. The increased contact of man with rural or sylvatic environments by tourism and increased leisure time and the increase in domestic pets in urban and suburban areas are a measure of this. In part, it is due to the increasing urbanization, and the need for companion animals, and in part, it is due to factors inimical to economic development, such as the migration of rural populations or refugees to cities, political unrest and natural disasters. Finally, in part, it is due to modifications of the environment wrought by man.

The parasitic zoonoses are represented in the spectrum of the epidemiological situations above and involve considerations related to all aspects of biomedical investigation.

Such considerations, in the past, have provided focal points for conferences of the World Association for the Advancement of Parasitology. This was the situation with the 6th International Conference of the W.A.A.V.P. which provided a forum for discussion on recent research and development in the field of Parasitic Zoonoses.

The core of the conference, and of this volume, are the invited papers by distinguished experts, who have reviewed the present knowledge in their fields of interest. Supporting these are contributions, selected from numerous short communications which are representative of the work in progress on parasitic zoonoses in various countries of the world.

As with the other International Conferences of the W.A.A.V.P., the local flavor of the venue and the hospitality of our hosts provided an added dimension to the meeting. Indeed, the "Parasitic Zoonoses" conference will be remembered by many as the Vienna Conference since the organization and hospitality provided by Professor Supperer and his staff are not likely to be forgotten.

PREFACE

I wish to thank the contributors to the volume for their cooperation in providing manuscripts, the majority of which were received on time. To the staff of Academic Press, Inc., I extend my special thanks for their patience during the preparation of the camera-ready copy. The production of such a volume requires diligence, industry and dedication on the part of secretarial and office staff. Mrs. Margo Bradford, Mrs. Karen Bell and Miss Cleola Taylor have performed outstandingly in producing this volume, and I extend to them my deepest thanks for their assistance.

Finally, to my wife, Annette, I thank her for her patience, forbearance and support during the task of editing and indexing.

E. J. L. Soulsby

Introduction
to the

Sixth International Conference of the
World Association for the Advancement of Veterinary Parasitology

on

Parasitic Zoonoses
Clinical and Experimental Studies

Dr. Georg Lämmler, President
Institute of Parasitology and Parasitic Diseases of Animals
Justus Liebig University, Giessen
Federal Republic of Germany

Magnifizenz, Distinguished guests, Ladies and Gentlemen:

It is my special duty and high honor to call this session to order, and thus open the Sixth International Conference of the World Association for the Advancement of Veterinary Parasitology.

The subject of this conference in Vienna, "Parasitic Zoonoses," was selected in Mexico City, two years ago, with the aim of bringing this important group of diseases to the forefront of scientific interest, public discussion and public awareness.

Zoonotic diseases are problems of considerable magnitude in every country, particularly where domestic animals are the principal reservoirs of infection since man comes into closest contact with such animals. Though once considered to be diseases of rural and sylvatic environments, the zoonoses now occur in the dense urban areas of large cities, often being associated with pet or companion animals such as the dog and cat and also with more exotic pets such as monkeys, reptiles and other animals.

Research in the field of zoonoses in the last few years (e.g., in toxoplasmosis, sarcocystosis and larva migrans) has been extremely dynamic and this conference provides an opportunity to present, discuss and analyse the recent advances in the field. Since the zoonoses represent a field of research involving both human and veterinary medicine, this conference is of interest and significance not only to comparative medicine, but also it emphasizes the need for the concept of "One Medicine" especially "One Experimental Medicine" in biomedical research on disease by veterinary, medical and natural science disciplines.

More than 150 zoonoses are now recognized in the world. On a world wide basis, therefore, zoonoses are the most frequent disease risks to which mankind is exposed. This is particularly true in the tropics and subtropics where arthropod vectors play an important role in the transmission of these communicable diseases. Of these zoonoses, about 100 are of major public health importance, and a considerable number of them are caused directly by parasites or are transmitted by arthropods.

The Joint FAO/WHO-Expert Committees in 1959 and 1967 defined zoonoses as *"those diseases and infection, which are naturally transmitted between vertebrate animals and man."* It has been argued that this definition is too wide and includes not only infections that man acquires from animal, but also diseases produced by non-infective agents, such as toxins and poisons, as well as infections that animals acquire from man, even if they are purely incidental infections and of no public health importance.

Despite these criticisms, the definition has been widely accepted, and is at present recommended by the World Health Organization. On the basis of this definition therefore *"Parasitic Zoonoses are parasitic diseases and infections which are naturally transmitted between vertebrate animals and man."*

Parasitic zoonoses consist predominantly of protozoal and helminthic infections. Opinions differ whether infestations with ectoparasites should be considered as zoonoses. The Expert Committee on Zoonoses of the World Health Organization concluded that if ectoparasites burrow into, or otherwise penetrate the body of the host, they should be considered as zoonoses. However, since there are no specific ectoparasites of man, except the human louse, and arthropods such as insects, ticks and mites which attack man are primarily parasites of animals, it could be debated that these are also zoonotic parasites. Regardless of this, ectoparasites are important vectors of disease, zoonotic or otherwise, and their intimate association with this is sufficient justification for their inclusion in this conference.

Parasitic zoonoses include *obligate zoonoses* which are transmitted from vertebrates only to man and *facultative zoonoses* which will generally be transmitted from man to man or animal to animal respectively, but may infect human beings occasionally.

Zoonoses may also be classified in terms of their reservoir hosts, whether these are man or lower vertebrate animals. The term *anthropozoonoses* has been applied to infections transmitted from man to lower vertebrates and the term *zooanthroponoses* to infections transmitted from lower vertebrate animals to man. Both terms have been used interchangeably for all diseases found in both animals and man, and these terms have served to confuse, rather than clarify. The term "zoonoses" is to be preferred.

The hazards of zoonotic diseases are faced by persons in most walks of life. Traditionally, they are especially serious in agriculturists, animal handlers, meat processors and laboratory workers. Nevertheless, the city dweller may be equally exposed to entities such as toxoplasmosis and visceral larva migrans, either through direct contact with companion animals or through contamination of public places such as parks and playgrounds by domestic pets. Further, the advent of modern advances in medicine such as the immunosuppressive therapy and drugs for transplantation, cancer and allergic disorders has identified the importance of subclinical infections of entities such as toxoplasmosis, babesiosis and malaria to the well being of the immunosuppressed patient.

Therefore, there is much to discuss in this conference. The stage will be set by eight "Invited Papers" by distinguished international experts who will discuss the major parasitic zoonoses. Within this framework, the "Short Communications" will contribute a variety of research findings and epidemiological investigations.

SOME ASPECTS OF TOXOPLASMOSIS, A WORLD WIDE ZOONOSIS

J. K. A. Beverley

Division of Pathology, University of Sheffield, England

The protozoan parasite *Toxoplasma gondii* was discovered in 1908 by Nicolle and Manceaux in generalised fatal infections of captive North African rodents called gondis. At about the same time Splendore (1909) found it in a rabbit. In the ensuing years it was shown to occur in many other animal species but it was not until 1939 that it was first recognised in man by Wolf *et al*. A parasitic cyst was seen in sections of an eye of a blind infant by Janku in 1923. This is now regarded as a toxoplasma cyst. The human infection described by Castellani in 1913 is unlikely to have been toxoplasmosis. Probably the first human infection to be described even though it was not recognised as toxoplasmosis but considered to be atypical sarcosporidiosis, was one reported by Darling (1909, 1910).

Recognition of human infections was an impetus to the development of serological tests. Of the many types of test which were evolved that which has proved to be of greatest use is the "dye test", described by Sabin and Feldman in 1948. Many surveys, both serological and parasitological were then done. These indicated that *T. gondii* had little host specificity, that any warm blooded animal including birds could be infected and that toxoplasmosis was a world wide zoonosis. While infection has been shown to be very common, only relatively rarely is it known to cause ill health.

During this period, therapeutic agents were sought. Sabin and Warren (1942) showed that sulphonamides were of use and Summers (1949) that sulphones were effective. Eyles and

Coleman (1953) discovered the synergy between sulphonamides and pyrimethamine. Garin and Eyles (1958) found spiramycin to be of value while the latest useful agent in experimental infections is clindamycin (McMaster *et al*, 1973).

No historical account, however short, should fail to mention the recent discovery of the role of the cat in transmission of infection, but more of this later.

THE PARASITE

Trophozoites

Toxoplasma trophozoites were the first forms of the parasite to be recognised. When mature these are elongated lemon shaped, are often flattened on one side and one end is more pointed than the other. They measure approximately 5.0μ x 1.5-2.0μ. The nucleus is situated nearer the rounded end. Electron microscopy shows that there are numerous sub-cellular organelles and a micropyle.

Multiplication

Multiplication occurs only in the cytoplasm of a nucleated host cell, usually close to the nucleus. Any cell will serve for this, most commonly it is a reticulo-endothelial cell, but it may even be an avian erythrocyte. A trophozoite actively penetrates the host cell wall using its more pointed end and becomes surrounded by a vacuole like structure (parasitophorous vacuole), inside which endodyogeny occurs. This is a form of internal budding in which the organelles of the parent become dismantled and then reconstructed as two smaller parasites still within the body of the parent. Eventually the original cell membrane of the parent splits open allowing the progeny to move to other parts of the vacuole, there to grow and each to have its twins.

Pseudocyst

By repetitions of this process the host cell cytoplasm becomes distended with parasites and is then known as a terminal colony or pseudocyst. This finally ruptures, liberating 16 or more parasites which tend to be more crescent or bow shaped than the mature forms. They swell in the extracellular fluids and each is then capable of invading another host cell. Spread may be local, across serous cavities, by the blood stream, or along lymphatics. In the first two of these instances the parasites are extracellular while in the last two they are more likely to be inside reticulo-endothelial cells.

Sequence of Events

Multiplication and spread continue until either the host dies or, much more usually, immunity is established. Extra-cellular parasites are then killed and intra-cellular multiplication is slowed. Concurrently with the development of immunity, but not necessarily because of it, tissue cysts develop. These probably arise as a result of the expulsion of a parasitophorous vacuole and its contained toxoplasma from the host cell. Such vacuoles have an elastic membrane which is made up of components from both host and parasite. Cysts enlarge slowly, taking about three weeks to double their volume and, presumbaly, to double the number of contained parasites. These are similar to, but smaller than, trophozoites and are known as zoites. A small cyst may contain only a few zoites but a large one many thousands. Intact cysts do not provoke an inflammatory reaction but should one rupture a local delayed hypersensitivity type reaction may develop. Cysts are found most frequently in the brain, less often in skeletal muscle and the heart and, more rarely, in the lung. They persist for many months or years, possibly even for the lifetime of the host.

Strain differences

Strains of toxoplasma vary in their virulence. Some kill small laboratory animals such as mice, hamsters or rabbits in 7-10 days. Others do not, but cause a life-long infection even though the animal remains apparently healthy. Infection with a strain of low virulence causes immunity to a subsequent challenge with a high virulence strain. The immunity, however, is only partial for, while the animal survives the challenge, superinfection takes place.

CLINICAL MANIFESTATIONS IN MAN

These may be the result of congenital or post-natally acquired infections.

Congenital infection

Congenital infection occurs only when a woman has a primary infection during pregnancy. While this rarely causes the mother any harm she does have a temporary parasitaemia which may lead to placental infection. When this happens minute focal lesions develop and on rupture toxoplasms are discharged into the foetal circulation. Foetal infection is at first generalised and it may cause exudates (which may be blood-stained) in the body cavities, oedema of connective tissues, lymphadenopathy, hepato-splenomegaly with or without jaundice, and bone marrow dysfunction. If, as it often does, the foetus survives this stage the infection is cleared from the viscera and resolution of the pathological changes takes place. Even so, the infection then becomes localised in the central nervous system.

Abortion

The severity of clinical manifestations varies enormously and depends on the degree of foetal damage. This in turn depends partly on the virulence of the infecting strain and partly on the duration of gestation at the time of foetal infection. Thus, infection early in pregnancy probably leads to abortion and toxoplasma has been isolated from the products of abortion (Magnuson, 1951; Wildfuhr, 1954). This does not mean that toxoplasmosis is a common cause of abortion; Feldman and Eichenwald (1953) failed to find evidence of active toxoplasmosis in any of 95 women who had abortion and Kimball *et al* (1971) found that none of 260 abortions were due to toxoplasmosis. If infection occurs late in pregnancy the child may appear normal at birth only to develop signs of infection when 4-12 weeks of age. Between these extremes, infection leads to signs of active disease at birth, if infection has occurred earlier, to a live child with quiescent or even healed lesions, while if the infection is still earlier it may lead to intrauterine death. It is not uncommon for each of twins to be infected but only one of them to have signs; the reasons for this are unknown.

Pathological changes are found more frequently in the central nervous system than in the viscera and somatic tissues. By far the commonest site is the eye and the basic change is a focal infiltration with round cells which, in the case of a large focus, tends to undergo central necrosis. The foci vary in number as well as in size. They may be so numerous and so close together that they become confluent.

Ocular disease

Very occasionally infection spreads throughout the globe causing a panophthalmitis and leaving a useless microphthalmic eye which is generally noticed at or very soon after birth. Nearly always, however, the changes are confined to the posterior chamber and involve both the choroid and retina. One or both eyes may be affected and lesions may be multiple though commonly they are single. Areas of acute choroidoretinitis or areas of destroyed uveal tissue are readily seen with an ophthalmoscope. The former are irregular shaped yellowish raised areas with imprecise edges and are often found alongside or bridging the retinal vessels. Inflammatory exudates cloud the vitreous so making the view of the fundus hazy or even obscuring it. As the acute processes subside, the vitreous clears, destroyed retina and choroid are removed leaving the underlying white sclera clearly visible. Sometimes the ciliary vessels can be seen crossing such a scar and proliferation of choroidal pigment can be seen at the edges of the lesion or even straddling it.

When very large areas are destroyed, a white reflection instead of a red one may be noticed on shining a light into the eye and be seen by an observant mother or midwife. A smaller lesion involving the macula will cause a squint, often first noticed at about the time the child should be developing binocular vision. If both macular areas are affected, a searching nystagmus occurs instead of a squint. The squint may be convergent, divergent or vertical. Lesions near but not involving the macula may not be found until early school age when defective vision is first suspected. Others in more peripheral areas may not cause signs and symptoms until early adulthood when a reactivation may occur and cause exudates in the vitreous and cloudiness of vision. Such reactivations are commoner in women especially in relation to pregnancy and lactation. Other lesions may not be found until still later when a complication such as detachment of the retina develops or when the presbyopic age is reached and an ophthmoscopic examination is made for the first time.

Intracerebral calcification

Changes may also occur in the brain. While some of them are uncommon they are more dramatic. The lesion is basically the same round cell infiltration. Meningeal signs may develop but these are rarely a predominant feature. Much more often the principal change is in the brain. Here the infiltrations are focal, are accompanied by oedema and glial proliferation and tend to undergo necrosis. Healing is often accompanied by calcification which may be sufficiently dense to be visible on x-rays. A common site for these calcified lesions is the sub-ependymal tissues of the walls of the ventricles. Here calcium is deposited in thin sheets which in "end-on" views appear as curvilineal streaks in line with the ventricular walls. Elsewhere, calcified areas are of irregular shape. In x-rays of some patients, both types can be seen.

Hydrocephalus

Should flakes of necrotic tissue in the walls of the lateral ventricles be shed, reach the aqueduct of Sylvius and block it, or, should inflammatory lesions develop in the walls of the aqueduct an obstructive internal hydrocephalus with a large head and gaping sutures will develop. Sometimes there is so much loss of brain tissue as to cause a non-obstructive internal hydrocephalus with microcephaly. Hydrocephalus is present in only about 3 percent of congenital toxoplasmosis.

Oligosymptomatic

On the other hand, changes in the central nervous system may be relatively minor. The smaller they are the greater is the time lapse before they produce signs and symptoms. Some are not noticed until later childhood. Included in these are mental defect (usually high grade), fits, psycho-motor retardation, paraesthesiae and palsies. Thalhammer (1961) calls these lesser and delayed manifestations oligosymptomatic toxoplasmosis.

Congenital toxoplasmosis has been variously estimated as occurring as frequently as 1 per 500 to as few as 1 per 20,000 births. The incidence varies from country to country.

Acquired infection

Acquired infections in man are not so well known as congenital ones and are not so disabling. While they have been recognised for a much shorter time they are proving to be more common. There are four clinical types, three acute, and one chronic. The three acute varieties include lymphadenopathy, lymphadenopathy with involvement of one other organ, and generalised toxoplasmosis.

Lymphadenopathy - clinical

By far the commonest of these is lymphadenopathy. This was first recognised by Siim (1951). The severity may vary from one patient who has a solitary enlarged node, found by accident, to another who has a protracted pyrexial illness warranting a lengthy convalescence. Any node, group of nodes or groups of nodes may be affected. The number varies from one to a score or more. Those most frequently involved are the upper deep cervical and this may indicate that the nasopharynx is often the portal of entry. Those least often affected are the inguinal and then usually as part of a generalised lymphadenopathy. The nodes are tender but not painful and the larger ones may measure as much as 3.0 cm. They are always discrete and they always resolve spontaneously though this may take several weeks. Relapses are prone to occur when the same nodes re-enlarge or others become enlarged.

Not infrequently the toxoplasmic nature of a lymphadenopathy is doscovered unexpectedly as on examining lymph nodes found at laparotomy for suspected acute abdominal emergency, or on finding enlarged hilar nodes on x-rays taken on account of chest symptoms. If resolution is slow, Hodgkin's disease, or lymphosarcoma or even carcinoma of the axillary tail of the breast may be suspected. Histological examination of the consequent biopsy may then point to a toxoplasmic aetiology.

Approximately one half of patients have a low grade pyrexia, one half (not necessarily the same half) have a feeling of general malaise and fatigue, a third have muscle pains and a fifth sore throat and headache. Headache may be severe and when combined with neck muscle pain may suggest meningitis. Rashes are uncommon but when one is present it is usually measles-like. As a rule the spleen is not sufficiently enlarged to be palpable. Differential leucocyte counts rarely show a polymorphonuclear leucocytosis but quite often a moderate increase in lymphocytes with varying numbers of abnormal mononuclears. Eosinophilia is uncommon and the Paul Bunnell test is negative. Toxoplasmosis is proving to be the commonest diagnosed cause of non-suppurative, Paul-Bunnell negative lymphadenopathy.

Lymphadenopathy - laboratory diagnosis

The diagnosis can be established by finding high or preferably rising titres of toxoplasma antibodies, or, by isolating toxoplasma from lymph node biopsies. Often the possibility of toxoplasmosis is first considered as a result of histological examination of a lymph node biopsy. The changes seen are essentially reactive and were first described by Piringer-Kuchinka (1952). They include hyperplasia of the follicles with active germinal centres in which there are large pale histiocytes, often containing phagocytosed nuclear debris. In the interfollicular pulp are aggregates of palely eosinophilic cells. Plasma cells are present in variable numbers, most often in the cortex. While these changes are a strong indication of toxoplasmosis they are not pathognomonic. Confirmation by antibody tests or by isolation is necessary.

Lymphadenopathy with involvement of another organ

The second type, lymphadenopathy with involvement of another organ, is not nearly so common. The other organ may be lung, heart, liver, skeletal muscle or brain. The clinical presentation is due mainly to the pathological changes in the other organ, yet, quite often, toxoplasmosis is not suspected until the relatively minor lymphadenopathy is investigated. X-rays of the chest, taken because of chest symptoms, may disclose enlarged hilar nodes in the absence of lymphadenopathy elsewhere in addition to lung changes. Involvement of the heart usually shows as cardiac irregularity not as myocardial insufficiency. Hepatitis is generally accompanied by splenomegaly. Myositis can be severe enough to be disabling but it occurs more often in minor for as muscle pain or fatigue. Central nervous system manifestations are due more to encephalitis than to meningitis.

Generalised toxoplasmosis

Generalised toxoplasmosis is also rare. It may follow accidental laboratory infections with strains of high virulence or, more usually, be associated with primary or secondary immunological deficiency states or with immunosuppressive treatment. As yet it is not known whether these are due to primary infections in patients with defective immune systems or if they are due to recrudescences of long standing latent infections developing in patients when their immune systems reach a low level of efficiency. Pyrexia and symptoms pointing to involvement of several organs, particularly of the brain, should arouse suspicion in such patients.

Chronic toxoplasmosis

Chronic acquired toxoplasmosis is even more rare. A few authentic instances of choroido-retinitis are known. These can be distinguished from reactivations of congenital infections by the absence of old scars with characteristic deposits of choroidal pigment and by the presence of higher antibody titres than would be expected in a long standing congenital infection since titres do not rise as a result of reactivations. Cerebral granuloma has been described. Repeated abortion is postulated by some to be a manifestation of chronic toxoplasma infection but as yet the evidence for this is far from complete.

COMPARATIVE PATHOLOGY

Parasitaemia occurs early and it is probable that all organs become infected. Histological changes can be found in many but not all organs in the majority of host species. They occur only very rarely in the kidneys of any species and only rarely in any organ of rats. The changes develop irrespective of the virulence of the infecting strain except that in high virulence infections (causing death of susceptible animals in 7-10 days) there may not be sufficient time for them to develop fully. They even occur when the infection is a symptomless experimental one, or one deemed to be subclinical. The changes are of two types, inflammatory and reactive.

Inflammatory changes

Inflammatory changes occur in non-lymphoid organs and consist of round cell infiltrations, mainly of lymphocytes but with some plasma cells and macrophages. Eosinophils are rare. The infiltrations tend to be focal in such tissues as brain (Fig. 1 & 2), lung and liver (Fig. 3), or interstitial in the heart (Fig. 4) and skeletal muscle (Fig. 5). The larger focal lesions in brain and liver tend to undergo central necrosis while the large interstitial ones are associated with fibre necrosis. In the lung, resolution does not take place in the larger lesions (Fig. 6). Instead there is organisation with eventual fibrosis. Fibrosis also occurs in the heart, skeletal muscle and liver. Healing may be accompanied by calcification as in the human brain, lamb brain and ovine placenta. The foci may be so numerous in part of an organ as to become confluent and are then visible to the naked eye (Figs. 7 & 8).

Reactive changes

Reactive changes are found in the lymph nodes, spleen and thymus of mammals. Those seen in the lymph nodes are similar to those which occur in man. They consist of follicular hyperplasia with active germinal centres in which there are large pale actively phagocytic macrophages and the development of variable numbers of plasma cells mainly in the medulla (Fig. 9). In the spleen there are hyperplastic follicles with active germinal centres (Fig. 10). Between the follicles there is dilation of the sinusoids, proliferation of sinus-lining cells and plasma cells. The cell cords show groups of darkly staining lymphocytes. During the first few weeks of infection, especially in young animals, depletion of lymphocytes occurs in the thymic cortex, but, repopulation takes place towards the end of the second and during the third month.

The reactive changes in birds are somewhat different. There is follicular hyperplasia in the spleen and lymphoid deposits in various organs are the equivalent of the lymph nodes of mammals. Reactive follicles with pale histocytes develop in such deposits (Fig. 11). Similar active follicles also develop in the bursa of Fabricius (Fig. 12).

Sequence of change

The inflammatory changes develop 7-14 days after infection and are usually maximal in the third and fourth weeks. The infiltrating cells are mainly lymphocytes with some macrophages and some plasma cells. Polymorphonuclear cells are rare. Thereafter inflammation gradually subsides so that at 12 weeks there is little activity. Fibrosis is then the main finding but residual stromal elements can be seen. The changes in lymph nodes and spleen likewise develop early and are usually maximal at about the same time as the inflammatory changes in non-lymphoid organs. It is possible that these changes are immunologically mediated and that the lymph nodes and spleen are concerned with the production of sensitized lymphocytes which are then taken to the site of the inflammatory changes. Further, the depletion of cortical lymphocytes which occurs in the thymus of young animals may be due to a heavy call for them at the site of the lesions, in the lymph nodes and in the spleen in order to cope with the cellular aspects of immunity needed to counter the infection.

These basic histopathological changes have been found in many species - man, chimpanzee, marmoset, pig, sheep, foetal lamb, guinea pig, rabbit, ferret, mouse, crow and pigeon. The degree of change and the organ preference vary somewhat with the host species and even within a single species the organ preference will vary from individual to individual. Whether signs and symptoms develop and the nature of these depends on the size and frequency of lesions and in which particular organ(s) they become prominent.

Histological diagnosis

Toxoplasma cysts do not provoke an inflammatory reaction and only rarely are they found near one. Even when they are, they still appear intact and unchanged by the inflammation unless there has been extensive necrosis. Intracellular aggregates of toxoplasma can be seen in some of the small inflammatory infiltrates before necrosis has occurred. These can be recognised with less certainty than cysts. On the other hand, intact extra-cellular forms are conspicuous by their absence after the first week or 10 days. Immunofluorescent techniqeus may not reveal them, but these do show non-particulate toxoplasma antigen in the cytoplasm of host reticulo-endothelial cells.

Serological responses

Titres of toxoplasma antibody rise rapidly to a maximum in 4-6 weeks, are maintained at this level for a few weeks and then fall steadily. However, there are variations from this generalisation. Using the same test on sera from different species show that there are great differences in the peak titres. In the coypu, titers may be in several hundreds of thousands, in rabbits tens of thousands, in man, guinea pigs and sheep several thousands, in cats high hundreds, in dogs and pigs low hundreds, while in rats and birds often less than 100. Similarly, titres remain fairly high for many months and detectable for many years in those species which develop high peaks but may fall below the level of detection in a few months in pigs, rats and birds.

Clinical manifestations

The histopathological changes suggest a great variety of clinical manifestations in animals. Some of these are better known, possibly because they are more easily noticed. Enteritis may result from extensive invasion of the mucosa following large scale ingestion of parasites. There may even be ulceration. Pneumonitis is common and tends to be much more severe when in association with virus infection. Disabling myositis is being quite frequently shown to be due to toxoplasmosis. Perhaps the most readily appreciated or the most clamant clinical manifestation is due to brain involvement. Encephalomyelitis occurs in new born lambs, cats, dogs and many other smaller animals.

Pigs

Pigs are part of this anthroprozoonosis and while infection is common in this species in many parts of the world, reported instances of clinical manifestations are rare. Attempts at producing clinically manifest infections with either highly or lowly virulent strains in sero-negative pigs have often failed, as have attempts at producing congenital infection comparable with that in sheep. These experimental findings could be taken to indicate a species resistance similar to that which is found in rats but this speculation would be contrary to the findings that naturally occurring infection is very common. Three other apparently unrelated observations may be relevant. Firstly, isolations of toxoplasma are frequently made from healthy sero-negative pigs at the time they are killed in the abattoirs. Secondly, while antibodies develop following infection, titres fall rapidly to low levels during the ensuing year. Thirdly, Janitschke and Wormuth (1970), using piglets delivered by Caesarian section and reared in near sterile surroundings, found them to develop clinical illness after experimental infection, even with lowly virulent cyst producing strains. One could deduce from this that natural infection is very common in pigs, that antibodies soon fall below the level of detection but that cellular immunity is still retained and this this is of more protective value than humoral immunity.

Sheep

Sheep also are part of the zoonosis. Primary infection of pregnant ewes does not harm the ewe itself but leads to congenital infection. The severity of this depends on the duration of gestation at the time of infection. Early, at about 45-55 days, it causes death of the foetus and the expelled products of conception are so small that they are unlikely to be seen by shepherds and the ewe is therefore presumed to be barren. Such small foetuses may be resorbed instead of being expelled. Most of the expelled foetuses which are submitted for examination are of at least 90 days development. They may be in good condition or macerated depending on the time interval between foetal death and expulsion. Infection of the ewe at 120 days or later will cause foetal infection but not death. The lambs are usually born alive and if, as most of them do, they survive the first few days they continue to grow and develop normally.

The main pathological change is in the placenta so much so that even though there are changes in the foetus we believe that foetal death is due to placental insufficiency. The inter-cotyledonary parts are not affected. Foci of necrosis are present in the villous part of the cotyledons and are uniformly distributed within a cotyledon - they are not predominantly near either the maternal or the foetal aspects. The size of the lesions varies from microscopic to 2.0 mm and they may be so numerous as to be confluent. In the same placenta, some cotyledons are markedly affected while others have only microscopic changes. Ewes having aborted in one year generally lamb normally in subsequent years, indicating a persistence of effective immunity similar to that in man, but this is in contrast to some rodents. In rodents congenital infection can occur in each of successive pregnancies, even though the mother is not re-infected.

Factors influencing outcome of infection

There are several factors which may adversely affect the outcome of toxoplasma infections. Among these are captivity, malnutrition, exposure to cold, extremes of age, endocrine disorders, pregnancy, lactation, concurrent malignancy and concomitant infections. One of the most interesting of these is concomitant infection. The association between distemper and toxoplasmosis in dogs and between respiratory distress and toxoplasmosis in cats are both well known. If focal hepatitis is found in a dog with distemper search should be made for evidence of toxoplasmosis. We have observed many instances of canine toxoplasmosis when investigating supposed breakdown of distemper vaccination, both with measles and with distemper derived live attenuated vaccines. In most of these the illness has started within 4-6 weeks of vaccination. The relation between measles and distemper viruses is also well known. Measles and some other virus infections are known to depress cellular immunity and even cause a tuberculin positive individual to become temporarily tuberculin negative. Live attenuated measles vaccine will also cause a reversion to the tuberculin negative state. Thus such infections or vaccinations may have an adverse effect on concurrent toxoplasma infection since it is believed that immunity to toxoplasma is dependent more on cellular factors than on humoral ones.

EPIDEMIOLOGY

General

Perhaps the most exciting of recent developments in our knowledge of toxoplasmosis is the discovery of the role of the cat in the transmission of infection. Prior to this, it was known that sources of infection were numerous since the infection is widespread in many animal species. It was also known that different strains of toxoplasma show no species specificity. Two forms of the parasite were recognised, zoites inside cysts and trophozoites. The former are present mainly in brain and skeletal muscle and to a lesser extent in the heart of many healthy as well as sick animals, whatever the cause of the sickness. Trophozoites are present in relatively small numbers in the tissues of healthy animals with subclinical infections and then only for a few days; they are present abundantly in most tissues, exudates and in some excretions of animals acutely ill or dying from toxoplasmosis but such severe infections are not common. One source worthy of special mention is the products of ovine conception when ovine abortion or still birth has been caused by toxoplasmosis. The placenta alone may contain many thousands of infectious doses.

It was also known that toxoplasma can enter by almost any portal - conjunctival, nasal, pharangeal, respiratory and percutaneous. They can even enter by the intestinal mucous membrane, though trophozoites require protection from the action of the gastric juices. This is achieved when infected tissue is consumed in contra distinction to exudates and other fluids. Experiments have shown that the minimal infecting dose for both cysts and trophozoites is much less by the upper respiratory route than by the alimentary one.

But, little was known about the mode of transfer except in congenital infections, accidental laboratory infections, those in predators, carnivors and scavengers, and those man due to consumption of raw or grossly undercooked meat. One other circumstance was known, vertical transmission through several generations in some rodents. This could maintain a nidus of infection for predatory animals. There were still many unexplained infections as in herbivores, in vegetarians and in human beings who eat only well cooked meat. The main difficulty seemed that neither cysts containing zoites nor trophozoites are resistant to even mildly adverse conditions.

Intestinal cycle in cats

Then came the discovery that on gaining the cat intestine exogenous toxoplasma undergo a coccidian cycle (Frenkel *et al*, 1970; Galuzo and Kriskova, 1970; Hutchison *et al*, 1970; Overdulve, 1970; Sheffield and Melton, 1969; Wieland and Kuhn, 1969; Witte and Pierkarski, 1970; and Zaman, 1970). Briefly, in the cytoplasm of epithelial cells at or near the tips of villi and usually near the brush border, the parasite multiplies by schizogony. On rupture of the host cell the released merozoites either invade other adjacent epithelial cells or penetrate the mucous membrane. Those which penetrate become what we have in the past called trophozoites and initiate a systemic infection. Those which invade other surface cells develop either into more schizonts or into gametes. After fertilization macrogametes develop into oocysts which are shed into the lumen of the gut and passed in the faeces without further development.

Oocysts

Within 48-72 hr of being voided, depending on the temperature, oocysts become sporulated with the formation of two sporocysts each containing four sporozoites. These are infective for all the warm blooded hosts so far tested. Ingestion is not necessary for excystment since it will follow injection. As would be expected, sporulated oocysts are much more resistant than are tissue cysts and trophozoites.

The pre-patent period and the patent period vary depending on the initial infecting form of the parasite (Wallace, 1973). If this is as zoites in cysts the prepatent period is 4-5 days and the patent period about 2 weeks. If it is as sporulated oocysts the periods are 3-7 weeks and about 1 week respectively. For trophozoites the two periods are each intermediate between those for the other two forms. Peak production develops within the first two days and continues for 4-5 days. The daily output of oocysts at the peak period has been estimated from 10^5 to 10^7.

So far, excretion of toxoplasma oocysts has been observed

only in the family Felidae and within this family only in two genera - Lynx and Felis. The species are European lynx, domestic cat, Bengal cat, ocelot and jaguar (Janitschke and Wemer, 1972; Jewell *et al*, 1972; Miller *et al*, 1972).

Oocyst production does not always follow infective feeds. It occurs in most domestic cats when they are fed tissue cysts (zoites), in about half when fed trophozoites and in only a quarter of those given oocysts, even when these are given in large doses (Wallace, 1973). This relative resistance of cats to infection by oocysts suggests that other animals which are likely to be a source of infected food for cats are necessary intermediate hosts.

Re-feeding toxoplasma tissue cysts to cats soon after the end of the patent period does not cause a further production of oocysts but re-feeding after an interval of several months will do so. Dubey and Frenkel (1972) have observed the persistence of gametes in the intestinal mucosa after the end of the patent period and Chessum (1972) has described what appears to be an interesting re-activation of toxoplasma oocyst production. A toxoplasma infected cat had a patent period from day 5 to day 14. Subsequent feeding of *Isopora felis* oocysts 110 days after the original toxoplasma infected feed was followed by production not only of *I. felis* oocysts but also *T. gondii* oocysts. The latter were found on days 119-122 and days 132-134.

Riuz, Frenkel and Cerdas (1973) have isolated toxoplasma from soil in a yard frequented by numerous cats while Fleck *et al* (1972) has found evidence of toxoplasma infection in a child's sandpit. Earthworms have been shown to tranport oocysts (Dubey, Miller and Frenkel, 1970). Cockroaches (Wallace, 1972) and filth flies (Wallace, 1971) have also been shown to have a potential mechanical role in the dissemination of oocysts. Another probable instance of mechanical transport has been reported by Pampiglioni *et al* (1973). They found sporulated oocysts in freshly voided faeces of a cat passed on the third day after feeding it with sporulated oocysts.

Population surveys

All this work stimulated many population surveys, most of them serological. These were based on the premise that following toxoplasma infection, and irrespective of whether this caused disease or not, antibodies to toxoplasma develop and persist for many years, possibly for life. Another assumption and one with which most will agree is that toxoplasma antibody tests are specific. The surveys were designed to assess the extent of the part played by cats in the spread of toxoplasmosis. Wallace (1969) has shown that human infection was virtually absent on Euripik, a Pacific atoll on which there were no cats but was present on two nearby ones where there were cats. He and his colleagues (Wallace *et al*, 1972) also showed the absence of infection in rats on the cat free island of Umap and its presence on two other islands of the group on which there were cats. Munday (1972) found that sheep bred on cat free islands in the Bass Strait were free of infection whereas it was present in those bred on cat infested islands. Peterson *et al* (1972) found that the risks of infection due to cat ownership, to living on a farm and to eating raw meat were not inconsiderable. Baruzzi (1970) found that a half of 254 Indian villagers of the Upper Xingu River, Central Brazil, had toxoplasma antibodies even though there were no cats in the villages. This contrary evidence was soon countered by Jewell *et al* (1972) who suggest that infection was derived by contact with soil contaminated by oocysts disseminated by wild felines.

Wallace (1973) examined 1,604 stray or unwanted cats over a two year period on the island of Oahu, Hawaii and found in the faeces of 12 of them oocysts which were proved to be toxoplasma oocysts and, in another 11, toxoplasma-like oocysts which were not proven to be toxoplasma. The incidence of toxoplasma oocyst excretion was higher in young cats of 6 or more months old. None was found in cats younger than this nor in any cats in the period of January to June. He suggests that this is related to the cat breeding season and to young cats being more prone to primary infection and consequent oocyst production during the early months of their search for wild life food. Dubey (1973) found a higher prevalence of antibodies in stray cats than in domiciled ones and that there was no oocyst excretion in any of 510 domiciled cats from Kansas City. However, he did isolate toxoplasma from the tissues of 8 kittens aged 12-16 wk out of 11 which were suspected of having active toxoplasmosis because they had dye test antibody titres of 1:64 or more.

Non-cat transmission

On the other hand, instances of non-cat transmission to man are well known. Desmonts *et al* (1965) showed that when a group of children in an institution were given a new diet including additional raw or undercooked meat, this change was followed by a rise to 9 percent per month in the conversion rate from sero-negative to sero-positive. Kean *et al* (1969) have reported a minor outbreak of toxoplasmic lymphadenopathy in a group of students and attributed this to eating raw beefburgers. However they were not certain that the meat was entirely beef; it may have contained either pork or mutton or both.

Statistics in Britain

In Britain, the main known problem caused by toxoplasmosis in the veterinary field is ovine abortion and still birth. Six surveys from 1958 to 1968 indicate that from 9.5 to 25 percent of these are due to this infection. On the basis of these surveys we estimate that annual lamb losses in Britain due to toxoplasmosis are 80,000 to 100,000. Even now we do not know how infection is transmitted to a flock. Contact between hill sheep and cats must be very remote.

The frequency of human clinical grade toxoplasmosis in Britain has been estimated on the basis of high toxoplasma dye test antibody titres. The total number of patients in 1963 was 347, in 1967, 609, in 1969, 762 and in 1971, 1,071. Approximately one half of these had ocular complaints and one third lymphadenopathy or pyrexia of uncertain origin. The gradual rise in numbers is probably due to increased clinical awareness and the consequent increased use of laboratory diagnostic facilities.

CONCLUSION

Despite the recent observations on the cat cycle there remain many unanswered questions in the epidemiology of human and animal toxoplasmosis. While the "dye test" is a specific and a sensitive test, it is both a difficult and an expensive test. Were a simple, reliable, specific and sensitive test to be discovered, it would prove a boon in epidemiological investigations. One of the major deficiencies of our present knowledge is the lack of any clear understanding of the diverse clinical presentations of toxoplasmosis in its many hosts. When these two needs have been met we can look forward to many interesting advances in our understanding of this zoonosis.

Acknowledgements

I wish to thank my many colleagues, both medical and veterinary, for all their help, interest and readiness to invite me to participate in clinical situations. In particular I wish to thank my colleague in the Division, Dr. Laurence Henry, for his major share in the histopathological investigations. The Photographic Department of the United Sheffield Hospitals gave much willing help.

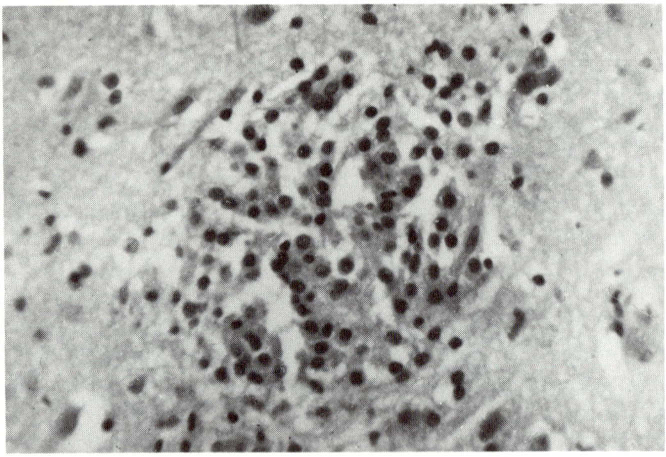

Fig. 1. Focus of lymphocytic infiltration in grey matter of cat brain.

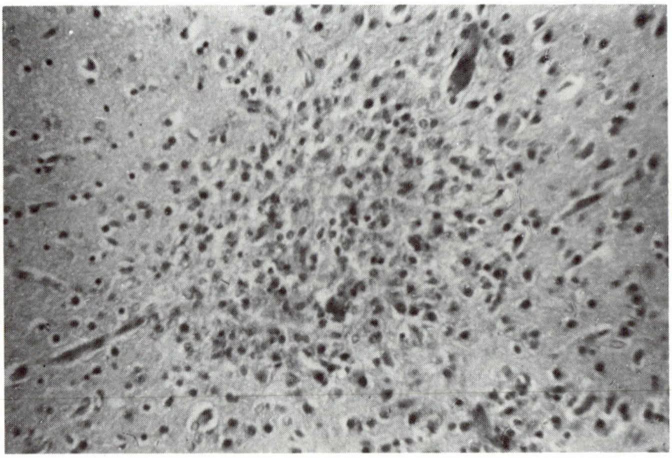

Fig. 2. Focus of lymphocytic infiltration in foetal lamb brain. This focus is larger than that in Fig. 1, and it is undergoing central necrosis. Immunologically mediated inflammatory responses do occur in the foetus of some species.

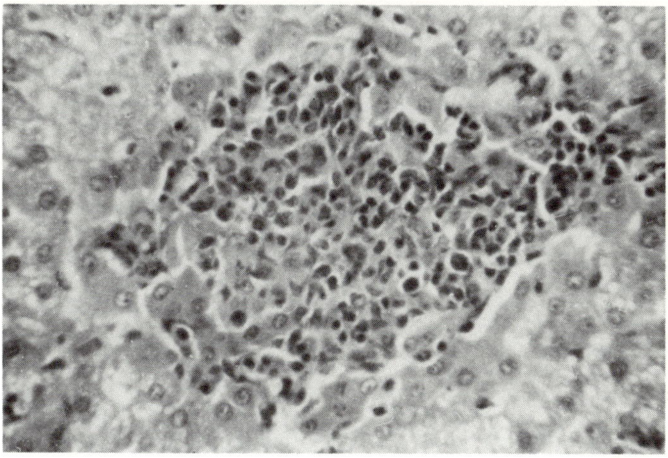

Fig. 3. Focus of lymphocytic infiltration in sheep liver with necrosis of liver cells.

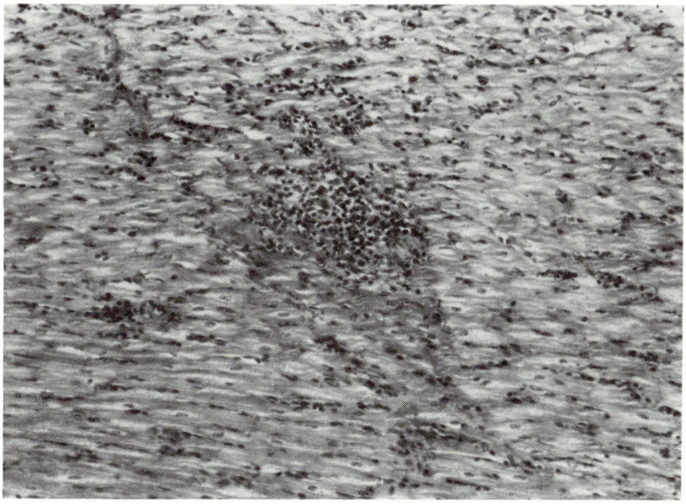

Fig. 4. Interstitial lymphocytic infiltration in rabbit myocardium.

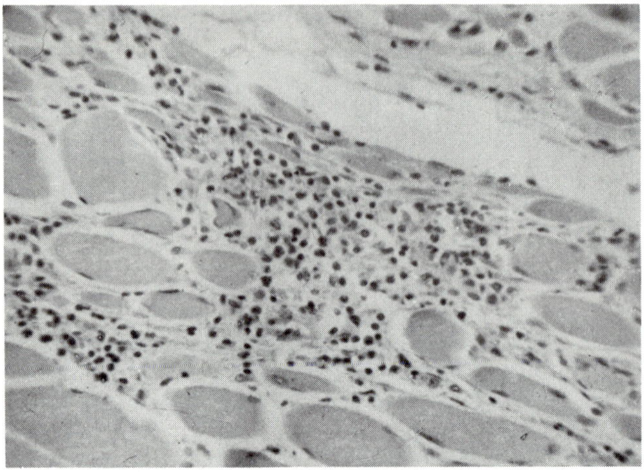

Fig. 5. Interstitial lymphocytic infiltration and fibre necrosis in dog skeletal muscle.

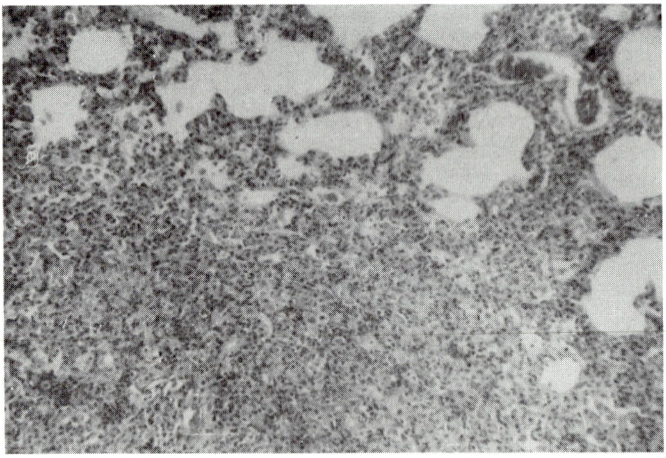

Fig. 6. Edge of organising focus of penumonitis in guinea pig.

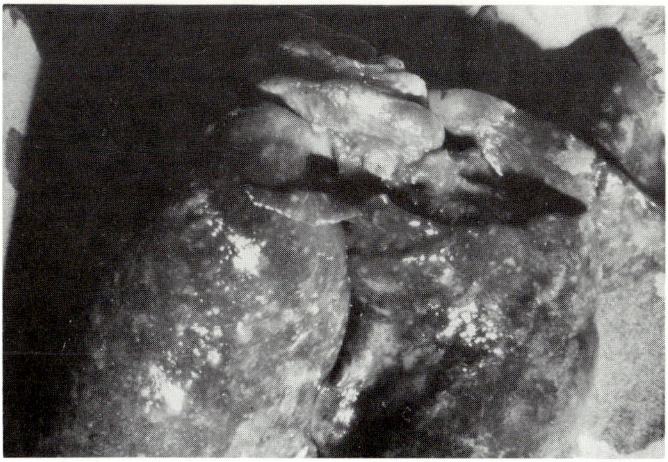

Fig. 7. Macroscopic foci of pneumonitis in dog.

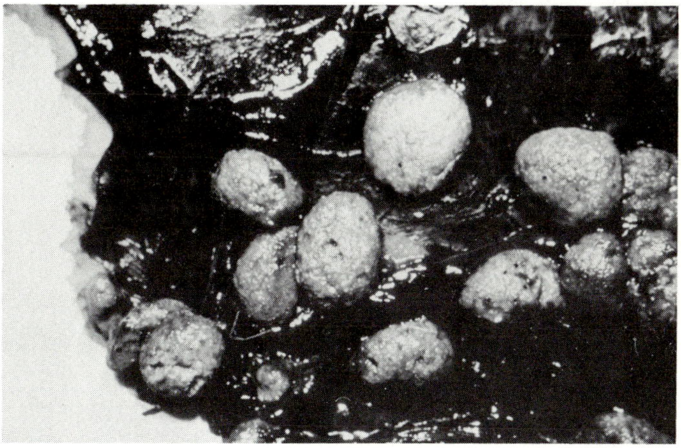

Fig. 8. Almost confluent macroscopic foci of necrosis in sheep cotyledons.

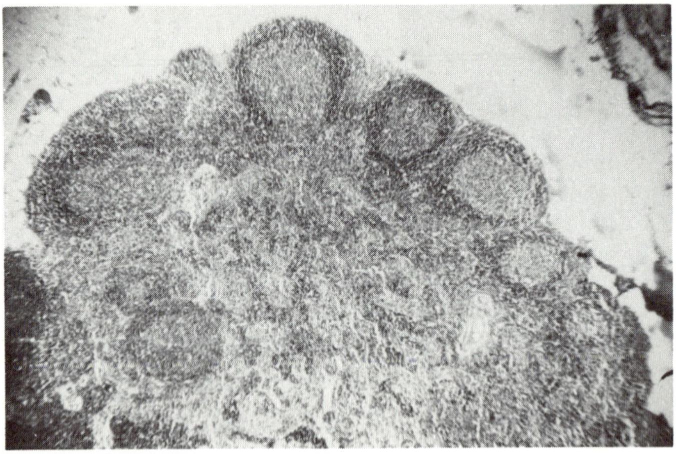

Fig. 9. Reactive follicles and medulla in ferret lymph node.

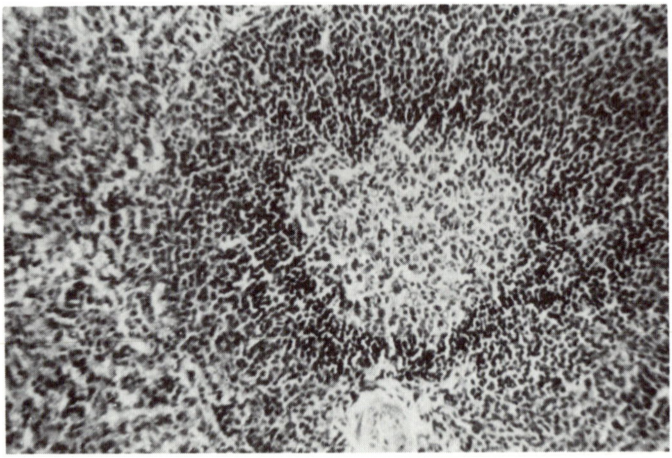

Fig. 10. Active germinal centre in follicle of sheep spleen.

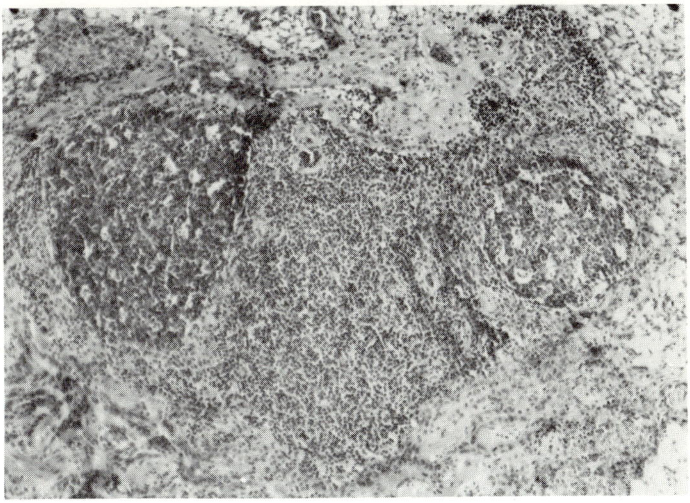

Fig. 11. Reactive follicles in lymphoid tissue of pigeon lung.

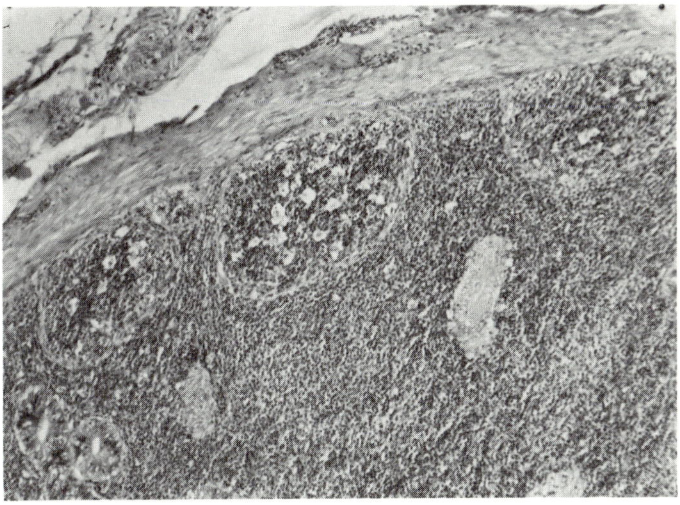

Fig. 12. Reactive follicles in bursa of Fabricius of crow.

REFERENCES

Baruzzi, R.G. (1970). *Rev. Ibst. Med. Trop.*, *12*, 93.

Castellani, A. (1913). *J. Ceylon. Br. Brit. Med. Assoc.*, *10*, 20.

Chessum, B.S. (1972). *Brit. Vet. J.*, *128*, 23.

Darling, S.T. (1909). *Arch. Int. Med.*, *3*, 183.

Darling, S.T. (1910). *J. Exp. Med.*, *12*, 19.

Desmonts, G., Couvreur, J., Alison, P., Baudelot, J., Gerbaux, J. and Lelong, M. (1965). *Rev. Franc. Etud. Clin. Biol.*, *10*, 952.

Dubey, J. P. (1973). *J. Am. Vet. Med. Ass.*, *162*, 873.

Dubey, J. P. and Frendel, J.K. (1972). *J. Protozool.*, *19*, 155.

Eyles, D.E. and Coleman, N. (1953). *Antibiot. Chemother.*, *3*, 483.

Feldman, H.A. and Eichenwald, H. (1953). Cited by Sabin, A.B. *in Am. J. Trop. Med. Hyg.*, *2*, 360.

Fleck, D.G., Chessum, B.S. and Perkins, M. (1972). *Brit. Med. J.*, *iii*, 111.

Frenkel, J.K., Dubey, J.P. and Miller, N.L. (1970). *Science*, *167*, 893.

Galuzo, I.G. and Kriskova, A.M. (1970). *Bull. Acad. Sci., Kazach. SSR*, *5*, 38.

Garin, J.-P. and Eyles, D.E. (1958). *Presse Med.*, *66*, 957.

Hutchison, W.M., Dunachie, J.F., Siim, J. Chr. and Work, K. (1970). *Brit. Med. J.*, *i*, 142.

Janitschke, K. and Werner, H. (1972). *Z. Parasitk.*, *39*, 247.

Janitschke, K. and Wormuth, H.J. (1970). *Zentbl. Bakt. I. Orig.*, *215*, 123.

Janku, J. (1923). *Cas. Lek. Ces.*, *62*, 1021, 1054, 1081, 1111, 1138.

Jewell, M.L., Frenkel, J.K., Johnson, K.M., Reed, V. and Riuz, A. (1972). *Am. J. Trop. Med. Hyg.*, *21*, 512.

Kean, B.H., Kimball, A.C. and Christenson, W.N. (1969). *J. Am. Med. Ass.*, *208*, 1002.

Kimball, A.C., Kean, B.H. and Fuchs, F. (1971). *Am. J. Obstet. Gynaecol.*, *111*, 219.

McMaster, P.R.B., Powers, K.G., Finerty, J.F. and Lunde, M.N. (1973). *Am. J. Trop. Med. Hyg.*, *22*, 14.

Magnuson, H.J. (1951). *Nordsk. Med.*, *45*, 344 (Abst). *Trop. Dis. Bull.*, (1951), *48*, 674.

Miller, N.L., Frenkel, J.K. and Dubey, J.P. (1972). *J. Parasit.*, *58*, 928.

Munday, B.L. (1972). *Res. Vet. Sci.*, *13*, 100.

Nicolle, C. and Manceaux, L. (1908). *C. R. Acad. Sci. (Paris)*, *147*, 763.

Overdulve, J.P. (1970). *Proc. k. Ned. Akad. Wet.* Ser. C., *73*, 129.
Pampiglione, S., Poglayen, G., Arnone, B. and Lalia, F. de (1973). *Brit. Med. J.*, *ii*, 306.
Peterson, D. R., Tronca, E. and Bonin, P. (1972). *Am. J. Epidem.*, *96*, 215.
Piringer-Kuchinka, A. (1952). *Verh. dt. Path. Ges.*, *36*, 352.
Ruiz, A., Frenkel, J.K. and Cerdas, L. (1973). *J. Parasit.*, *59*, 204.
Sabin, A.B. and Feldman, H.A. (1948). *Science*, *109*, 660.
Sabin, A.B. and Warren, J. (1942). *Proc. Soc. Exp. Biol. Med.*, *51*, 19.
Sheffield, H.G. and Melton, M.L. (1969). *Science*, *164*, 431.
Siim, J. Chr. (1951). *J. Am. Med. Ass.*, *147*, 1641.
Splendore, A. (1909). *Bull. Soc. Path. Exot.*, *2*, 462.
Summers, W.A. (1949). *Am. J. Trop. Med. Hyg.*, *29*, 889.
Thalhammer, O. (1961). *Wiener Klin. Woch.*, *73*, 885.
Wallace, G.D. (1969). *Am. J. Epidem.*, *90*, 103.
Wallace, G.D. (1971). *Am. J. Trop. Med. Hyg.*, *20*, 411.
Wallace, G.D. (1972). *J. Inf. Dis.*, *126*, 545.
Wallace, G.D. (1973). *Am. J. Trop. Med. Hyg.*, *22*, 313.
Wallace, G.D., Marshall, L. and Marshall, M. (1972). *Am. J. Epidem.*, *95*, 475.
Wieland, G. and Kuhn, D. (1969). *Tierärztl. Wschr.*, *82*, 401.
Wildfuhr, G. (1954). *In* "Toxoplasmose", p. 62, Gustav Fischer, Jena.
Witte, H.M. and Piekarski, G. (1970). *Z. Parasitk.*, *33*, 358.
Wolf, A., Cowen, D. and Paige, B. (1939). *Science*, *89*, 226.
Zaman, V. (1970). *S. E. Asian J. Trop. Med. Pub. Hlth.*, *1*, 329.

TOXOPLASMOSIS IN CATTLE AND SHEEP IN THE COTE D'OR

Y. Campana-Rouget, F. Levitte & A. M. Assmann

Laboratoire de Parasitologie, Faculte de Medicine de Dijon, France

INTRODUCTION

Examination for toxoplasmosis in the prenatal clinics of the Maternity Hospital of the Regional Medical Center of Dijon is a routine procedure in the Laboratory of Parasitology.

Statistics on human toxoplasmosis obtained in the laboratory have proved to be comparable to those in the rest of France in that approximately 80% of the adult population, between 20 and 30 years of age, shows positive serodiagnosis for toxoplasmosis.

Because of the serodiagnostic facilities in the Laboratory of Parasitology, a study on the prevalence of *Toxoplasma* antibodies in slaughter animals was possible, and was considered appropriate, since it was believed that such animals are the principal source of human infection in this region of France.

We have chosen to examine only herbivors (cattle and sheep) in which the method of infection with *Toxoplasma* should be identical and hence such a study should provide comparable results.

REVIEW OF PREVIOUS STUDIES OF TOXOPLASMOSIS IN HERBIVORS

The majority of previous studies on toxoplasmosis in herbivors have been conducted prior to the discovery of the life cycle of *Toxoplasma gondii* in the cat, and consequently do not evaluate the potential pathways of infection in herbivors. Nevertheless they indicate that toxoplasmosis is woldwide in distribution. It may be apparent as in the case of epizootics associated with abortion in sheep (in the Netherlands and New Zealand) or inapparent as indicated by the isolation of cysts from animals showing positive serodiagnostic tests.

The prevalence of infection varies considerably, both according to country and author. Thus Boch *et al.* (1965), in a summary of toxoplasmosis in cattle, states that the prevalence varies from 0 to 100% when the Sabin-Feldman dye test is used for diagnosis discounting the extreme figures and those obtained from small groups of animals, the prevalence in cattle varies from 30 to 70%, though in Germany is varies from 7 to 93%. More recent studies show comparable results. Thus in Scandinavia Work (1967) found that 58% of sheep and 11.43 of cattle showed positive dye-tests. Catar *et al.* (1969) estimated 18.8% of the cattle in Czechoslovakia to be the complement fixation test and Lievig (1968) in Kazakstan, found rates varying from 4.2 to 52.1 per cent depending on the herd of cattle and in sheep 60% of of animals were positive.

In France, few studies have been undertaken on toxoplasmosis in animals. Guillo and Desmonts (1960) found rates of infection of 72% in sheep (115 tested) and 4% in cattle (64 tested). Unfortunately, these authors did not know the age nor the origin of their animals and these factors, together with the small number of animals examined indicate that the study cannot represent a statistical evaluation of toxoplasmosis in France.

In 1970, Callot *et al.* examined samples from 326 cattle and 180 sheep from slaughterhouses in Strasbourg which draw animals from the Lower Rhine district. Using the indirect fluorescence technique, 35.52% of adult cattle, 6.19% of calves and 30.54% of sheep were positive for toxoplasmosis.

In summarizing the various studies it is seen that the serum titers , regardless of the serodiagnostic test used, are fairly homogenous for a given species. Thus, precluding epizootic situations, in sheep the range of titers are comparable to those of man. In immune animals they range from 1 in 20 to 1 in 100, in chronic infections, 1 in 1,000 to 1 in 2,000 and may reach 1 in 8,000 in the acute phase of the disease. Titers may remain high for some time. In cattle titers are lower, generally from 1 in 10 to 1 in 100. A titer of 1 in 256 in cattle has been noted in Europe while one of 1 in 1,000 has been seen in the U.S.A.

Congenital toxoplasmosis seems rarer in cattle than in sheep; indeed most of the severe epizootics are reported among the sheep.

The distribution of high titers may be uneven and where the origin of animals is known, it may be possible to identify the herd or flock concerned. For example, in an epizootic situation in the Netherlands, Roever-Bonnet (1963) identified a farm on which all the animals had much higher serological titers than elsewhere. Stepanova (1968) reported a similar situation in the U.S.S.R.

Most authors conclude that the serolgoical rate in animals is directly proportional to age. Work (1967) discounts this relationship, however, his results are based on a small number of animals.

STUDIES IN THE COTE D'ÔR

The indirect immunofluorescence technique was used employing specific conjugated antiglobulin serum from the Pasteur Institute in Paris.

Serum was obtained from two sources. The first was the slaughterhouses of Dijon and consisted largely of sheep serum. The address of the breeder and the approximate age of the animal was known for each sample. The second source was the Laboratory of the Regional Veterinary Service, which provided serum samples, originally sent to the Regional laboratory for examination for brucellosis or other infections. Only sera negative for these infections were exmained for toxoplasmosis. These samples included sera from sheep (whose age and origin were known) and sera from cattle (whose origin was known, but not always the age).

In all, the sera of 583 sheep and 890 cattle were examined. The results are summarized in Table I.

TABLE I

Serological survey of toxoplasmosis in Burgundy

	Sheep (583 samples examined)						
	-	±	1/10	1/20	1/100	1/200	>1/1000
Number	66	97		353		60	7
%	11.3	16.5		60.5		10.3	1.3
Total Percent	27.8%			72.1%			

	Cattle (890 samples examined)						
	Negative or Doubtful		Positive at titers indicated				
	-	±	1/10	1/20	1/100	1/200	>1/100
Number	89	166	127	458	51		
%	10	18.6	14.2	51.5	5.7		
Total Percent	28.6%		71.4%				

In sheep it was found that 16.3% of questionable responses at a dilution of 1 in 20 occurred in lambs. It is concluded that this represents reaction by residual maternal antibodies in the lambs. In sheep animals with the highest titers came from two farms in the region near Autun.

While the percentage of positive reactions was similar for cattle and sheep, the titers were lower in cattle. With the bovine sera there was a marked homogeneity for each lot of serum samples. The origin of these lots was known and they varied from 3 to 30 animals per lot, with a mean of 15. Animals in each lot were all negative, all doubtful or all positive with remarkable regularity. This suggests that in survey work for toxoplasmosis it is more valuable to study a large number of small groups of animals (10 to 15 animals per lot) than to study a small number of groups each containing a large number of animals. If, as has been shown in this study, the animals in each lot react in a homogenous manner then the differences among herds of flocks in an area are more readily identified

Further work is necessary to determine whether such differences remain constant. In addition work is necessary to determine the reason for the differences.

DISCUSSION

Many studies have contributed to our knowledge of *Toxoplasma* and its biology. Those relating to the mode of transmission are considered here.

In 1958, Lainson studied the cystic forms of *T. gondii* and demonstrated the successive appearance of pseudocysts and of true cysts. The pseudocysts appear rapidly, during an acute infection, in the cells of most of the tissues (liver, lungs, peritoneal exudates, etc.), they do not possess a membrane, are poorly resistant, and are not infectious orally. The true cysts appear slowly, in the course of chronic infection in the brain, the lungs and the muscles. They possess their own membrane, and contain numerous trophozoites which continue to divide by endodyogeny until about 3000 forms are produced. They are orally transmissible and survive in the tissue for at least five years.

The discovery of the sexual cycle in the cat by Hutchison *et al.* (1970) has been confirmed by many authors and represented a major advance in the knowledge of toxoplasmosis.

Piekarski and Witte (1971) and Piekarski *et al.* (1971) have studied the different developmental stages of *Toxoplasma*, with the electron microscope and have confirmed the relation of the parasite to the Coccidia, and, in particular its affinities for the genus *Isospora*. They considered that reporduction in the intestine of the cat was by endopolygeny, a form of endodyogeny, rather than by schizogony.

Some authors, for example Ben Rachid (1970) think that *T. gondii* is, in fact, synonym of *Isospora bigemina*, a well known coccidia of the cat. This is not impossible, but others, such as Senaud (1972), are not sure of this point

However, the life cycle in the cat does not explain all the problems associated with the transmission of toxoplasmosis. The existence of oocysts in the feces of the cat facilitated an understanding of the mode of transmission in the herbivores. However, Lainson (1958) has speculated that pulmonary cysts might be expectorated to produce contamination of herbage.

Numerous transmission experiments have been performed in the mouse. It is a very sensitive animal, which can be infected orally or peritoneally, by cysts or oocysts. Mice die in 4 to 5 days if inoculated with a virulent strain such as the RH strain, but they can survive for several months with less virulent strains, then having cysts in their brain.

Piekarski and Witte (1971) infested cats with different strains, and they observed that the elimination of the oocysts took place between the second and the seventh day after ingestion of cysts, a little later after ingestion of oocysts. The production of oocysts lasted for 3 to 15 days, depending on the strain. Fecal material remained infective for several months. In addition, the cats became immune and eliminated the infection and subsequently infection was present only in those cats which were either serologically negative or weakly positive.

With herbivores, few experiments have been attempted and a limited number of animals have been used. Garnham *et al.* (1960) inoculated five sheep with cysts originating from the brain of mice. Four of them which were innoculated either intraperitoneally, intravenously or intratrachially became infected, but an oral infection of a sheep did not produce infection. Similarly, Stepanova (1968) infected 29 sheep by the oral or subcutaneous routes with two different strains of the organism. In the subcutaneously infected sheep, animals became infected, but none became infected by the oral route. These resutls are an insufficient basis on which to conclude that cysts cannot infect ruminants by the oral route, but the possibility exists that this is so. It is possible that cysts do not survive the digestive process in ruminants.

Though experimentally several species of animals can be infected by various routes with cysts it is considered that, under natural conditions men and animals are hardly ever infected by the oral pathway, occasionally they may be infected by inhalation or by contamination of a wound. However, carnivors and omnivors are an exception to this since they may be infected either by cysts or oocysts since infection can occur in them regardless of the mode of infection.

In ruminants, transmission by oocysts is the only realistic mode of transmission. Nevertheless, it is difficult to envisage how contamination by cat feces can explain the occurrence of infection in an entire herd or flock of animals. The habits of cats, which bury their feces in predetermined places, do not favor the widespread dissemination of oocysts. In addition, an infected cat produces oocysts for a limited time once in its life-time.

The possibility has been considered that during the winter season, when animals in stables are in closer contact with cats, that the risk of infection would be increased during this period. However, we have not been able to demonstrate this serologically, on the contrary, the rates of infection were, in general, lower in winter than in the spring time.

Other modes of transmission require investigation. For example, the existence of a sexual cycle in animals other than the Felidae should be further investigated, though to date no other definitive host has been identified. The transfer of oocysts, for example, by coprophageous beetles or wild rodents may play a part, though recent studies with rodents would not suggest they have a role in the epidemiology of toxoplasmosis of ruminants. Recent studies in Czechosolvakia by Pavlik *et al.* (1971) have shown that the sensitivity of field mice and voles to *T. gondii* is inferior to that of the white mouse, but, nevertheless, infection in these rodents is sufficient to provide a source of infection. However, according to Pavlik *et al.* (1971) it is exceptional to find such rodents infected naturally, though Hubner and Uhlikova (1970) in Poladn have reported finding cysts of *T. gondii* in the salivary gland of a vole.

The present authors have attempted to demonstrate the dessimination of unsporulated oocysts by voles, but such oocysts apparently were destroyed in the digestive tract and none were found in the feces.

In summary, therefore, several aspects of the transmission of *T. gondii* remain to be elucidated. Knowledge of these would permit more effective control measures.

REFERENCES

Ben Rachid, M.S. (1970. *Arch. Inst. Pasteur Tunis, 47*, 33.
Boch, J., Janitschke, K., Rommel, M. and Sommer, R. (1965).

Wien. Tierarzt. Montschrift, 52, 1029.
Callot, J., Kremer, M., Gbreto, L. and Cranz, G. (1970). *Rev. Techn. Vet. Abattoir Hyg., 69,* 30.
Catar, G., Bergendi, L. and Holkova, R. (1969). *J. Parasit., 55,* 952.
Garnham, P., Lund, M. and Lainson, R. (1960). *Lancet,* July 9, 71.
Guillo, B. and Desmonts, G. (1960). *Rev. Med. Vet., 136,* 385.
Hubner, J. and Uhlikova, M. (1970). *Folia Parasit. (Praha), 17,* 126.
Hutchison, W., Dunachie, J., Siim, J. and Work, K. (1970). *Brit. Med. J., i,* 143.
Lainson, R. (1958). *Trans. Roy. Soc. Med. Hyg., 52,* 396.
Lievig in Stepanova (1968).
Overdulve, J.P. (1969). *Koninkl. Nederl. Akad. van Wetenschappen (Amsterdam) Proc. Series C., 73,* 129.
Pavlik, B., Dymon, K. and Slowiakiewicke, E. (1971). *Biol. Cracov. Ser. Zool., 14,* 38.
Piekarski, G. and Witte, H. (1971). *Z. Parasitenk, 36,* 95.
Piekarski, G., Plester, B. and Witte, H. (1971). *Z. Parasitenk., 36,* 122.
Roever-Bonet, de H (1963). *Trop. Geogr. Med., 15,* 431.
Senaud, J. (1972). *Bull. Inst. Pasteur, 70,* 3.
Stepanova, N. (1968). *Trav. Inst. Exp. Vet. l'URSS, 35,* 211.
Work, K. (1967). *Acta Path. Microb. Scand., 71,* 296.

COOMBS POSITIVE PHENOMENON ON ERYTHROCYTES OF RATS EXPERIMENTALLY INFECTED WITH *TOXOPLASMA GONDII*

Naoyoshi Suzuki*, Susumu Makimura*, Yoshitako Omata* Isamu Tomoda** and Toshio Ishii***

Universities of *Obihiro, Hokkaido and **Tokyo, Tokyo and ***Nippon Institute for Biological Science, Tokyo, Japan

INTRODUCTION

Blood changes in human clinical toxoplasmosis have been reported by Kalderon, (1964), Olbing, (1963), Barlotta *et al.*, (1964), Connolly, (1963), Keel *et al.*, (1963), Goodman and Maher, (1966), and Remington, (1970).

However, there is little information on the kinetic aspects of the blood changes in toxoplasmosis.

In previous studies on experimental toxoplasmosis, we have reported the pathophysiological changes in acute and chronic toxoplasmosis in mice and rats, infected with the various strains of *T. gondii* (Suzuki *et al.*, 1969; 1971; 1973abc; Tomoda *et al.*, 1969). In these experiments, an inoculum of a few parasites of the virulent strain of *T. gondii* killed mice within 10 days. Rats survived inoculation with millions of organisms of the same strain, showing only a slight reaction in the acute stage of the infection, and they had a tendency to enter a subclinical phase of infection about the 18th week post-infection. It has been observed that the morphology and the functional capabilities of erythrocytes was altered in the subclinical form of rat toxoplasmosis.

MATERIALS AND METHODS

Wistar strain, female, adult rats or ICR-JCL SPF mice were inoculated intraperitoneally with 1 x 10^5 or 1 x 10^2 parasites of the RH or Beverley-Shimizu (Shimizu *et al.*, 1967) strains obtained from the peritoneal fluid of 2-day infected mice. Mouse peritoneal fluid was centrifuged at 2,000 rpm for 15 minutes and the sediment was washed two times with physiological saline. The organisms were resuspended in the saline solution and adjusted to contain approximately 1 x 10^5 organisms in 1.0 ml.

Erythrocytes were washed 3 times in 0.15 M NaCl at 4°C by centrifugation and the buffy coat was removed. An aliquot of cells was lysed in distilled water at 4°C and the resultant lysate was assayed for erythrocyte enzymes. Determinations of the activities of lactate dehydrogenase (LDH), glutamic oxalacetic and glutamic pyruvic transaminases (GOT and GPT) (Reitman and Frankel, 1957), alkaline phosphatase, glucose-6-phosphate dehydrogenase (G6PD) (Beutler, 1966), reduced glutathione (GSH) (Beutler *et al.*, 1963) and concentration of pyruvate and lactate (Tada, 1966) were done using commercially prepared substrate solutions and test kits (Böhringer, Calbiochem and Sigma). The erythrocyte survival rate was measured by the method of labelling red cells with chromium (Miwa, 1967).

Antibody titers to *Toxoplasma* were examined by the dye test and indirect immunofluorescence (Kobayashi *et al.*, 1968). Separation of immunoglobulins G and M (IgG and IgM) from serum was done by liquid microcolum chromatography (Suzuki *et al.*, 1973b).

The direct Coombs test, using macroscopical and immunofluorescent examinations, was carried out by mixing the 3 times washed erythrocytes from *Toxoplasma* infected rats with sera from rabbits immunized to rat-whole serum, rat-globulins, rat-IgG and rat-IgM. These anti-rat sera were conjugated with fluorescein isothiocyanate (FITC), and then were inactivated at 56°C for 30 minutes. Before the tests, rabbit anti-rat sera were absorbed with washed rat erythrocytes.

RESULTS

Blood changes

Mice infected with a virulent strain of *T. Gondii* showed a macrocytic hyperchromic anemia in the terminal stages of the infection. The total leukocyte count declined sharply, and shortly before death there was a transient decrease of lymphocytes and an increase of neutrophils. In the serum, the albumin fraction decreased while alpha-2 and beta globulins showed a tendency to increase through the 9th day post-infection. The levels of LDH, GOT, GPT and SDH in the serum increased markedly on the 7th and 9th day post-infection (Suzuki *et al.*, 1973a).

In the rats infected with the same strain of *T. gondii*, mean corpusclar hemoglobin and mean corpusclar volume decreased slightly through the 8th week post-infection. The total leukocyte count increased slightly, being accompanied by a transient increase and decrease in neutrophiles and lymphocytes respectively. An abrupt increase of monocytes in the acute stage was noted, these cells appearing as degenerated forms with some vacuoles. Serum albumin showed a slight decrease, and alpha and gamma globulins, the enzymes LDH, GOT and GPT showed an increase during acute infection, although they approached the preinfection values by the 8th week post-infection. In the bone marrow, a slight hyperfunction of erythropoiesis was found at the 8th week post-infection (Suzuki *et al.*, 1971).

Activities of GSH, GOT and GPT in the erythrocytes showed a slight tendency to increase through the 8th week post-infection, which the activity of erythrocyte G6PD decreased gradually to the 8th week. The concentration of lactate in the erythrocytes decreased on the 1st week but showed slightly higher values by the 8th week post-infection. Lactate, produced when erythrocytes were incubated at 37°C for 2 hours, decreased markedly on the 3rd and 8th weeks post-infection and showed an overall decrease over the 8 week period.

Erythrocyte survival rates in 2 non-infected rats and 3 *Toxoplasma*-infected rats in the 8th week post-infection, were determined by measuring the radioactivity of blood at 10 minutes and 10 days after an intravenous injection of erythrocytes labeled with radioactive chromium. The average percentage of surviving erythrocytes on the 10th day after injection was 50.4 for non-infected rats, and 41.4 for *Toxoplasma*-infected rats. No radioactive chromium was found in the plasma of the non-infected rats on the 10th day after injection, but such activity was found in the plasma of each of the 3 *Toxoplasma*-infected rats on the 10th day after injection.

Antibody responses

The dye test titers obtained in the rats are shown in Table 1. The antibody occurred only in the IgM fraction on the 5th day after infection but by the 7th day antibodies were present in both the IgM and the IgG fractions. From the 21st to the 140th day after infection, antibodies occurred only in the IgG fraction.

Foetuses taken from 3 rats on the 83rd day of infection showed antibody by the dye test technique, but *T. gondii* was not found in the foetuses or in the placentas. In newborn rats antibodies were present in the IgG fraction of serum and the titres remained at the same level as that in the foetuses until 21 days after birth (Table 1). Thereafter titres gradually decreased and were minimal at 56 days after birth.

To determine whether erythrocytes were coated with globulin in rat toxoplasmosis, the erythrocytes were examined by the direct Coombs test, and antibody titers to *Toxoplasma* were assessed by the indirect immunofluorescent method.

Table 2 shows that the erythrocytes of infected rats showed Coombs' positive reactions with rabbit anti-whole rat serum, anti-rat-globulin and anti-rat IgG from the fourth week of infection onwards. The Coombs' positive reactions were demonstrable both macroscopically and by immunofluorescence, but nevertheless, they were weak. Material eluted from infected rat erythrocytes also reacted with the anti-globulin sera.

Table 1

Immunoglobulin Location of Antibody in Rats Infected with T. gondii

Days after infection	Days after delivery	Mother			Foetus or Infant		
		Sabin-Feldman Dye Test			Sabin-Feldman Dye Test		
		Whole Serum	IgM (Pool 9)	IgG (Pool 1)	Whole Serum	IgM (Pool 9)	IgG (Pool 1)
3		<1: 4	-	-			
5		1: 16	+	-			
7		1: 256					
		1:1024	+	+			
21		1: 256					
		1:1024	-	+			
56		1: 256	-	+			
83	- 1				1: 64	non-examined	
87	3	1: 256	-	+	1: 64	-	+
91	7	1: 256	-	+	1: 64	-	+
105	21	1: 256	-	+	1: 64	-	+
					1: 4		
119	35	1: 256	-	+	1: 16	-	-
140	56	1: 256	-	+	1: 4	-	-

The direct Coombs' test with rabbit anti-rat IgG and erythrocytes from newborn rats born of mothers in the 7th week after infection, was negative in all cases, through the 5th week after birth.

Absorption of the rabbit anti-rat globulin sera with rat IgG abolished the positive Coombs' reaction with the erythrocytes of infected rats. Consequently it was concluded that the material on the surface of erythrocytes which reacted with rabbit anti-rat IgG was antigenically related to rat IgG.

DISCUSSION AND CONCLUSIONS

From these results, we propose that slight changes of morphology and function of erythrocytes occur in subclinical toxoplasmosis of rats by the 8th week post-infection. A positive result with the direct Coombs' test indicates the presence of an abnormal protein factor on the surface of the erythrocytes and suggests the presence of an auto-immune acquired hemolytic process.

The origin of the material producing the Coombs positive phenomenon is not yet clear. However, it might be caused by the production of "incomplete" antibody against the erythrocyte after infection with *Toxoplasma*.

Table 2

Antibody Response in Rats Infected with T. gondii

	Infection ↓	1	2	3	4	Animals Mated ↓	5	6	7	Parturition ↓	8	9	10	11	12	>25
WEEKS AFTER INFECTION																
Toxoplasma Antibody																
SF Dye test	<4	256*			4096						4096				4096	4096
IgG		256			16000						>4096				>4096	4096
IgM		256			< 16						< 16				< 16	< 16
Direct Coombs Test																
Mother																
Whole serum	-	-	-	±	+						+		+		+	+
Globulin	-			-	+						+		+		+	+
IgG	-				+						+		+		+	+
IgM	-				-						-				-	-
Eluate From R.B.C.					+						+		+		+	+
Neonate																
Globulin											+		-		-	
IgG											-					
Eluate from R.B.C.											-					

Note: Antibody titers in IgG and IgM to toxoplasma were measured in the indirect immunofluorescent method.

* Reciprocal of titer.

REFERENCES

Barlotta, F.M., Ochoa, M. and Neu, H.C. (1969). *Ann. Intern. Med. 70*, 517.

Beutler, E., Duron, O. and Kelly, B.M. (1963). *J. Lab. Clin. Med. 61*, 882.

Beutler, E. (1966). *Blood, 28*, 553.

Connolly, C.S. (1963). *Arch. Intern. Med. 112*, 393.

Goodman, M.I. and Maher, E. (1966). *J. Amer. Med. Ass. 198*, 1129.

Kalderon, A.E. (1964). *Arch. Intern. Med. 114*, 95.

Keel, H.J. Roth, W., Keiser, G., Reutter, F. and Martz, G. (1963). *Schweiz. Med. Wochen. 93*, 1465.

Kobayoshi, A., Kumada, M. and Tsunematsu, Y. (1968). *Jap. J. Parasit. 17*, 81.

Miwa, S. (1967). *Jap. J. Clin. Med. 25*, 50.

Olbing, H. (1963). *Zeit. Kinderheilk. 87*, 459.

Reitman, S. and Frenkels (1957). *Am. J. Clin. Path. 28*, 56.

Remington, J.S. (1970). *Ann. Rev. Med. 21*, 201.

Shimizu, K., Kito, S. and Shirahata, T. (1967). *Jap. J. Vet. Sci. 29*, 71.

Suzuki, N., Tomoda, I., Makimura, S. and Ishii, T. (1969). *Jap. J. Vet. Sci. 31*, 104.

Suzuki, N., Piekarski, G., Janssen, P. and Viswanathan, R. (1971). *Res. Bull. Obihiro Univ. 7*, 55.

Suzuki, N., Piekarski, G., Janssen, P. and Viswanathan, R. (1973a). *Res. Bull. Obihiro Univ. 9*, 15.

Suzuki, N., Makimura, S., Tomoda, I and Ishii, T. (1973b). *Jap. J. Vet. Sci. 35*, 279.

Suzuki, N., Makimura, S., Tomoda, I and Ishii, T. (1973c). *Res. Bull. Obihiro. Univ. 9*, 369.

Tada, K. (1966). *Clin. Pediat. 29*, 647.

Tomoda, I., Suzuki, N. and Ishii, T. (1969). *Jap. J. Parasit. 18*, 368.

ZOONOSES CAUSED BY HEMOPROTOZOA

Miodrag Ristic and Ronald D. Smith

College of Veterinary Medicine, University of Illinois, Urbana, Illinois 61801

INTRODUCTION

The definition of zoonoses being "those diseases and infections which are naturally transmitted between vertebrate animals and man" (WHO, 1959) does not do justice to the complexity of the zoonotic phenomenon in the biosphere. A further classification of zoonoses offered by the Expert Committee on Zoonoses of the Food and Agricultural Organization and World Health Organization of the United Nations (WHO, 1967) was an effort to emphasize the epidemiologic features of zoonoses. According to the report, zoonoses were grouped into 4 categories:

Direct zoonoses which are transmitted from one vertebrate host to another by contact, fomite, or mechanical vector (rabies, trichinosis and brucellosis).

Cyclo-zoonoses in which more than one vertebrate host species are required to complete the developmental cycle of the agent (echinococcosis, taeniasis).

Meta-zoonoses which are transmitted biologically by invertebrate vectors with an agent being able to develop in these vectors (spotted fever, arbovirus infections, malaria).

Sapro-zoonoses which have both a vertebrate host and a non-animal reservoir (larva migrans).

In this paper we will be concerned with the *meta-zoonosis* or, more specifically, with zoonoses caused by various species of trypanosomes, plasmodia, and babesiae.

It will become apparent from the subsequent discussion that the chance of contact between man and vector, the latter harboring the agents maintained in an animal reservoir, will determine the frequency of occurrence of respective zoonoses. This in turn will indicate actual field importance of hemoprotozoan diseases shown to be transmissible between man and animals under laboratory conditions. Distinction between field and laboratory situations is clearly demonstrated in the case of monkey malaria where infected mosquitos reside in areas usually not easily accessible to man, thereby possibly minimizing practical importance of malarial zoonoses. In addition, the behavior of carrier monkeys is such to avoid contact with man. Similar concepts exist in the case of Rhodesian sleeping sickeness where man is infected by exposure to arthropod vectors feeding on game animals. Exposure thus takes place through invasion of the natural wildlife ecosystem of bush, wild animals and tsetse flies.

In contrast to the above somewhat chance field exposure, American trypanosomiasis (Chagas' disease) exists in human populations where man provides optimal conditions for the entrance, reproduction, and feeding of triatome vectors in his own dwellings. Obviously, socio-economic conditions are most important in the predisposition of man to this type of trypanosomal infection.

Babesiosis, the most recent zoonosis, has been known as a disease affecting a variety of animals and causing severe losses among cattle for over 80 years (Smith and Killborne, 1893). The first 3 recognized human cases were in persons whose spleens had been removed (Skrabalo and Deanović, 1957; Scholtens *et al.*, 1968; Fitzpatrick *et al.*, 1968). The finding indicated partial susceptibility of man to *Babesia* species and reinforced general concepts that erythrocytic parasites commonly restricted to certain species of host can cause infections in other hosts when the protective effects afforded by the presence of the spleen are removed. Recent recognition of babesiosis in two human beings with spleen *in situ* (Western *et al.*, 1970; Ristic *et al.*, 1971; Cassady *et al.*, 1973) has widened the zoonotic implication of babesiosis considerably and has introduced disturbing practical implications for those engaged in the control of falciparum malaria. Few places in the world are free of babesia parasites; their presence may present a hazard to splenectomized persons and to those whose susceptibility to the disease may be enhanced by unknown disease precipitating factors.

Information gained from studies of babesiosis in domestic animals indicates that for every clinically demonstrable case, there are hundreds of cases of latent infection. The human health impact of latent babesiosis might thus be much greater than anticipated on the basis of 5 documented acute cases of the disease.

Thus, future epidemiological research must place special emphasis on improvement of methods for identification of hemoprotozoa in human beings and lower animals; determination of feeding habits (vertebrate host spectrum) of arthropod vectors of zoonotic hemoprotozoa; and detection of subclinical human and animal carrier infections.

In 1968 Bray summarized our knowledge of the zoonotic blood protista, including protozoa. We will, therefore, briefly review current knowledge of each of the zoonotic hemoprotozoa, and cite more recent findings that may help to clarify the zoonotic potential of these agents in the field.

TRYPANOSOMIASIS

A distinction must be drawn between African trypanosomiasis (sleeping sickness) and American trypanosomiasis (Chagas' disease) on both geographic and epidemiologic grounds. Man falls prey to African trypanosomiasis (*T. brucei rhodesiense* and *T. brucei gambiense*) most frequently during the day, away from the home, through the bite of the tsetse fly (*Glossina sp.*). In contrast, American trypanosomiasis (*Trypanosoma cruzi*) is the most commonly contracted in man's home at night while asleep through the feeding behavior of reduvid bugs (WHO, 1969a).

In addition, the number and identity of species of animal reservoirs, and their importance in the maintenance of trypanosomes in endemic areas are much better established in the case of Chagas' disease than Rhodesian or Gambian sleeping sickness. Research designed to elucidate the role of wild and domestic animals as reservoirs of *T. rhodesiense* and *T. gambiense* is still in the early stages.

African Trypanosomiasis

The major obstacle to a better understanding of the importance of animal reservoirs of human trypanosomes and/or infections of man with trypanosomes of lower animals continues to be the accurate identification of trypanosome species. The identification of *T. brucei* subgroup organisms, which are morphologically identical, has been based upon cultural, drug sensitivity and physico-chemical tests, susceptibility to infection and the disease produced in various vertebrate hosts, geographic distribution, species of fly involved in transmission and infectivity for man (Gray, 1969).

These somewhat unrealistic and artificial barriers erected between species and subspecies, "demes" or nosodemes" (Hoare, 1972a) have been questioned by a number of recent findings. The species of vector is no longer a valid criterion upon which to distinguish the type of trypanosome causing a case of human infection (WHO, 1969b). Palpalis-group tsetses have transmitted rhodesiense-like human infections and morsitans-group tsetses have transmitted gambiense-like infections. However, the efficiency with which these flies transmit infections is unknown and merits further investigation (WHO, 1969b). Ford (1971) has pointed out that simply knowing the species of fly transmitting trypanosomes to man does not indicate the original source of the infective agent. *Palpalis*-group flies, which do not ordinarily feed upon game animals, may transmit wild animal trypanosomes to man from domestic animals (bovine) which were infected earlier *via Glossina* spp. feeding on both wild and domestic animals. Omerod (1967) has pointed out that the reported characteristics of *T. rhodesiense, gambiense,* and *brucei* relative to epidemiology, clinical aspects, and host-parasite relationships are not the exclusive properties of either of these species. He referred to a chronic form of Rhodesian sleeping sickness (usually an acute disease in man) occurring in the Zambezi basin as "Zambian" sleeping sickness and considered *T. brucei* the ancestral form of the 3 strains, or demes, causing Rhodesian, Gambian, and Zambian sleeping sickness, whose biological and clinical features in man were integrated.

Reports by Heisch *et al.*, (1958) and Onyango *et al.*, (1966) and more recently by Geigy *et al.*, (1973) of *T. rhodesiense* in game and domestic animals have further eroded the earlier divisions erected between human and non-human trypanosomes. In spite of early reports of naturally occurring *T. gambiense* in the ox and the dog (Yorke and Blacklock, 1915; Hoof, 1947) only circumstantial evidence has linked *T. gambiense* outbreaks in man to animal reservoirs of *T. brucei* subgroup trypanosomes (Gray, 1969).

Thus, more than ever before, it is important to determine the identity of *brucei* subgroup trypanosomes isolated from domestic animals and man, assess the infectivity of animal trypanosomes of the *brucei* subgroup for man, and establish the extent to which wild and domestic animals are reservoirs of human infection.

Isolation and identification of brucei *subgroup trypanosomes.*

A description of diagnostic techniques for human and animal trypanosomiases is beyond the scope of this chapter. Suitable references are available on this subject (WHO, 1969b; Díaz-Ungría and Maldonado Alvarex, 1970; Schindler and Sachs, 1970; Cunningham *et. al.*, 1967; Ross, 1971; Lucasse, 1970; Woo and Soltys, 1972). Improved techniques are needed for detecting trypanosomes in patients with low parasitemia, often a problem in *T. gambiense* infections and an obstacle to efficient detection of human and animal trypanosome carriers. The appearance of constant and variable antigens during the course of trypanosomal infections has proven to be a major difficulty to accurate serological identification of *T. brucei* subgroup trypanosomes. Gray (1969) has proposed the use of "predominant variant antigens" rather than "basic antigens" for the identification of trypanosomal strains. He indicated, however, that the mild infections occurring in most laboratory animals infected with *T. gambiense* may make it difficult to obtain antigens for agglutination tests.

Le Ray *et al.*, (1971) have described cross-absorption studies utilizing soluble precipitinogens from culture forms of a strain of *T. brucei*. Precipitating antibodies were absorbed out by antigens of *T. brucei* and *T. rhodesiense* but not by *T. gambiense* are distinct species.

The blood incubation infectivity test (BIIT) (Rickman and Robson, 1970a, b) as applied to animal trypanosomiasis is a novel procedure designed to distinguish between *T. brucei* and *T. rhodesiense* or strains of *T. brucei* infective or not infective for man (Fig. 1). This test has been used in field surveys of animal trypanosomes (Geigy and Kauffman, 1973) and may eliminate the need for inoculation of human volunteers with animal isolates.

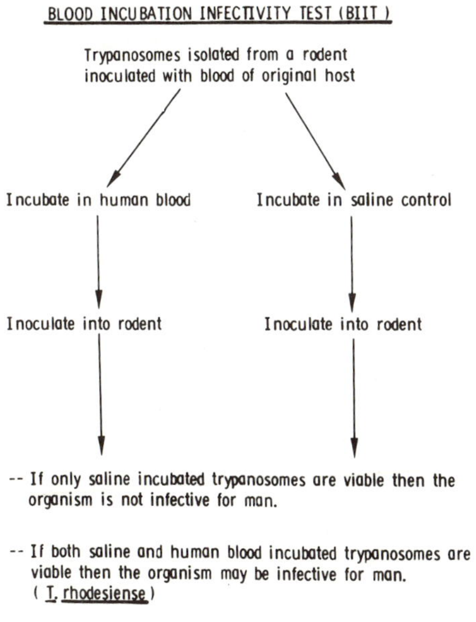

←*Fig. 1. Diagram of procedure for the Blood Incubation Infectivity Test for the identification of trypanosomes.*

From this discussion it should be clear that serological and other tests for distinguishing the *T. brucei* subgroup trypanosomes of actual or potential zoonotic importance are far from perfect. It is also clear that the efficacy of all such tests may be helped by the establishment of a world reference bank of trypanosomes as recommended by the World Health Organization (WHO, 1969b).

Infectivity of brucei *subgroup trypanosomes for man.*

Earlier identifications of *T. rhodesiense* in animals have been confirmed by inoculation of human volunteers (Heisch *et al.*, 1958; Onyango *et al.*, 1966). Recently Geigy *et al.*, (1973) recovered 2 more isolants of *T. rhodesiense* from a hartbeest in Serengeti National Park and a cow in Ikoma, Misumo District, Tanzania. Although final identification resided ultimately in human inoculation, it is noteworthy that the BIIT was used to screen all animal isolants recovered in their study and was positive in both cases. This, and the earlier work of Rickman and Robson (1970a, b) lend support to the value of this test in the search for *T. rhodesiense* in epidemiologic surveys among animal populations. Rickman and Robson (1972) reported that some strains of *T. congolense* have retained their infectivity for rodents after incubation in human blood. This might indicate zoonotic potential of another trypanosome species.

In comparison with *T. rhodesiense*, the zoonotic potential of *T. gambiense* is difficult to ascertain due to the mild infection induced in man and the difficulty of detecting low grade, chronic infections. Lumsden (1972) discussed possible existence of clinically healthy human carriers of *T. brucei* subgroup trypanosomes and Onyango (1969) described atypical clinically mild cases of *T. rhodesiense* and assessed the importance of healthy carriers in the epidemiology of Rhodesian sleeping sickness. In light of the occurrence of asymptomatic infections of man with *T. brucei* sub-group trypanosomes, subclinical human infections with animal trypanosomes in endemic areas may be more common than currently believed, as suggested for human babesiosis.

Wild and domestic animal reservoirs of human infection.

Not unexpectedly, the discovery of *T. rhodesiense* in wild and domestic animals has directed the attention of epidemiologic investigations to animal reservoirs and fly feeding habits. Onyango (1969) has pointed out that in the past it was felt that outbreaks of Rhodesian sleeping sickness were due to the entrance of a human carrier into a clean area. In view of the domestic and wild animal carriers, it is likely that animals have played a role in the introduction of disease into disease-free areas. The next question is the extent to which various animal species have served as reservoirs of human infection and under what conditions was man exposed. Several studies have been carried out to determine the extent to which wild and domestic animals are infected with trypanosomes, including the *T. brucei* subgroup, and their importance as a source of infection for man (Moloo *et al.*, 1971; Mwambu and Mayende, 1971; Onyango *et al.*, 1971; Geigy and Kauffman, 1973; Mwambu and Woodford, 1972).

Geigy and Kauffman (1973) found that of 95 animals examined in the Serengeti National Park, 78% were infected with trypanosomes. Forty out of 74 isolates belonged to *T. brucei* subgroup and 4 of these gave *T. rhodesiense*-like reactions in the BIIT. On the other hand, Mwambu and Woodford (1972) found only 11% of 72 animals in the Queen Elizabeth National Park, Western Uganda, to be infected with trypanosomes. Differences in infection rate reported in these 2 studies undoubtedly reflect differences in species susceptibility, diagnostic tests used, geographical locale, and other factors. Onyango (1969) pointed out the complexity of the problem of wildlife reservoirs as evidenced by conflicting reports by authors on the occurrence of *T. rhodesiense* in game animals.

The question of epidemiologic importance of animal reservoirs is further complicated by factors peculiar to tsetse flies. Wilson *et al.*, (1972) have studied the relative importance of different species of tsetse flies in the transmission of trypanosomes to the vertebrate host. The efficiency of infection of tsetse flies by *T. brucei* with reference to the percent parasitemia in the vertebrate host was studied by Page (1972). Yesufu (1971) has reported that despite very low parasitemia in dogs, he was able to transmit *T. gambiense* to certain species of tsetse flies. Relative to these studies, Mshelbwala (1972) has reported that survival of trypanosomes in the haemocoel of tsetse flies means that the examination of salivary glands alone for the detection of infection is not adequate.

Geigy *et al.*, (1973) and Onyango (1969) agree that although cattle may serve as reservoirs of Rhodesian sleeping sickness, game animals are probably more important since they occupy the same ecological setting as the tsetse fly. Cattle are only incidental reservoirs.

American Trypanosomiasis

The epidemiology of Chagas' disease, caused by *T. cruzi*, has little in common with the African trypanosomiases. Although Chagas' disease occurs primarily in rural areas, as does African trypanosomiasis, man-vector contact is not the result of invasion of vector habitats, but rather the provision of a habitat favorable for maintenance of the vector. Poor socioeconomic and sanitary conditions associated with dirty, dark houses made of mud, grass and cane provide an excellent breeding ground for *Triatoma* and *Panstrongylus* spp., another triatomid vector of Chagas' disease, often lays its eggs on the leaves of palm trees which are subsequently incorporated into the roofs of huts, thus providing a mode of entry of this vector into the home (WHO, 1969a).

Chagas' disease may be transmitted from animal to man and

vice versa, animal to animal, and man to man. Our discussion of this zoonosis may be conveniently divided into (1) maintenance of *T. cruzi* in animal and human population, (2) transmission of *T. cruzi* from animals to man and, (3) recent advances in the study of the epidemiology of Chagas' disease.

Maintenance of T. cruzi *in human and animal populations.* An outstanding characteristic of Chagas' disease in man is its chronicity. As might be expected, this form of the disease is difficult to detect, thus xenodiagnosis and complement fixation (CF) tests have been the most commonly used diagnostic techniques. Schenone *et al.*, (1968) showed that *T. cruzi* may be found in the blood of 60% of patients with chronic Chagas' disease using xenodiagnosis.

Transmission of *T. cruzi* by triatomid bugs is probably the most important means of interhuman transmission of the disease. Rohwedder (1969) considered transmission by blood transfusion to be the second most common means of interhuman transmission in Latin America. He reported frequencies of positive CF tests among blood donors in various Latin American countries to be between 4.7% and 9%. Huggins and Lucena (1969) found 4.4% positives in a similar study of blood donors in Brazil.

A third means of interhuman transmission is from mother to young. Although the possibility of infection acquired from milk exists (WHO, 1969a) a more likely route is transplacentally. Many cases of transplacentally acquired Chagas' disease have been noted but the importance of this route of infection in maintenance of the disease is not clear. Bittencourt *et al.*, (1972) and Bittencourt and Barbosa (1972) have studied this phenomenon in Brazil. From an examination of 500 premature births, 93 mothers were found to be positive for Chagas' disease. Approximately 10% of the infected mothers transmitted *T. cruzi* to the fetus, all of which died prior to or at delivery. It would seem that a large proportion of congenital infections with *T. cruzi* result in death of the fetus.

The list of animal reservoirs of *T. cruzi* is enormous. Soto (1971) and Barretto (1967) have published lists of animal reservoirs of the disease in the Americas. Although transmission among animals by triatomid bugs is common, it is not the only means for transmission of *T. cruzi*. *Trypanosoma cruzi* has been found in the milk of mice at the same time that it appeared in the blood (Disko and Krampitz, 1971) and transmission to suckling mice has been confirmed by Miles (1972).

Transplacental transmission may occur in some animal species but its importance is questionable. Werner and Egger (1971) found that while the musculature and endometrium of the uterus of mice contained *T. cruzi*, no infection was seen in the embryos or fetuses, although 1/3 of the embryos died.

The transmission of *T. cruzi* to dogs by ingested flies (*Musca domestica*) that have previously fed on feces of *R. prolixus* has been demonstrated with flies infected in the laboratory and those captured from huts containing *T. cruzi*-infected triatomes (Díaz-Ungría, 1969). Yaeger (1971) has infected opossums orally with *T. cruzi*.

The possibility of inter-triatomid infection with *T. cruzi* has been studied by Székely *et al.*, (1971). These workers were unable to demonstrate *T. cruzi* transmission between infected and uninfected 3rd and 5th instar triatome nymphs. Further studies along these lines are necessary, however, in light of the high incidence of infection among various riatome species (Sousa and Johnson, 1973).

Transmission of T. cruzi *from animals to man.*

Bray (1968) stated that the main reservoir of human infection with *T. cruzi* is man himself. In view of the influence of socioeconomic conditions, size, variety and proximity of infected wild and domestic animal populations to man, and species of triatomid vectors involved in different regions of the Americas, it would seem that the relative importance of human and animal reservoirs is variable, depending upon the geographic region under consideration.

The most common animal reservoirs of human infection are considered to be dogs, cats, armadillos and opossums (Bray, 1968; Soulsby, 1968; Zeledón and Ponce, 1972). The efficiency with which *T. cruzi* is transmitted from these animals to man by triatomid bugs appears to be quite variable. In spite of widespread infection of wild animals and triatomids by *T. cruzi* in southern Georgia, human infections have not been reported. Complement fixing antibody titers amont the human population in Georgia, even among patients with primary myocardial disease, were found to be low (Farrar *et al.*, 1972). The prevalence of titers to *T. cruzi* in Latin America countries is usually much higher than in the southern United States (Bruce-Chwatt, 1972).

It has been postulated that part of the observed difference in infection rates is due to the feeding and defecating habits of the triatomid vectors themselves (WHO, 1969a). Cerisola *et al.*, (1971a) have shown that certain triatome species differ markedly with respect to the efficiency of xenodiagnosis. This may also help explain differences in the degrees of triatomid and human infection in some areas, e.g., the southern United States. In the final analysis, Bray's constention that the human reservoir is the most important one in human *T. cruzi* infections may be the best explanation of the above-mentioned disparity.

Diagnostic methods in Chagas'disease epidemiology.

Xenodiagnosis and the CF test have long been the leading diagnostic techniques for *T. cruzi* infections (Bruce-Chwatt, 1972). A *T. cruzi*-like organism, *Blastocrithidia triatomae* has been described in laboratory bred *T. infestans* (Cerisola *et al.*, 1971b). Hoare (1972b) pointed out the importance of distinguishing this organism from *T. cruzi* and *T. rangeli* when xenodiagnosis is employed.

Other tests have been compared with xenodiagnosis and the CF test for use in diagnosis and screening large populations for Chagas' disease. Marsden *et al.*, (1970) have studied levels of immunoglobulins in people at risk to Chagas' disease and those withacute infections. When compared with xenodiagnosis and the CF test they concluded that IgM estimations were of no value as a screening technique for Chagas' disease.

Perruolo-Laneti (1971) compared a "dye test" using flagellate forms of *T. cruzi* with the CF test and concluded that the dye exclusion test was of value for the diagnosis of chronic Chagas' disease.

Cerisola *et al.*, (1970) compared the indirect fluorescent antibody (IFA), indirect hemagglutination (IHA) and CF tests during various phases of *T. cruzi* infection. The IFA test gave the earliest reactions, followed by the CF test which, during the first 2 months post-infection, appeared more sensitive than the IHA test. By 6 months after infection, the results of all tests were in agreement.

Collection of blood on filter paper may contribute to future more efficient application of sero-diagnostic tests for Chagas' disease. Alvarez *et al.*, (1971) compared the use of fresh serum samples and filter paper collected blood samples in the IFA test on 390 patients, 97 of whom had Chagas' disease. Both collection methods gave comparable results with the exception of 0.8% false positives obtained when the filter paper method for collecting sera was used. Filter paper collected blood samples were well preserved for as long as 80 days at room temperature.

Control of Chagas' disease is presently directed toward effective spray programs and identification of human infections early in life. Rocha E. Silva *et al.*, (1970) pointed out the value of estimating triatomid infestations of dwellings and serological surveys of children under 8 years of age in control of Chagas' disease.

Other Trypanosomes

Although *Trypanosoma rangeli* occurs in a wide variety of animals, including man, its non-pathogenic nature excludes it from this discussion of diseases caused by zoonotic haemoprotozoa.

MALARIA

In contrast to the problems facing trypanosome epidemiologists, identification of simian and human malaria parasites is possible on the basis of morphological criteria alone. An excellent book has been published by Coatney *et al.*, (1971) which depicts the developmental stages of primate malarial parasites in the vertebrate and arthropod hosts.

The first case of naturally acquired zoonotic malaria was an accidental mosquito-borne infection in the laboratory with *Plasmodium cynomolgii* (Eyles *et al.*, 1960). Since that time other reports of laboratory infections have appeared, the most recent being that of Most (1973). Three infections of man with simian parasites in the field under natural conditions have been reported. Two of these occurred in Malaysia and involved *Plasmodium knowlesi* (Chin *et al.*, 1965; Fong *et al.*, 1971) (Fig. 2). The third case occurred in Brazil and the parasite was identified as being *Plasmodium simium* (Deane *et al.*, 1966). Coatney (1971) has raised questions as to the identity of the organism, however, suggesting that the parasite may have been *P. vivax* and therefore not necessarily of simian origin.

Reports of the occurrence of simian malaria parasites in man have generated considerable research on the susceptibility of mosquito vectors and men to simian malarial parasites and of monkeys and their mosquitoes to human malaria (Collins and Contacos, 1969, 1972; Contacos and Collins, 1969; Young and Porter, 1969; Porter, 1970; Garnham *et al.*, 1971; Young *et al.*, 1971; Collins *et al.*, 1972; Bafort and Kageruka, 1972) and on the identification of simian malaria parasites and their vectors in the field (Warren *et al.*, 1970; Deane *et al.*, 1971; Ferreira Neto *et al.*, 1972). Most of this work has been reviewed and analyzed epidemiologically by various authors (WHO, 1969c; Juminer, 1970; Coatney, 1971).

An interesting concept relating to primate malaria has been introduced by Juminer (1970), Coatney *et al.*, (1971) and Coatney (1971). Sufficient similarity and/or identity exist between some simian plasmodia and those of man to raise the question of the original source of primate infection, i.e., is malaria a zoonosis (simian forms infecting man) or an anthroponosis (human forms infecting other primates).

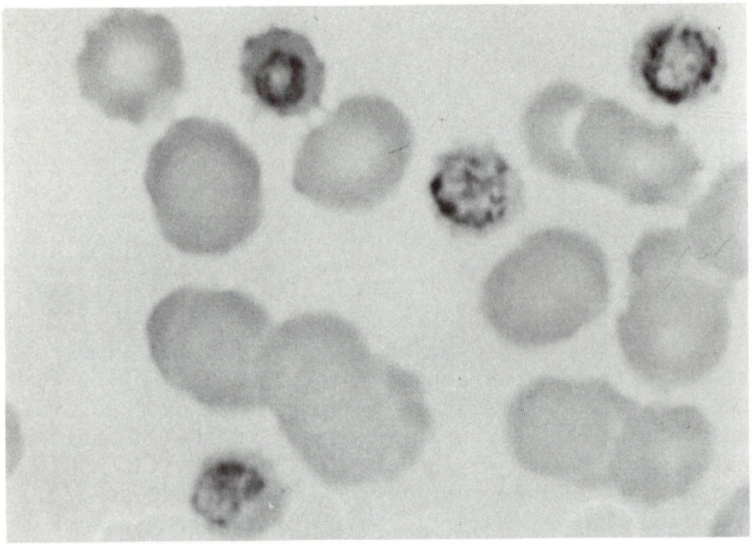

Fig. 2. Trophozoites of Plasmodium knowlesi *in erythrocytes of an experimentally infected monkey.*

Evidence most suggestive of the latter may be found in Central and South America where the only 2 simian malaria parasites identified thus far (*P. simium* and *P. brasilianum*) have direct counterparts in man and apparently did not exist in these areas until after 1492, when the first Europeans entered the New World.

In reviewing the subject of simian malaria in man, Coatney (1971) proposed that *P. cynomolgi*, *P. knowlesi*, *P. inui*, and *P. schwetzi* were true zoonotic agents. *P. schwetzi*, as *P. ovale* may be anthropozoonotic agents, and *P. malariae* and *P. rodhaini* are probably synonyms for the same organism, which may be zoonotic or anthropozoonotic in nature. The author further suggested that *P. brasilianum* and *P. simium* may be synonyms for *P. malariae* and *P. vivax*, both species being arthropozoonotic or possibly only zoonotic in the case of *P. brasilianum* (Table 1).

As with vectors of African trypanosomes, the taxonomic identification of malaria vectors does not always indicate their role in malaria epidemiology. Rutledge *et al.*, (1970) described differences among and within species of anopheline mosquitoes with reference to their susceptibility to infection with malarial parasites. These differences extended even to colonies of mosquitoes derived from the same laboratory stock. Differences in niche and host selection among

Table 1

Zoonotic and anthropozoonotic plasmodium species and their geographic distribution. Adapted from Coatney, G.R., (1971). Am. J. Trop. Med. Hyg. 20, *795.*

SIMIAN MALARIA IN MAN

Organism	Geographic Region	
P. cynomolgi	Asia	True zoonotic agents (Simian forms infecting man)
P. knowlesi	Asia	
P. inui	Asia	
P. schwetzi	Africa	Anthropozoonotic agents (Human forms infecting other primates)
P. schwetzi (P. ovale)	Africa	
P. rodhaini (P. malariae)	Africa	
P. brasilianum (P. malariae)	South America	Zoonotic, possibly anthropozoonotic agents
P. simium (P. vivax)		

individuals of the same species of mosquitoes are influenced by geographic locale, have been described for *Anopheles cruzi* in Brazil (WHO, 1969c). It is hoped that newer techniques designed to identify the host species from which arthropod blood meals were obtained (Tempelis and Rodrick, 1972) will facilitate future work in primate malaria epidemiology.

The development of techniques for characterizing plasmodia on the basis of deoxyribonucleic acid (DNA) (Gutteridge *et al.*, 1971) and isoenzymes (Carter and Voller, 1973) may eventually supplement the morphological criteria presently used for identifying primate malaria parasites.

The World Health Organization (WHO, 1969c) has pointed out that the primary factors to be considered in assessing the importance of human infection with plasmodia of simian origin are (1) contact between man, vector, and simian hosts, (2) vector susceptibility to simian and/or human plasmodia and (3) the presence and levels of gametocytes in the vertebrate host's blood. The evidence accumulated thus far suggests that simian malaria represents little or no danger to man or malaria eradication programs except during the rare occurrence of human exposure to vectors of simian plasmodia.

BABESIOSIS

In 1888, Babes first observed *Babesia* parasites in the blood of African cattle showing hemoglobinuria. In 1893, Smith and Kilborne demonstrated tick transmission of *Babesia bigemina*, the causative agent of bovine babesiosis, "Texas fever." This was the first pathogenic protozoan shown to be transmitted by an arthropod vector. Since then, 17 distinct species of *Babesia* have been found in various vertebrate hosts (Riek, 1968). The organism may be transmitted by various blood-sucking arthropods but ticks are the main vectors. Recent electron-microscopic studies of bovine, ovine, and equine species of babesia, including erythrocytic and tick phases of development, have shown that the organism is structurally similar to sporozoa (Riek, 1964a, Riek, 1964b; Ristic, 1966; Friedhoff and Scholtyseck, 1968a, 1968b, 1969; Holbrook *et al.*, 1968; Holbrook, 1970). Unlike plasmodium, however, babesia does not leave residual hemozoin pigment following ingestion of food vacuole-stored hemoglobin (Rudzinski and Vickerman, 1968). Now, some 80 years after discovery of the first case, babesiosis remains one of the most important bovine hemotropic diseases which occurs in tropical and semitropical regions of the world. Clinical symptoms of acute babesiosis are characterized by fever, anorexia, hemolytic anemia, and occasional hemoglobinuria (Ristic, 1970, 1972).

Until recently, the various *Babesia* strains were considered to be host specific. However, 5 confirmed human cases of babesiosis have been described indicating the zoonotic potential of certain babesial species. Three of the patients had been splenectomized prior to the onset of the disease; 2 of these individuals died. The fourth case involved an intact (spleen *in situ*) human patient (Western *et al.*, 1970; Ristic *et al.*, 1971).

While this manuscript was in preparation, the fifth human case of acute babesiosis was reported (Cassady *et al.*, 1973). This represented the second human case with spleen *in situ* and occurred in the same geographical location as the previous case.

Babesiosis in splenectomized individuals

In 1957 Skrobalo and Deanović reported the first case of acute babesiosis in man. A 33-year-old farmer living on the outskirts of Zagreb, Yugoslavia had suffered internal injuries in a car accident 11 years earlier and his spleen had been removed. In June, 1956, he was admitted to a hospital ill with fever, anemia, jaundice, and hemogloginuria. His blood contained numerous intraerythrocytic "rings" which were later identified as *Babesia bovis*. The patient died 8 days later. Cattle in pastures where the patient tended his animals had been affected by babesiosis.

The second case occurred in 1966 in California in a 46-year-old man who, because of hereditary spherocytosis, was splenectomized 2 years earlier (Scholtens *et al.*, 1968). The patient had visited remote coastal areas near San Francisco during the months preceding illness. He was admitted to a hospital with chills and fever, diagnosed as a case of malaria placed on 250 mg. of chloroquine weekly for about 15 weeks, and recovered. The case was later diagnosed as babesiosis when "Maltese-cross"-type intraerythrocytic organisms were observed in his blood. The organism in question was suspected of being of equine origin.

The indirect fluorescent antibody test of the patient's serum was negative to *Plasmodium* antigens, but *Babesia* antibodies were demonstrated in both complement fixation and latex tube agglutination tests.

The third case occurred in Ireland in 1967 (Fitzpatric *et al.*, 1968; Fitzpatrick *et al.*, 1969). A deep-sea fisherman became ill with fever, jaundice and anemia. An intraerythrocytic parasite found in his blood shortly before death was later identified as *Babesia divergens*. The patient was splenectomized 4 months before the onset of illiness. Epidemiologic investigation showed that the patient had presumably contacted the disease from bites of infected ticks during the holiday in the country.

Babesiosis in persons with a spleen

The fourth human case occurred on Nantucket Island off the coast of Massachusetts, in a previously healthy, 59-year-old widow whose spleen had not been removed. Thus, this was the first spleen *in situ* human case of babesiosis (Western, *et al.*, 1970). The patient was admitted to a New Jersey hospital on July 13, 1969, with a 2-week history of fever, headache and crampy abdominal pain. A Wright-stained peripheral blood smear obtained on admission showed numerous ring-like structures within erythrocytes that resembled *Plasmodium falciparum* trophozoites. Since malaria was suspected, oral therapy with chloroquine phosphate was initiated on the evening of July 14. A total of 1.5 g was given in the initial 24 hours. When the diagnosis of babesiosis was made on the 3rd hospital day, it was decided to continue chloraquine in a daily dose of 0.5 g for the next 30 days. By the 7th day, the patient was afebrile and had no systemic complaints.

Epidemiologic investigations revealed that before her illness, the patient's dog was frequently infested by ticks, and often chased, killed and returned mice and other small rodents to the house. In mid-May the patient found a tick deeply embedded in her own suprasternal notch and removed it with some difficulty.

A babesia strain was isolated in hamsters (Gleason *et al.*, 1970) and splenectomized monkeys (Ristic *et al.*, 1971) from the blood of the patient. Van Peenen and Healy (1970) studied infections with the organism in laboratory reared prairie voles. Three consecutive passages of the parasite were made in splenectomized monkeys, and it was transmitted from the monkeys to hamsters, but not to dogs. Intraerythrocytic parasites appeared as spherical, ameboid or elongated bodies, 1.5 to 2.5 μ in size. The parasite was limited by a single membrane, and its ultrastructural features were similar to those described for *Babesia microti*. Indirect fluorescent-antibody tests showed that the stain was serologically related but not identical with *Babesia canis*. A capillary tube agglutination test, with an antigen prepared from the blood of a dog infected with *B. canis*, detected antibody in serum of infected monkeys, of the patient, and of her dog, but not her horse and donkey (Ristic *et al.*, 1971) (Fig. 3).

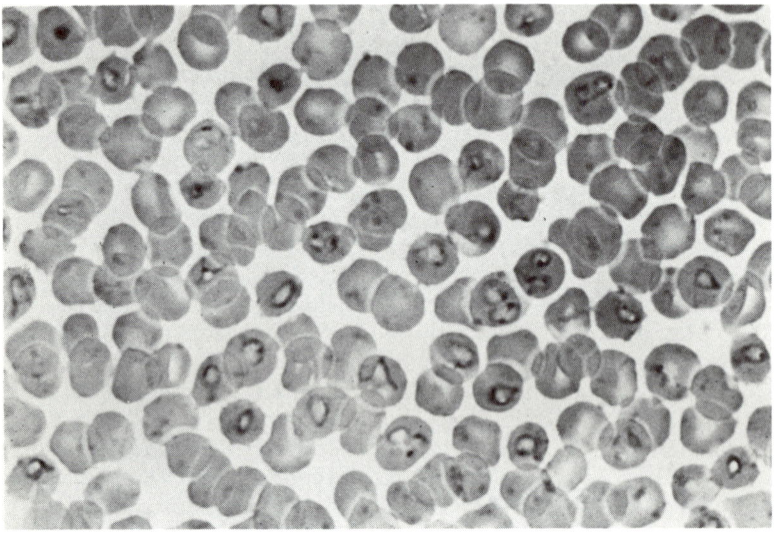

Fig. 3. Giemsa stain blood film from a hamster infected with Babesia microti *isolated from a human.*

The second human case of acute babesiosis with spleen *in situ* was a 48-year-old woman also residing in Nantucket Island, Mass. (Cassady *et al.*, 1973). Medical history of the patient showed that she had received a tick bite in mid-August, 1973, which became inflamed. On August 17, the patient's physician excised the local abscess containing the tick head. The patient was admitted to the hospital on September 6 with temperature of 104 F, symptoms of chills and myalgia in her legs and side, and depression. Intraerythrocytic parasites identified as *Babesia microti* were found upon examination of the patient's Giemsa-strained blood smears. The patient's serum was positive to *B. microti* using the indirect fluorescent antibody test at a titer of 1:1024. The organism was recovered in gerbils inoculated with the blood of the patient. As in the case of the other patient with spleen *in situ*, this person had not traveled outside the United States since 1971 and had lived in southeast Nantucket Island with her son since June, 1973. She had no history of recent blood transfusion or parenteral drug use. Rats and ticks were abundant on the Island.

Significance of human babesiosis

The pathogenic potential of babesia for human beings has been documented by the 5 cases described herein. Three of these individuals had been splenectomized prior to the disease while the most recent patients were persons with spleen *in situ*. Lacking further knowledge of the virulence of *Babesia* species for intact human beings, one should consider deficient splenic function and concomitant infectious or non-infectious disease syndromes (metabolic and endocrinologic) as possible co-factors which could enhance the virulence of the agent. With these stipulations in mind, babesiosis may present a hazard to numerous splenectomized persons and to an unknown number whose splenic function is deficient or who possess "disease precipitating co-factors." Susceptibility of splenectomized chimpanzees to infections with *Babesia divergens* was experimentally shown by Garnham and Bray (1959). The fact that the last two cases occurred in the same geographic region (Nantucket Island) and involved persons who had not been splenectomized, raises speculation regarding the role of the virulence of certain *Babesia* species in the pathogenesis of human babesiosis. In both instances the organism was identified as *B. microti*, a species of rodent origin. It is thus possible that this particular organism may be more virulent for man than similar *Babesia* organisms. One must, however, take into consideration the role of the vector (tick) in the completion of the cycle of infection. It is well established that differences exist among different tick species with respect to their ability to invade man.

The human health impact of the latent form of babesiosis, which is the major concern of this study, might be greater than generally anticipated. Information gained from studies of babesiosis in domestic animals indicates that for every clinically demonstrable case there are hundreds of cases of latent infection. According to Nicolle (1961), inapparent or latent infections are a common feature in many microbial infections of man and can be detected only by employing special techniques. Aside from the frequency of latent human babesiosis, acquisition of the knowledge regarding manifestations of this form of babesiosis is medically important. Latent human babesiosis may be manifested by symptoms not commonly ascribed to this disease. On the subject, Garnham *et al.*, (1969) suggested that babesia may be the etiologic agent of multiple sclerosis, particularly among farm workers. Babesial infections are known to affect nervous and other extravascular tissues, thus symptoms may be variable and many.

There are only a few places in the world that are free of babesiosis. In many tropical and subtropical regions, babesiosis is endemic. Undoubtedly, agricultural workers and people who spend much time in rural endemic areas frequently come in contact with *Babesia*-infected ticks. Various babesial species have been incriminated as potential human pathogens. Four, and possibly 5, species of babesiae have been the cause of the 5 human cases of babesiosis. Under these circumstances one may anticipate that the latent form of human babesiosis is frequent in endemic areas.

In each of the above described cases the initial diagnosis was falciparum malaria. This is because the trophozoites of *P. falciparum* resemble morphologically certain forms of babesia parasites. Serologic diagnosis is even more complicated, particularly in view of suggested cross-reactions between certain babesia antigens and antibodies to a malaria parasite antigen present in both *P. falciparum* and *P. vivax* (Ludford and Hall, 1972).

SUMMARY

The zoonotic potential of trypanosomes, both African and American types, has been established. The role of wild and domestic animals as reservoirs of human infection with African trypanosomes needs further study. Progress is being made toward development of more practical methods for identification of zoonotic trypanosome species.

Current evidence indicates that simian malaria poses little danger to man and to the malaria eradication programs. The question of certain plasmodial species being true zoonotic and/or anthropozoonotic agents needs further study.

Babesiosis, the most recent zoonosis, is intriguing and the least scientifically understood. Public health importance of babesiosis may be anticipated because (1) the disease is widespread among domestic and wild animals and infected tick vectors occur in most tropical and subtropical regions of the world; (2) at least 4 and possbly more species of babesia have been shown to cause acute human infections.

In view of the morphologic resemblance between *Babesia* parasites and *P. falciparum*, and because of possible antigenic relationships between certain malarial and bebesial species, the occurrence of human babesiosis may have disturbing practical implications for those engaged in the control of malaria.

REFERENCES

Alvarez, M., De Rissio, A.M., De Martini, G.J.W., Abramo Orrego, L., and Cerisola, J.A. (1971). *Bol. Chil. Parasit. 26*, 2.

Babes, V. (1888). *Compt. Rend. Hebdomadaires des Sênac. de L'Academ. des Scien., 107*, 692.

Bafort, J.M. and Kageruka, P. (1972). *Ann. Soc. Belg. Méd. Trop. 52*, 235.

Baretto, M.P. (1967). *Revsta. Soc. Bras. Med. Trop., 1*, 167.

Bittencourt, A.L. and Barbosa, H.S. (1972). *Revsta. Inst. Med. Trop. S. Paulo 14*, 257.

Bittencourt, A.L., Barbosa, H.S., Rocha, T., Sodré, I., and Sodré, A. (1972). *Revsta. Inst. Med. Trop. S. Paulo 14*, 131.

Bray, R.S. (1968). *In Infectious Blood Diseases of Man and Animals.* (D. Weinman and M. Ristic, Eds.), Vol. I, pp. 123-136.

Bruce-Chwatt, L.J. (1972). *Trop. Dis. Bull. 69*, 825.

Carter, R. and Voller, A. (1973). *Br. Med. J.* Jan. 20, 149.

Cassady, P., Anderson, A.E., and Fiumura, N.J. (1973). *US DEW NO. (CDC) 74-8017*, 331.

Cerisola, J.A., Alvarez, M., And Rissio, A.M. (1970). *Revsta. Inst. Med. Trop. S. Paulo 12*, 403.

Cerisola, J.A., Rohwedder, R.W., and Del Prado, C.E. (1971a). *Bol. Chil. Parasit. 26*, 57.

Cerisola, J.A., Del Prado, C.E., Rahwedder, R., and Bozzini, J.P. (1971b). *J. Protozool. 18*, 503.

Chin, W., Contacos, P.G., Coatney, G.R., and Kimball, H.R. (1965). *Science, 149*, 865.

Coatney, G.R. (1971). *Am. J. Trop. Med. Hyg. 20*, 795.

Coatney, G.R., Collins, W.E., Warren, McW., Contacos, P.G. (1971). Supt. of Documents, U. S. Gov't. Printing Office, Washington, D. C.

Collins, W.E. and Contacos, P.G. (1969). *J. Parasit. 55*, 1253.

Collins, W.E. and Contacos, P.G. (1972). *Trans. Roy Soc. Med. Hyg. 66*, 371.

Collins, W.E., Contacos, P.G., Krotoski, W.A., and Howard, W.A. (1972). *J. Parasit. 58*, 332.

Contacos, P.G. and Collins, W.W. (1969). *Science, 165*, 918.
Cunningham, M.P., Bailey, N.M., and Kimber, C.D. (1967). *Trans. Roy Soc. Trop. Med. Hyg. 61*, 688.
Deane, L.M., Deane, M.P., and Neto, J.F. (1966). *Bull. Wld. Hlth. Org. 35*, 805.
Deane, L.M., Deane, M.P., Ferreira Neto, J.A., and Almeida, F.B. (1971). *Revsta. Inst. Med. Trop. S. Paola 13*, 311.
Díaz-Ungría, C. (1969). *Revsta. Univ. Zulía. Supl. Científico, No. 44/47*, 114.
Díaz-Ungría, C. and Maldonado Alvarez, C. (1970). *Revsta. Ibér. Parasit. 30*, 659.
Disko, R. and Krampitz, H.E. (1971). *Z. Tropenmed. Parasit. K. 22*, 56.
Eyles, D.E., Coatney, G.R., and Getz, M.E. (1960). *Science, 131*, 1812.
Farrar, W.E., Jr., Gibbins S.D., and Whitfield, S.T. (1972). *Am. J. Trop. Med. Hyg. 21*, 404.
Ferreora Neto. J.A., Deane, L.M., and Almeida, F.B. (1972). *Revsta. Inst. Med. Trop. S. Paulo, 14*, 231.
Fitzpatrick, J.E.P., Kennedy, C.C., McGeown, M.G., Oreopoulos, D.G., Robertson, J.H., Soyannwo, M.A.W. (1968). *Nature, 217*, 861.
Fitzpatrick, J.E.P., Kennedy, C.C., McGeown, M.G., Oreopoulos, D.G., Robertson, J.H., and Soyannwo, M.A. O. (1969). *Brit. Med. J. 4*, 770.
Friedhoff, K. and Scholtyseck, E. (1968a). *J. Parasit. 54*, 1246.
Friedhoff, K. and Scholtyseck, E. (1968b). *Z. Parasit. 30*, 347.
Friedhoff, K. and Scholtyseck, E. (1969). *Z. Parasit. 32*, 266.
Frong, Y.L., Cadigan, F.C., and Coatney, G.R. (1971). *Trans. Roy Soc. Trop. Med. Hyg. 65*, 839.
Ford, J. (1971). *In The Role of the Trypanosomiases in Africa Ecology. A Study of the Tsetse Fly Problem.* Clarendon Press, Oxford University Press, London.
Garnham, P.C.C. and Bray, R.S. (1959). *J. Protozool., 6*, 352.
Garnham, P.C.C.,Donnelly, J. Hoogstraal, H., Kennedy, C.C., and Walton, G.A. (1969). *Brit. Med. J., 4*, 768.
Garnham, P.C.C., Warren, Mc.W., and Killick-Kendrick, R. (1971). *J. Trop. Med. Hyg. 74*, 32.
Geigy, R. and Kauffmann, M. (1973). *Acta. Tropica, 30*, 12.
Geigy, R., Kauffmann, M., Mayende, J.S.P., Mwambu, P.M., and Onyango, R.J. (1973). *Acta. Tropica, 30*, 49.
Gleason, N.N., Healy, G.R., Western, K.A., Benson, G.D., and Schultz, M.G. (1970). *J. Parasit. 56*, 1256.
Gray, A.R. (1969). *Bull. Wld. Hlth. Org. 41*, 805.

Gutteridge, W.E., Trigg, P.I., and Williamson, D.H. (1971). *Parasitology, 62,* 209.
Heisch, R.B., McMahon, J.P., and Manson-Bahr, P.E.C. (1958). *Brit. Med. J. 3,* 1203.
Hoare, C.A. (1972a). *In: The Trypanosomes of Mammals. A Zoological Monograph.* Blackwell Scientific Publ., Oxford.
Hoare, C.A. (1972b). *Trop. Dis. Bull. 69,* 188.
Holbrook, A.A., Anthony, D.W., and Johnson, A.J. (1968). *J. Protozool. 15,* 391.
Holbrook, A.A. (1970). *Miscellaneous Publications 6,* 345.
Hoof, L.M.J.J. van (1947). *Trans. Roy Soc. Trop. Med. Hyg. 40,* 728.
Huggins, D. and Lucena, D.T. (1969). *Anals Escola Nac. Saúde Publ. Med. Trop. 3,* 97.
Juminer, B. (1970). *Arch. Inst. Pasteur Tunis 47,* 229.
Le Ray, D., Afchain, D., Jadin, J., Capron, A., and Fameree, L. (1971). *Ann. Parasit Hum. Comp. 46,* 523.
Lucasse, C. (1970). *Trop. Geogr. Med. 22,* 227.
Ludford, C.G. and Hall, W.T.K. (1972). *Expt. Parasit. 32,* 317.
Lumsden, W.H.R. (1972). *Brit. Med. Bull. 28,* 34.
Marsden, P.D., Seah, S.K.K., Mott, K.E., Prata, A., and Platt, H. (1970). *J. Trop. Med. Hyg. 73,* 157.
Miles, M.A. (1972). *Parasitology, 65,* 1.
Moloo, S.K., Steiger, R.F., Bran, R., and Boreham, P.F.L. (1971). *Acta. Trop. 28,* 181.
Most, H. (1973). *Am. J. Trop. Med. Hyg. 22,* 157.
Mshelbwala, A.S. (1972). *Trans. Roy Soc. Trop. Med. Hyg. 66,* 637.
Mwambu, P.M. and Mayende, J.S.P. (1971). *Acta. Trop. 28,* 181, parts I-V.
Mwambu, P.M. and Woodford, M.H. (1972). *Trop. Anim. Hlth. Prod. 4,* 152.
Nicolle, C. (1961). Geneva, Alliance Culturelle du Livre.
Omerod, W.E. (1967). *J. Parasit. 53,* 824.
Onyango, R.J. (1969). *Bull. Wld. Hlth. Org. 41,* 815.
Onyango, R.J. Van Hoeve, K., and De Raadt, P. (1966). *Trans. Roy Soc. Trop. Med. Hyg. 60,* 175.
Onyango, R.J., Geigy, R., Mwambu, P.M., and Moloo, S.K. (1971) *Acta. Trop. 28,* 181.
Page, W.A. (1972). *Trop. Anim. Hlth. Prod. 4,* 41.
Perruolo-Lanetti, G.J. (1971). *Kasmera. 3,* 343.
Porter, J.A., Jr. (1970). *J. Protozool. 17,* 361.
Rickman, L.R. and Robson, J. (1970a). *Bull. Wld. Hlth. Org. 42,* 650.
Rickman, L.R. and Robson, J. (1970b). *Bull. Wld. Hlth. Org. 42,* 911.
Rickman, L.R. and Robson, J. (1972). *Bull. Wld. Hlth. Org.*

46, 403.
Riek, R.F. (1964a). *Aust. J. Agr. Res. 15*, 802.
Riek, R.F. (1964b). *Aust. J. Agr. Res. 40*, 261.
Riek, R.F. (1968). *In Infectious Blood Diseases of Man and Animals*, (D. Weinman and M. Ristic, eds.), Vol. II, Academic Press, New York. pp. 219-268.
Ristic, M. (1966). *In Biology of Parasites*, (E.J.L. Soulsby, ed.), Academic Press, New York. pp. 127-141.
Ristic, M. (1970). *In Bovine Medicine and Surgery*. (W.J. Gibbons, E.J. Catcott, J.F. Smithcors, eds.), Am. Vet. Publ. Inc., Wheaton, Ill. pp. 208-209.
Ristic, M., Conroy, J.D., Siwe, Sandra, Healy, G.R., Smith, A.R., and Huxsoll, D.L. (1971). *Am. J. Trop. Med. Hyg. 20*, 14.
Ristic, M. (1972). *In Equine Medicine and Surgery*. (E.J. Catcott, J.F. Smithcors, eds.), Am. Vet Publ. Inc., Wheaton, Ill. pp. 137-155.
Rocha E. Silva, E.O., Maluf, J., and Correa, R.R. (1970). *Revsta. Saúde Publ. 4*, 129.
Rohwedder, R.W. (1969). *Bol. Chil. Parasit. 24*, 88.
Ross, J.P.J. (1971). *Ann. Trop. Med. Parasit. 65*, 327.
Rutledge, L.C., Hayes, D.E., and Ward, R.A. (1970). *Expt. Parasit. 27*, 53.
Rudzinska, M.A. and Vickerman, K. (1968). *In Infectious Blood Diseases of Man and Animals*, (D. Weinman and M. Ristic, eds.), Vol. I, Academic Press, New York. pp. 217-306.
Schenone, H., Rubinstein, P., Knierim, F., Sandoval, J., and Rojas, A. (1968). *Bol. Chil. Parasit. 23*, 83.
Schindler, R. and Sachs, R. (1970). *Z. Tropenmed. Parasit. 21*, 339.
Scholtens, R.G., Branff, E.H., Healy, G.R., and Gleason, N. (1968). *Am. J. Trop. Med. Hyg., 17*, 810.
Smith, T. and Killborne, F.L., (1893). *U.S. Dept. Agr., Bureau Anim. Ind. Bull, 1*, 1.
Skrabalo, Z. and Deanović, Z. (1957). *Doc. Med. Geogr. 9*, 11.
Soto, S.T.G. (1971). *Kasmera. 4*, 5.
Soulsby, E.J.L. (1968). *Helminths, Arthropods & Protozoa of Domesticated Animals* (6th Ed. of Mönnig's Veterinary Helminthology & Entomology) Williams & Wilkins Co., Baltimore
Sousa, O.E. and Johnson, C.M. (1973). *Am. J. Trop. Med. Hyg. 22*, 18.
Székely, R., Rojo, M., and Reys, H. (1971). *Bol. Chil. Parasit. 26*, 17.
Tempelis, C.H. and Rodrick, M.L. (1972). *Am. J. Trop. Med. Hyg. 21*, 238.
Van Peenen, P.F.D. and Healy, G.R. (1970). *J. Parasit. 56*, 1029.

Ward, R.A. (1969). *Parasitologia 11,* 135.
Ward, R.A. (1970). *Trop. Dis. Bull. 67,* 6.
Warren, M., Cheong, W.H., Fredericks, H.K., and Coatney, G.R. (1970). *Am. J. Trop. Med. Hyg. 19,* 383.
Werner, H. and Egger, I. (1971). *Z. Tropenmed. Parasit. 22,* 224.
Western, K.A., Benson, G.D., Gleason, Neva N., Healy, G.R., and Schultz, M.G. (1970). *New England J. Med. 383,* 854.
Wilson, A.J., Dar, F.K., and Paris, J. (1972). *Trop. Anim. Hlth. Prod. 4,* 14.
Woo, P.T.K. and Soltys, M.A. (1972). *Z. Tropenmed. Parasit. 23,* 166.
Wld. Hlth. Org. Techn. Rep. Ser. (1959). No. *169.*
Wld. Hlth. Org. Techn. Rep. Ser. (1967). No. *378.*
Wld. Hlth. Org. Techn. Rep. Ser. (1969a). No. *411.*
Wld. Hlth. Org. Techn. Rep. Ser. (1969b). No. *434.*
Wld. Hlth. Org. Techn. Rep. Ser. (1969c). No. *433.*
Yaeger, R.G. (1971). *J. Parasit. 57,* 1375.
Yesufu, H.M. (1971). *Ann. Trop. Med. Parasit. 65,* 341.
Yorke, W., and Blacklock, B. (1915). *Ann. Trop. Med. Parasit. 9,* 383.
Young, M.D. and Porter, J.A., Jr. (1969). *Trans Roy Soc. Trop. Med. Hyg. 63,* 203.
Young, M.D. Baerg, D.C., and Rossan, R.N. (1971). *Trans. Roy Soc. Trop. Med. Hyg. 65,* 835.
Zeledón, R. and Ponce. C. (1972). *J. Parasit. 58,* 180.

ZOONOSES IN LEISHMANIASIS

R. S. Bray

MRC Laboratories, Fajara, nr. Banjul, The Gambia

INTRODUCTION

Leishmania species primarily parasitize animals and only secondarily man. They infect lizards, marsupials, rodents, carnivores, edentates, insectivores and man. They may be restricted to lizards or to man but usually they infect a wild animal and are transmitted occasionally to dogs and/or to man. Occasionally they may be transmitted from dog to dog or man to man. They may infect only a small area of skin or they may spread through the whole macrophage system. There is a large number of species but here I will confine myself to those with the potentiality of infecting man.

THE SPECIES OF LEISHMANIA *IN MAMMALS*

Leishmania donovani

L. donovani donovani, the Indian sub-continent and Burma, largely Assam and Bengal.

No reservoir, an anthroponosis; transmitted by *P. argentipes*.

L. donovani sensu lato (s.l.), Kenya, Southern Ethiopia, Somalia and Uganda.

Probably an anthroponosis. There may be some involvement of rodents (ground-squirrels *Xerus rutilans*, gerbils *Tatera robusta*) as reservoirs (Heisch, 1963); transmitted by *P. martini*, and possibly *P. vansomeranae* and *P. celiae* (Minter and Wijers, 1963).

L. donovani s.l., Sudan, Western Ethiopia, Chad, Niger, Republique Centrafricaine, Gabon.

Reservoir: carnivores (*Felis serval phillipsi*, *Genetta genetta senegalensis*) and rodents (*Arvicanthis niloticus luctuosus*, *Acomys albigena*); transmitted by *P. langeroni orientalis* (Hoogstraal and Heyneman, 1969).

L. chagasi

L. chagasi, North-east Brazil (Ceara State).	Reservoir: the "fox" (*Lycalopex vetelus* and *Cerdocyon thous*), (Deane and Deane, 1954a, 1955; Lainson *et al.*, 1969), domestic reservoir the dog; transmitted by *Lutzomyia longipalpis* (Deane and Deane 1954b).
L. chagasi s.l., Venezuela and other South American and Central American states.	Reservoir: the crabeating fox, (Cerdocyon), possibly others, the domestic dog may be more important: transmitted by *Lu. longipalpis* (Pifano *et al.*, 1962) and possibly other *Lutzomyia* species.
L. infantum, North China, South Soviet Asia, Iran, Iraq, Syria, Jordan, Lebanon, Arabia, Turkey, the Mediterranean area and islands, Portugal, North Africa.	Reservoir: fox, (*Vulpes vulpes*), wolf (*Canis lupus*), jackal (*Canis aureus*) and porcupines (*Histrix hirsutirostris satunini*) (Laytchev *et al.*, 1951; Maruashvili and Bardzhadze, 1966; Petrisceva, 1954; Rioux and Golvan, 1969), domestic reservoir: the dog; transmitted by *P. ariasi*, *P. chienensis*, *P. major syriacus*, *P. kandelakii*, *P. simici* and *P. papatasi*, *P. perfiliewi*, *P. perniciosus tobbi*, *P. chienensis sspp.*, *P. longicuspis*, *P. caucasicus*, *P. mongolensis* (Lewis, 1971).

L. tropica

L. tropica, urban Middle East, urban South Soviet Asia, urban Iran, Mediterranean area, urban North India, urban Afghanistan, North Africa oases.	Reservoir: unknown; domestic reservoir: possibly the dog and to a lesser degree the cat (Chadwick and McHattie, 1927); transmitted by *P. papatasi*, *P. sergenti*, *P. perfiliewi* (Lewis, 1971).

L. tropica s.l., West Africa particularly Senegal, Mali, Upper Volta, Niger, Northern Nigeria, Sudan.	Reservoir: the Nile grass rat (*Arvicanthis niloticus*) (Larivière *et al.*, 1965); transmitted possibly by *P. duboscqi* or *Sergentomyia clydei* (Larivière *et al.*, 1961).
L. tropica s.l., rural Israel, Jordan, Syria and Arabia.	Reservoir: the sand rat (*Psammomys*) and a gerbil (Gunders *et al.*, 1969); transmitted by *P. papatasi* (Adler and Theodore, 1957).
L. major, rural S. Soviet Asia and Iran.	Reservoir: in descending order of importance, the giant gerbil (*Rhombomys opimus*), other gerbils (*Meriones libycus erythrourus, M. meridanianus, M. tamariscinus*), the suslik (*Spermophilopsis leptadactylus*) and the hedgehog (*Hemiechinus auritus*) (Petrescheva *et al.*, undated; Zvyagintseva, 1965); transmitted by *P. caucasicus, P. papatasi, P. mongolensis, P. ansarii*, possibly *S. arpaklensis* (Lewis, 1971).
L. aethiopica, highland Ethiopia and Mt. Elgon, Kenya.	Reservoir: rock hyraxes (Ashford *et al.*, 1973); transmitted by *P. longipes* and *P. pedifer*.

L. mexicana

L. mexicana mexicana, South Mexico, British Honduras (Belize), North Guatemala.	Reservoir: the tree rat (*Ototylomys phyllotis*), the pocket mouse (*Heteromys desmarestianus*), the vesper rat (*Nyctomys sumichrasti*) and the cotton rat (*Sigmodon hispidus*). (Lainson and Strangways-Dixon, 1964; Williams, 1970); transmitted by *Lu. olmeca* (Williams, 1970).

L. m. amazonensis, Amazonia (Brazil).	Reservoir: Cricetid rodents (*Oryzomys spp.*, *Proechimys spp.*, *Neacomys spinosus amoenus*, *Diplomys labilis*, *Nectomys squamipes*, *Kannabateomys amblyonyx*, *Zygodontomys microtinus*, opossums (*Marmosa spp.*) paca (*Cuniculus paca*), agouti (*Dasyprocta azarae*). (Forattini, 1960; Nery-Guimarães and Costa 1964; Lainson and Shaw, 1968; Lainson and Shaw, 1970; Herrer *et al.*, 1971; Kerdel-Vegas and Essenfield-Yahr, 1966); transmitted by *Lu. flaviscutellata*. (Lainson and Shaw, 1968).
L. peruviana, Peru highlands.	Reservoir unknown, domestic reservoir: the dog (Herrer, 1948); transmitted probably by *Lu. verrucarum* and *Lu. peruensis*. (Adler and Theodore, 1957; Lainson and Shaw, 1972).

L. braziliensis

L. b. braziliensis, Brazil, Venezuela, Columbia, Equador, Peru, Paraguay, Bolivia.	Reservoir: forest rodents (*Oryzomys concolor*) (Lainson and Shaw, 1972); transmitted by *Lu. paraensis* and *Lu. wellcomei* (Fraiha *et al.*, 1971) and probably by *Lu. migonei*, *Lu. whitmani* and by *Lu. anduzei*. (Lainson and Shaw, 1972; Lewis, 1971).
L. braziliensis panamensis, Panama, Costa Rica, Honduras.	Reservoir: sloths (*Choloepus hoffmanni*, *Bradypus infuscatus*), kinkajous (*Potos flavus*), porcupine (*Coendu rothschildi*) and rodents (*Proechimys semispinosus*, *Hoplomys gymnurus*) (Herrer and Telford, 1969; Thatcher *et al.*, 1965; Herrer *et al.*,

	1966); transmitted by *Lu. trapidoi* and perhaps *Lu. gomezi*, *Lu. sanguinaria*, *Lu. panamensis* and *Lu. ylephiletrix*. (McConnell, 1963; Johnson *et al.*, 1963).
L. b. guyanensis, Guyana, Surinam, French Guyana.	Reservoir: unknown; transmitted probably by *Lu. anduzei*. (Wijers and Linger, 1966).

For a summary of the phlebotomid vectors of leishmaniasis see Lewis (1971).

ASPECTS OF TRANSMISSION

I intend to deal mostly with the factors controlling transmission of the organism as these factors largely control the nature of the zoonosis both as an enzootic and an endemic. It is also this area which is most lacking in hard facts.

The distribution and course of infection of Leishmania *in the mammal host.*

In order to be an effective reservoir a host must present its parasites to the vector in a readily available manner. In dogs with visceral leishmaniasis the whole of the skin may be heavily parasitized causing hair loss, so that not only are the organisms easily available but also a barrier to biting, the hair is removed. Dedet (1971) demonstrated that 13 of 16 dogs infected with *L. infantum* showed depilation.

The incubation time of infection in a reservoir may also be important if the animal is out in the open in an environment frequently hostile to the sandfly. Most transmission occurs in a mircoclimate suitable for both reservoir and vector but the dog is an exception to this. While the dog may be only a "liaison host" (Garnham, 1965) between the wild host and man it may nonetheless be an important and possibly irreplaceable link. So to complete the zoonosis it may be that a sandfly infected by a fox or a jackal must seek out and infect a dog to bring the parasite into the domestic situation. If sandfly flights outside burrows or earths are restricted to certain times of the year as happens in Tunisia or Iraq and if the incubation time in the dog is greater than this period then the dog must retian the infection for at least 9 to 10 months in order to act as a domestic reservoir in the following year.

Dedet (1971) estimates that the incubation period is not

less than one month and symptomatic incubation may be 6 months. Nothing is known about the incubation period between infective bite and infectivity to new sandflies. However it seems almost certain that the dog is a significant reservoir of *L. infantum* mostly in the following year as in most areas of *L. infantum* sandfly flight in open areas is restricted to the summer months. This is reinforced by the knowledge that infection of sandflies increases with the infection of the dog's skin (Adler and Theodore, 1957).

It would be advantageous to the parasite if the wild reservoir were to have a long-lasting infection and it is significant that the jackal infected by Dedet (1971) had a milder and longer infection than is usual in dogs. On the other hand the jackal showed little depilation.

In the reservoirs of cutaneous leishmaniasis the little understood immune mechanisms confine or help to confine the organisms to the site of the infecting bites. Sandflies will tend always to bite the same piece of exposed skin. In the rock hyrax *L. aethiopica* is confined almost absolutely to the very tip of the nose which is where the sandfly both delivers and picks up the infection (Ashford *et al.*, 1973). The same applies to the ears of the great gerbil in the Kara-Kum desert (Eliseev and Kellina, 1964; Dubrovsky *et al.*, 1968) and the base of the tail of cricetid and heteromyid rodents of the Americas (Lainson and Strangways-Dixon, 1964; Lainson and Shaw, 1968; Kerdel-Vegas and Essenfeld-Yahr, 1966; Herrer *et al.*, 1971).

In many cases the organism will not survive at the higher temperatures of hirsute areas of the body (as in *L. enriettii* infection, Bryceson *et al.*, 1970) and these areas are also unavailable to the delicate sandfly which cannot easily probe through hair. The organisms thrive at the lower temperatures of bare skin where the fly is able to bite.

The pick-up of Leishmania *by sandflies*

The sandfly survives and breeds most often in highly confined microclimates and sometimes these microclimates also support the reservoir. In fact, the reservoir host may even contribute significantly to the microclimate essential for the sandfly. Most sandflies breed in soil with critical amounts of organic material and this may be contributed directly or indirectly by the reservoirs' wastes. The giant gerbil in Soviet Asia constructs burrows and provides the faeces and food remains necessary for the breeding of sandflies and also contributes significantly to the necessary high humidity (Petrisceva, 1971).

Of course other factors also contribute towards a microclimate suitable for either reservoir or sandfly or both. One of the most important is sub soil- water and Pringle (1952) has shown that a high water table around Baghdad favors the development of the larvae of *P. sergenti*. Petrischeva (1971) notes two consequences of greater infiltration of the sandy soil of the Turkmen SSR desert area caused by irrigation. The water may become excessive around human habitation causing the giant gerbil to move away in which case human disease is greatly reduced. On the other hand conditions near large rivers or in irrigation schemes may provide the right amount of water for the giant gerbil and the sandfly vector to thrive together and give rise to intense epizootics with a consequent rise in human disease in the immediate vicinity. (See also Neronov and Gunin, 1971).

When the reservoir host and sandfly occupy the same habitat the transmission of leishmaniae between reservoir hosts may be intense. The intensity of transmission, given stable microclimatic conditions in the shared habitat will be directly proportional to the inhospitality of the outside environment. At 2600 m. in Ethiopia for much of the year dusk and night temperatures and humidities are so low that *P. longipes* do not leave the cliff cracks and caves which they share with the rock hyraxes and hyrax feeding by the vector and therefore transmission is intense. Hyraxes are about 25% infected and *P. longipes* about 4% (Ashford *et al.*, 1973). In the gerbil burrows in the USSR steppes or deserts such as the Kara-Kum temperatures fluctuate by only 2°C at the most and relative humidity by no more than 10% (Petrisceva, 1971). Outside, over the year shade temperatures fluctuate from well below 0°C to over 40°C and the soil surface may be 80°C, the relative humidity may drop below 10% and strong winds are a common feature. The sandflies remain below ground feeding almost exclusively on gerbils. There, conditions facilitate pick-up and up to 25% of sandflies may be infected from which up to 100% of gerbils may acquire infections in some situations (Petrisceva, 1971).

Another environment in which reservoir and vector may coexist is forest, particularly in the New World where the conditions of temperature and humidity below the canopy alter little through the day and the year. Near Belem at the mouth of the Amazon the relationship between *Lu. flaviscutellata* and the cricetid *Oryzomys capito* is also close. Using rodent baited traps Lainson and Shaw (1968) found that 99.15% of sandflies coming to feed on rodents were *Lu. flaviscutellata*. The rodents are about 18% infected. The sandflies however are only 0.3% infected which must reflect to some degree the "open" situation of the forest as compared to the gerbil burrow or hyrax cave. *Lu. flaviscutellata* is fairly catholic in its tastes, feeding upon monkeys, chickens and marsupials as well as rodents when these animals are used as bait in traps (Shaw and Lainson, 1968).

Much less is known about the shared environment between reservoir and sandfly in visceral leishmaniasis. However sandflies are known to colonize jackal and porcupine holes readily and both are known reservoirs (Petrisceva, 1971; Ashford *et al.*, 1973); as many as 33% of jackals have been shown to be positive (Petrischeva *et al.*, undated). The vector of Kenya kala-azar is *P. martini* which lives in the air shafts of termite hills but no reservoir is known (Minter, 1963). One "open" situation is known where in the Sudan *P. langeroni orientalis* occupies the system of cracks which appears in the black cotton soil in the dry season. The reservoirs are burrowing rodents, non-burrowing rodents and two hunting carnivores. The contact between reservoirs and sandflies seems to be adventitious in this "open" woodland situation. Even so 2.5% sandflies were infected; much higher than in Amazonia (Hoogstraal and Heyneman, 1969).

When the sandfly probes it seems able to take up tissue juice as well as blood and therefore it seems probable that it slashes and breaks cells (Adler and Theodore, 1957). This would obviously facilitate the ingestion of the intracellular leishmaniae. It also seems probable that it requires only very few organisms to establish an infection in sandflies. We have seen infections with 2 or 3 flagellates in guts of nulliparous sandflies which also contained whole red cells (i.e. less than 24 hrs after feeding). The source of the flagellates - the nose of a hyrax - commonly contains only very few organisms (Ashford *et al.*, 1973).

In the reservoir of both visceral and cutaneous leishmaniasis, the parasites usually occur in the macrophages of the dermis. It is unlikely that parasites in circulating monocytes or reservoirs other than man play any great part in maintaining the species.

THE INFECTION IN SANDFLIES

For the establishment of the infection in the mid-gut of the sandfly it seemsthe gut must be sterile (Adler and Theodore, 1957), which is usually the case though occasional infection with bacteria can be seen. For the infection to be transmitted it seems it must move anteriorly and flagellates must be found anterior to the proventriculus and probably in the pharynx and mouth parts. This tends to restrict a particular species or sub-species of *Leishmania* to a particular species or sub-species of sandfly. For instance Sudanese *L. donovani* infects the local vector *P. l. orientalis* progressively and the infection moves into the anterior portions of the gut. However in another sandfly *P. papatasi*, a known vector elsewhere, the infection is not progressive and the anterior portions are either not infected or the infection there dies out (Heyneman, 1963).

Transmission to man

The next step in the zoonotic pathway is the seeking out of man by the sandfly. So obviously the sandfly must be anthropophilic but far from exclusively so. Obviously divergence away from man as a host will have a profound effect upon the extent of a zoonosis. *P. argentipes* once a manbiter *par excellence* and the vector involved in the great pandemics of kala-azar in Bengal and Assam is now almost exclusively feeding on cattle. In this case it would be interesting to know if *P. argentipes* has been diverted to cattle-feeding or if *P. argentipes* was a species complex containing a distinct anthropophilic and a distinct zoophilic species. In the former case the divergence would be due to irritability towards antimalarial DDT in houses and in the latter DDT has eradicated the anthropophilic species.

P. longipes near Addis Ababa becomes infected from rock hyrax but is primarily a cattle feeder when near human habitation so the incidence of disease in man is very low.

More important perhaps is the effect of the triad - temperature, humidity and wind - upon flight range. Pifano *et al.*, (1962) have pointed out that sandflies will venture forth from their microclimate only if the outside tempature and humidity approximate to that of their microclimate. While this may commonly be the case in humid warm forest it is only rarely so in savannah or highlands.

In savannah, desert or highlands sandflies may be confined to the microhabitat for most or all of the day and much of the year. In the Uzbek SSR Zvyagintseva (1968) showed that in August *P. papatasi* is 4.9% infected near gerbil burrows but only 1.5% infected 800 m. from the burrows. Ashford *et al.*, (1973) showed that at an altitude of 2600 m. in Ethiopia *P. longipes* could not be taken with any regularity using human bait more than 1 m. from the cliff face which was the hyrax-sandfly habitat. In this area prevalence of the human disease was below 1%. At 1800 m. altitude and further south (warmer) in the Ethiopian highlands *P. pedifer* flew freely in a village at dusk and the prevalence rate of human diseases was 40%. Any amount of wind will also cause sandflies to cease biting man. Hoogstraal *et al.*, (1962) found that sandflies in the Sudan ceased biting even when winds were relatively light. Dr. Ashford and I have found that in gullies at 1800 m. in the Ethiopian highlands *P. l. orientalis* will cease to bite man when the wind is sufficient to rustle dry leaves on the ground.

Finally man himself may induce the biting process by disturbing the sandflies. Wijers and Linger (1966) found that *Lu. anduzei* was more prone to bite when disturbed from its resting place in tree buttresses by the entomologists searching for it. Williams (1970) considers that *Lu. olmeca* transmits *L. m. mexicana* to man largely when man disturbs the leaves of the forest (its resting place) early in the morning.

Assuming the vector is heavily infected in the pharynx and hypopharynx and has reached a suitable mammal it is able to transmit the organism. But we do not know how or whether it will. The salivary glands are not infected and the salivary duct meets the alimentary canal so anteriorly that the passage of saliva cannot flush the organisms into the wound. The mode of delivery is known to be inefficient both because of the enormous number of failures of laboratory transmission and on epidemiological grounds where, although reservoir animals may be bitten almost daily to infected sandflies, relatively few animals are infected (Ashford *et al.*, 1973). In the laboratory the only successful transmissions have involved tricks like intermediate feeds on raisins or feeding the sandflies on blood diluted with saline (Adler and Theodore, 1957).

On one occasion infection of man was achieved by a sandfly which merely probed and it may be that the relaxation of the muscles used in probing at the time of an unsuccessful probe may force some flagellates from the hypopharynx into the wound. Obviously slapping and crushing the sandfly would also force flagellates into the wound but this would not explain infantile kala-azar or the infection of most reservoirs.

How the flagellate is innoculated into the vertebrate remains the major mystery in leishmaniasis. This lack of an essential piece of knowledge is the major reason why a mathematical epidemiological formula cannot be produced for leishmainisis as has been attempted by MacDonald (1957, 1965) for malaria and schistosomiasis. So long as it cannot be calculated what proportion of a population of infected sandflies can deliver the organism into a vertebrate, the attack rate cannot be calculated thus nullifying any attempt to predict epidemiological factors. This is compounded by a lack of knowledge of the number of flagellates necessary to achieve a continuing infection in the new vertebrate host. At present it is impossible to approach the epidemiology of leishmaniasis with any preconception of the prevalence to be expected among reservoirs, sandflies or man.

There has been a discussion on the sandfly seeking out man but of probably more importance is man's activity in relation to the sandfly. Leishmaniasis is to a considerable degree an occupational disease as it is frequently man's occupation which brings him within range of the sandfly. In Ethiopia where very close proximity to the reservoir-vector habitat may be necessary to acquire the disease the occupation of herding goats on the rocky slopes brings the pre-teenage children into the orbit of *P. longipes*.

In the Americas any occupation taking man to the forest carries with it the hazard of cutaneous leishmaniasis. The chichle gatherer of British Honduras, the farmer clearing land in Panama and the road builder in Amazonian Brazil are all at high risk to cutaneous leishmaniasis. In Kenya the boy sitting on a termite hill watching his cattle at dusk is at risk to visceral leishmaniasis because *P. martini* rests in the air shafts of the termitary. In the arid steppes of Uzbek and Turkmen SSR's the irrigation of soil may bring gerbils and the attendant sandflies closer to human habitation and greatly increase the prevalence of cutaneous leishmaniasis.

Once inoculated a variety of fates awaits the promastigote. Some temperature sensitive organisms may have been inoculated into dermis at too high a temperature and will therefore die. Any one flagellate may not reach its goal, which is a histiocyte of the dermis, and may either perish in the tissue spaces, be ingested by a neutrophil or even meet antibody and be immobilized. If the flagellate reaches the histiocyte and invades it, then the flagellum is lost and the organism rounds up prior to division. If the person is immune, competent cells will reach the area within 48 hours and deal with the parasitized cell in a manner not clear at present. If the parasite is in any way defective then the histiocyte's lysosomes quickly kill and digest it. Only if the parasite manages to run the gamut of all these hazards will the new vertebrate contract leishmaniasis.

REFERENCES

Adler, S. and Theodore, O. (1957). *Ann. Rev. Entom.*, *2*, 203.

Ashford, R.W., Bray, M.A., Hutchinson, M.P. and Bray, R.S. (1973). *Trans. R. Soc. Trop. Med. Hyg.*, *67*, 568.

Bray, R.S. (In Press). *In: Trypanosomiasis and Leishmaniasis with special reference to Chagas Disease.* CIBA Foundation London.

Bryceson, A.D.M., Bray, R.S., Wolstenholme, R.A. and Dumonde,

D.C. (1970). *Clin. Exp. Immunol.*, *7*, 301.
Deane, L. and Deane, M.P. (1954b). *O Hospital*, *45*, 419.
Deane, L.M. and Deane, M.P. (1955). *O Hospital*, *48*, 61.
Deane, M.P. and Deane, L.M. (1954a). *O Hosptial*, *45*, 679.
Dedet, J.P. (1971). "Epidemiologie de la Leishmaniose Viscerale en Tunisie. Etude des reservoirs de Virus. Incidence et Repartition de la Leishmaniose Canine." These presentée à Université des Sciences et Techniques du Languedoc. Montpellier. 163 pp.
Dubrovsky, Y.A., Neronov, V.M., Belova, E.M. and Komarova, L.V. (1968). *Medskaya Parasit.*, *37*, 60.
Eliseev, L.N. and Kellina, O.I. (1964). *Med. Parasit. Parasit. Dis.*, *33*, 101.
Forattini, O.P. (1960). *Revta. Inst. Med. Trop. S. Paulo*, *2*, 195.
Fraiha, H., Shaw, J.J. and Lainson, R. (1971). *Mems. Inst. Oswaldo Cruz*, *69*, 485.
Garnham, P.C.C. (1965). *Am. Zool.*, *5*, 141.
Heisch, R.B. (1963). *East Afr. Med. J.*, *40*, 359.
Herrer, A. (1948). *Rev. Med. Exp. Lima*, *7*, 62.
Herrer, A. and Telford, S.R. (1969). *Science*, *164*,1419.
Herrer, A., Thatcher, V.E. and Johnson, C.M. (1966). *J. Parasit.*, *52*, 954.
Herrer, A., Telford, S.R. and Christensen, H.A. (1971). *Ann. Trop. Med. Parasit.*, *65*, 349.
Heyneman, D. (1963). *Am. J. Trop. Med. Hyg.*, *12*, 725.
Hoogstraal, H., Dietlein, D.R. and Heyneman, D. (1962). *Trans. R. Soc. Trop. Med. Hyg.*, *56*, 411.
Hoogstraal, H. and Heyneman, D. (1969). *Am. J. Trop. Med. Hyg.*, *18*, 1091.
Johnson, P.T., McConnell, E. and Hertig, M. (1963). *Exp. Parasit.*, *14*, 107.
Kerdel-Vegas, F. and Essenfeld-Yahr, E. (1966). *Trans. R. Soc. Trop. Med. Hyg.*, *60*, 563.
Lainson, R. and Shaw, J.J. (1968). *Trans. R. Soc. Trop. Med. Hyg.*, *62*, 385.
Lainson, R. and Shaw, J.J. (1970). *Trans. R. Soc. Trop. Med. Hyg.*, *64*, 654.
Lainson, R. and Shaw, J.J. (1972). *Brit. Med. Bull.*, *28*, 44.
Lainson, R. and Strangways-Dixon, J. (1964). *Trans. R. Soc. Trop. Med. Hyg.*, *58*, 136.
Lainson, R., Shaw, J.J. and Lins, Z.C. (1969). *Trans. R. Soc. Trop. Med. Hyg.*, *63*, 741.
Larivière, M., Quenum, C. and Abonnenc, E. (1961). *Bull. Soc. Med. Afr. Noire. Lang. Franc.*, *6*, 431.
Larivière, M., Camerlynck, P., Ranque, P., Villod, M.T., Diagne, S., Raybaud, N. and Toury, M.F. (1965). *Bull.*

Soc. Med. Afr. Noire Lang. Franc., *10*, 237.
Latyshev, N.I., Kryukova, A.P. and Povalinshina, T.P. (1951). *Problems of Regional, General and Experimental Parasitology and Medical Zoology*, *7*, 35.
Lewis, D.J. (1971). *Bull. Wld. Hlth. Org.*, *44*, 535.
McConnell, E. (1963). *Exp. Parasit.*, *14*, 123.
MacDonald, G. (1957). "The Epidemiology and Control of Malaria" Oxford University Press, London, 201 pp.
MacDonald, G. (1965). *Trans. R. Soc. Trop. Med. Hyg.*, *59*, 489.
Maruashvili, G.M. and Bardzhadze, B.G. (1966). *Med. Parasit. Parasit. Dis.*, *35*, 462.
Minter, D.M. (1963). *Ann. Trop. Med. Parasit.*, *57*, 19.
Minter, D.M. and Wijers, D.J.B. (1963). *Ann. Trop. Med. Parasit.*, *57*, 24.
Neronov, V.M. and Ginin, P.D. (1971). *Bull. Wld. Hlth. Org.*, *44*, 577.
Nery-Guimarães, *F. and Costa, O.R. da (1964). O Hospital*, *66*, 287.
Petrisceva, P.A. (1954). "Field Methods of Studying Sandflies and Sandfly-Control Measures, Medgiz, Moscow, 785 pp. (In Russian)
Petrisceva, P.A. (1971) *Bull. Wld. Hlth. Org.*, *44*, 567.
Petrishcheva, P.A., Zasulkin, D. and Safyanova, V. (undated). *In* "Human Diseases with Natural Foci" (Y.N. Pavlovsky, ed). pp. 282-346. Foreign Languages Publishing House, Moscow.
Pifano, C.,F., Romero, M., J. and Alvarez, A. (1962). *Arch. Venez. Med. Trop. Parasit. Med.*, *4*, 17.
Pringle, G. (1952). *Bull. Ent. Res.*, *43*, 707.
Shaw, J.J. and Lainson, R. (1968). *Trans. R. Soc. Trop. Med. Hyg.*, *62*, 396.
Thatcher, V.E., Eisenmann, C. and Hertig, M. (1965). *J. Parasit.*, *51*, 1022.
Wijers, D.J.B. and Linger, R. (1966). *Ann. Trop. Med. Parasit.*, *60*, 501.
Williams, P. (1970). *Trans. R. Soc. Trop. Med. Hyg.*, *64*, 317.
Zvyagintseva, T.V. (1965). *Med. Parasit. Parasit. Dis.*, *34*, 347.

BABESIA GALAGOLATA N.SP. AND ITS HOST SPECIFICITY

H. K. Dennig and G. Hösl

Institut für vergleichende Tropenmedizin der Ludwig Maximilians-Universität München

Five species of *Babesia* have been isolated previously in subhuman primates. Their characteristics are summarized in Table 1. Another species, *Babesia galagolata*, has now been isolated and described in galagos (*Galago crassicaudatus*) which were caught in Tansania and brought to Germany (Dennig, 1973).

TABLE 1

The species of Babesia *in monkeys. The figures in parenthesis in the left column indicate size in microns.*

Babesia spp.	Morphology	Host	References
B. pitheci (1.2 - 3u)	round, oval, ameboid, piriform. Occasionally multiple infection of the erythr. (up to 20 parasites). Multiplication: probably binary fission.	*Cercopithecus* spp. *Cercocebus aterrimus* *Cynocephalus papio*	Ross (1905); Schwetz *et al.*, (1933); Tanguy (1937); Kikuth (1927).
B. cellii *(Theileria cellii)*	rod-shaped, piriform, adjacent to each other. Multiplication: ?	*Macacus pileatus*	Castellani and Chalmers (1910).
B. perodictici *(Theileria perodictici)* (1.5u)	anular, rod-shaped, small crossforms ("merozoites") Multiplication: ?	*Perodicticus potto ibeanus*	Berghe, van den, *et al.*, (1956; 1957).
B. propitheci (1.5 - 4u)	round, oval, piriform, occasionally up to 16 parasites in the erythr. Multiplication: binary fission.	*Propithecus verreauxi coquereli*	Uilenberg *et al.*, (1972).
B. cheirogalei *(Achromaticus cheirogalei* (1 - 2.5u)	round, oval, triangular, piriform, small crossforms. Multiplication: division into 4 daughter forms. Occasionally binary fission.	*Chirogaleus major Geoffroy*	Uilenberg (1970).
B. galagolata (0.8 - 1.9u)	round, oval, lancette shaped dividing angle about 180° occasionally up to 6 parasites in the erythr. Multiplication: binary fission.	*Galago crassicaudatus* rhesus monkey, mouse, rat, hamster, gerbil, guinea pig	Dennig (1973).

Morphology of B. galagolata

Figure 1 shows the most characteristic form of the parasite. Since the size ranges from 0.8μ - 1.9μ *B. galagolata* belongs to the small species of *Babesia*.

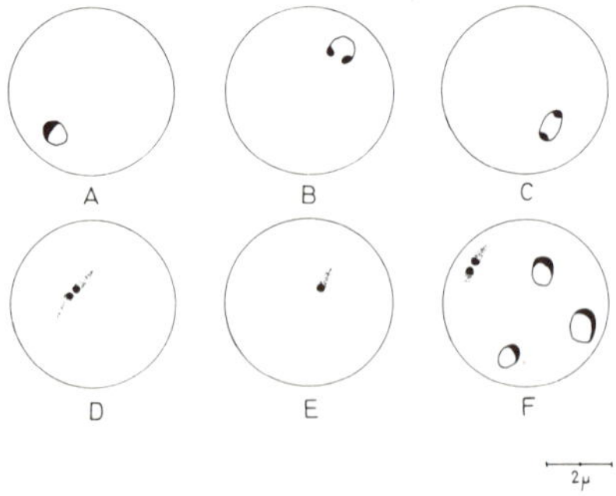

Fig. 1. The most common forms of B. galagolata.

Multiplication occurs by binary fission. Multiplication forms are narrow, lancet shaped, with round and opposite located nuclei (D). Dividing forms are mostly found at an angle of about 180°. Cross forms have never been observed. Angular forms differ little from those of the other small type of *Babesia*. They are round or oval and show mostly an excentric nucleus (A) and occasionally also 2 grains of chromatin (C). Besides this, open forms with 2 marginal chromatin bodies are found very often (B). At the climax of parasitemia single red cells can be infected with *Babesia* in various stages of development (F) or with single division forms (E).

Host-specificity of B. galagolata

The host specificity of *B. galagolata* is very wide. Multiplication can occur in the rhesus monkey (*Macacca mulatta*), in the mouse (*Mus musculus* var. *alb.*), in the rat (*Rattus ungniculatus*) and in the guinea pig (*Cavia porcelcus* L.). The parasitemia generally is much higher in splenectomized animals than in other ones. The following species were not susceptible: pig (*Sus scrota domesticans*), cat *(Felis domesticus*), rabbit (*Oryctolagus cuniculus*), chinchilla (*Chinchilla camigera*) and chicken (*Gallus domesticus*).

A species was considered to be susceptible when a multiplication of the parasites was evidenced in the blood. A species was considered to be resistent if the multiplication failed to take place or if blood from the animal failed to induce infection in splenectomized mice.

The course of parasitemia in the various host species showed clear differences.

Course of infection in the galago and rhesus monkey

In splenectomized galagos the average prepatent period, after intravenous inoculation was 8 days. The climax of parasitemia, with a rate of 7% - 31% infected red cells, was reached within about 3-4 weeks after infection. After this the rate of infection decreased up to a low level (< 0.1% - 5%), and increased again a few weeks later. This intermittent course of infection has been observed in several galagos over a period of 8 months (Fig. 2).

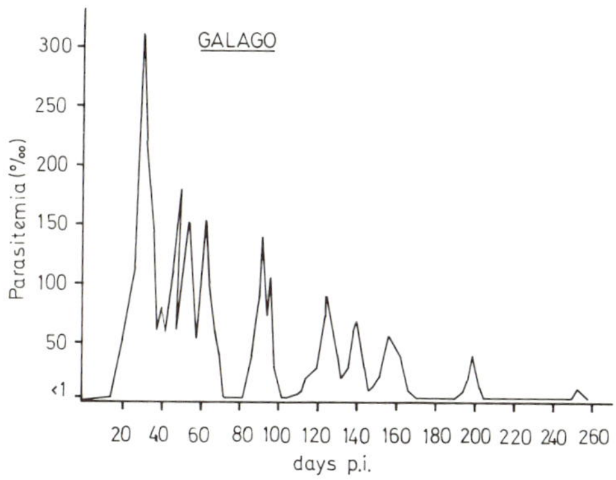

Fig. 2. Course of parasitemia of B. galagolata *in the galago.*

Galagos with intact spleens were not infected because, latent, natural infections could not be excluded in these animals. To evidence such inapparent infections some galagos in which no babesia could be found by microscopic examination were splenectomized. An average period of about 46 days (max. 61 days) elapsed between the splenectomy and the appearance of the first parasites in the peripheral blood. The disease and the level of parasitemia did not differ from that of experimentally infected galagos.

In rhesus monkeys the prepatent period was 3-25 days. A maximum parasitemia of 20% was reached in a period up to 59 days after infection. After this the parasitemia fell to levels comparable to those in galagos. In rhesus monkeys also a course of parasitemia was observed in which an increase, a decrease and an inapparent stage regularly followed each other. Exceptions to this have been seen occasionally.

Course of infection in mice and rats.

In splenectomized mice the average prepatent period after intraperitoneal infection was 20-30 days, exceptionally 1-51 days. At the climax the parasitemia reached the rate of 25%. In mice the sinusoid course of parasitemia was observed regularly (Fig. 3).

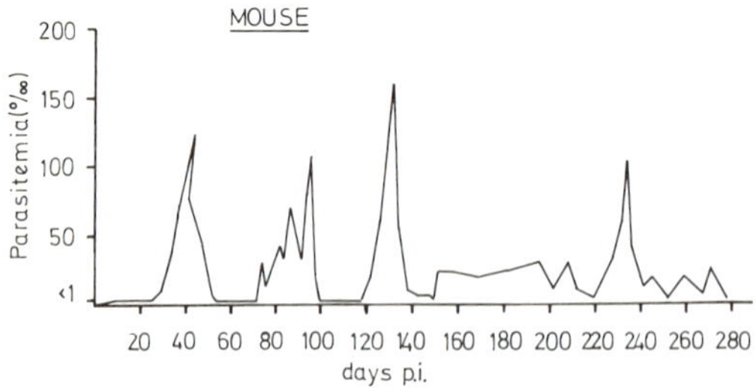

Fig. 3. Course of parasitemia of B. galagolata *in splenectomized mice.*

Eighteen passages of *B. galagolata* were carried out in splenectomized mice. A very similar course of the disease was produced on each passage with a constant dose of inoculum (8 mio/g/b.w.). Changes in the virulence of the parasites were not observed.

In non-splenectomized mice a very low level of parasitemia, of about 1% miximal value, was seen. Parasitemia was followed frequently by inapparent states.

A similar situation was observed in rats, though the sinusoidal course of infection in splenectomized rats was not as distinct as in mice. Autosterilisation was occasionally observed in splenectomized and in normal rats.

Course of infection in hamster, gerbil and guinea pigs.

Splenectomized and normal, hamsters and gerbils, were susceptible to infection with *B. galagolata*. The prepatent period lasted up to 35 days, at climax, the parasitemia reached maximal values of 0.3%. The parasites were found in hamsters for up to 140 days post infection and in gerbils for up to 14 days post infection (Fig. 4).

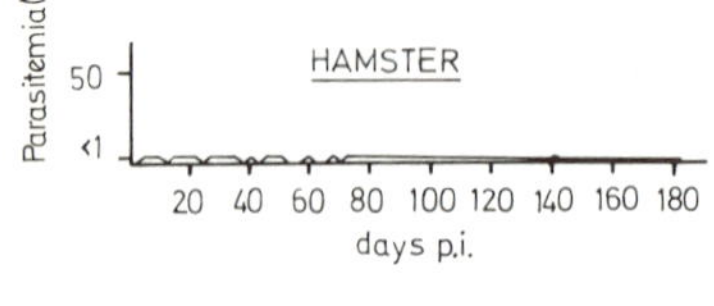

Fig. 4. Course of parasitemia of B. galagolata *in hamsters.*

Inoculation of blood from rats and hamsters, after parasitemia into susceptible mice failed to transmit the infection. *Babesia galagolata* could never be detected microscopically in guinea pigs after intraperitoneal infection. Backtransmission trials into mice carried out with material from 2 splenectomized guinea pigs 6 months after infection, resulted, in both cases, in transmission of the infection.

Clinical course of Babesia galagolata *infection.*
At the climax of the infection in splenectomized galagos clinical signs of the disease included: anemia, icterus and haemoglobinuria. In spite of very serious manifestations death occurred only exceptionally. In rhesus monkeys the disease was similar. In both species of monkeys, after the maximum of parasitemia, there was marked polychromasia, erythropenia, poikilocytosis, anisocytosis, basophile stippling and multiplication of the proerythroblasts, which lasted for a few days. The minimum count of red cells was generally found 3-5 days after the climax of parasitemia. In the other susceptible animals clinical signs were not observed, even with high parasitemias. In splenectomized mice and rats marked modifications of the blood picture were seen, and these were similar to those observed in monkeys (Fig. 5).

CONCLUSIONS

The results of these investigations have shown that *B. galagolata* is an interesting and diversified representative of the *Babesia* genus. It has a wide host-spectrum, being transmissable to at least 7 different host species, and hence it might be considered as one of the least host specific *Babesia* known to date. *Babesia galagolata* can be transmitted readily to new hosts and manipulations for adaptation are not necessary. The parasite shows basic differences in its behavior in different hosts and these hosts may provide suitable models for research on mechanisms pertaining to host specificity of *Babesia* spp.

It is evident that there are still significant gaps in the field of chemotherapy of *Babesia* infections in man. The availability of *B. galagolata* in primates as a model for human infection, will permit the evaluation of babesicidal drugs for human use.

Finally, since *B. galagolata* has a wide host spectrum, its potential as a zoonotic parasite requires evaluation.

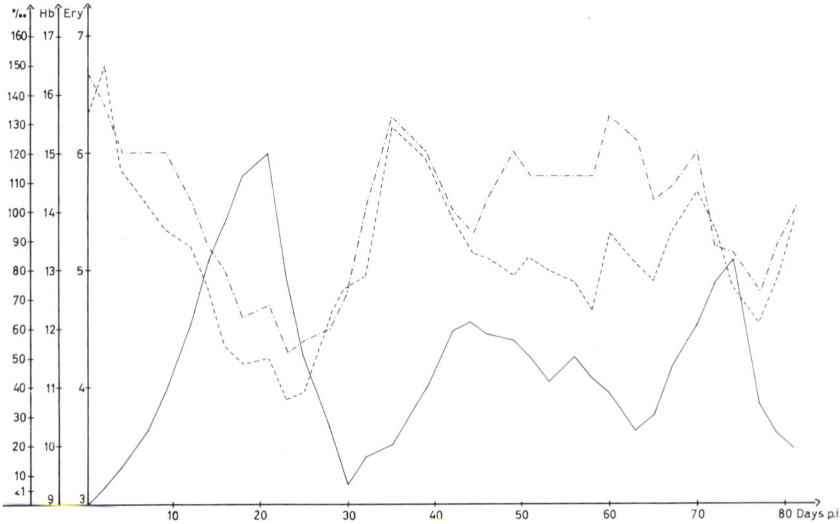

Fig. 5. The course of infection of B. galagolata *in mice. Ordinate: Left to right - parasitemia; haemoglobin; erythrocytes x* 10^6. *Abscissa: Days after infection. Solid line - Parasitemia; Dashed line - Erythrocytes; dashed and dot line - Haemoglobin.*

REFERENCES

Berghe, L. van den, Peel, E and Chardome, M. (1957). *Fol. Scient. Afr. Cent.*, *2*, 16.

Berghe, L. van den, Peel, E. and Chardome, M. (1957). *Fol. Scient. Afr. Cent.*, *3*, 87.

Castellani, A. and Chalmers, A.J. (1910). *Manual of Tropical Medicine.* 1st ed., Bailliere, Tindall & Cox, London.

Dennig, H.K. (1973). *Z. Parasitenk.*, *41*, 281.

Kikuth, W. (1927). *Arch. Schiffs. Tropenhyg.*, *31*, 37.

Ross, P.H. (1905). *J. Hyg.*, *5*, 18.

Schwetz, J., Droeshaut, G. and Peel, E. (1933). *Zbt. Bakt.*, *130*, 121.

Tanguy, Y. (1937). *Ann. Inst. Pasteur*, *59*, 610.

Vilenberg, G. (1970). *Ann. Parasit. Hum. Comp.*, *45*, 183.

Vilenberg, G.,Blancou, J. and Andrianjafy, G. (1972). *Ann. Parasit. Hum. Comp.*, *47*, 1.

THE SPECIFIC IMMUNE RESPONSE IN THE LYMPH NODES OF CATTLE UNDERGOING *THEILERIA PARVA* INFECTION, AS DETERMINED BY THE ROSETTE TEST

W.P.H. Duffus and G.G. Wagner

UNDP/FAO Special Fund Project (KEN 22), c/o Veterinary Research Laboratory, P.O. Kabete, and the U.S. Department of Agriculture Co-operative Research Project[1], c/o East African Veterinary Research Organisation, Muguga, P. O. Box 32, Kikuyu, Kenya

INTRODUCTION

East Coast Fever (ECF) is a severe often fatal disease of bovines, caused by the protozoan *Theileria parva (T. parva)*. Clinically the disease is characterized by a febrile reaction, hyperplasia of lymph nodes and by the presence of two intracellular stages of the parasite: a schizont stage within lymphoid cells and a piroplasm stage within erythrocytes.

Work has been published on the immunoglobulin response to *T. parva*, both to the live parasite (Löhr and Ross, 1969; Duffus and Wagner, 1973a), and to the isolated antigen (Wagner, *et al.*, 1973). In the latter publication it was found that high titres of specific *T. parva* antibody did not protect experimental animals from subsequent challenge with live *T. parva*. One possible explanation for this result could be that the mechanism of immunity is cell-mediated rather than humoral, as has been suggested by Hulliger, *et al.*, 1965.

In an initial study of ECF immune animals delayed hypersensitivity has been demonstrated amongst circulating leucocytes (Muhammed, *et al.*, 1973). It was decided that in conjunction with studies on leucocyte migration and intradermal reactions, attempts should be made to develop a specific rosette-forming cell (RFC) technique for *T. parva* infections. It was felt that a RFC technique developed for protozoal infections could act as a useful indicator of the cellular immune response in studies on parasitic zoonoses.

Since the early work on RFC (Nota, *et al.*, 1964) there have been numerous investigations involving the RFC technique.

---

[1]In collaboration with the UNDP/FAO Immunological Research on Tick-borne Cattle Diseases and Tick Control Project, (AFR REG 77) at EAVRO.

The majority of published work have either utilised the so-called "background" level of RFC in lymphoid tissue (Bach and Dormont, 1971) or with the RFC response to heterologous erythrocytes (Zaalberg, *et al.*, 1968; Duffus and Allan, 1971), both sets of data relying on normal erythrocyte surface antigens. However, a few publications have reported on RFC techniques where the indicator erythrocytes are sensitized with specific antigen (Cunningham, *et al.*, 1966; Duffus and Allan, 1969). In the present study sheep erythrocytes were sensitized with isolated *T. parva* piroplasm antigen (Duffus and Wagner, 1973b) and used to study the RFC response in the lymph nodes of cattle infected with ECF.

MATERIALS AND METHODS

Experimental animals and inoculation: Ayreshire cattle aged between 6-9 months were used throughout the experiment. Eight cattle were inoculated with a stabilate containing infective particles of *T. parva* (Muguga), (Purnell *et al.*, 1973), four of the cattle receiving 1.0 ml of a 1:10 dilution of the stabilate and four cattle 1.0 ml of a 1:100 dilution. The injection was given s/c in front of the left ear. Two other cattle were inoculated with 10.0 mgm protein *T. parva* piroplasm antigen (Wagner, *et al.*, 1973) in Freund's complete adjuvant (Difco); the injection being given s/c above the left prescapular lymph node. Two further cattle were given a similar injection of Freund's complete adjuvant and saline.

Observations: Daily rectal temperatures were taken. Starting at 6 days post inoculation (dpi) Giemsa stained blood smears and biopsies from the left prescapular lymph node were prepared and examined for *T. parva* parasites.

Lymph node biopsies and lymphoid cell suspensions: Biopsies were taken from the left prescapular lymph nodes of all cattle at the time of inoculation and then three times weekly until 63 dpi. The skin above the node was shaved, washed and then swabbed with ethyl alcohol. Using sterile 14 g. needles biopsies were withdrawn into 1.0 ml of Hanks tissue culture medium containing 30 I.U. heparin/ml. The tissue culture fluid contained 1.5 ml of a 4.4% solution of sodium bicarbonate per 100 ml, and 100 I.U. penicillin and 100 ng streptomycin/ml.

The biopsies were teased in fresh medium containing heparin and then homogenized gently with three strokes of a loose fitting glass homogenizer. The resulting cell suspension was filtered through stainless steel gauze and washed three times in tissue culture medium containing no heparin.

RFC technique: Washed sheep erythrocytes were treated with tannic acid and sensitized with isolated *T. parva* antigen as described by Duffus and Wagner (1973b). After the final wash the cells were resuspended in tissue culture medium at a concentration of 4.5 x 10^8 erythrocytes/ml, and then passed through a 26 g. needle approximately 20 times. The lymph node cell suspension was adjusted to 1.5 x 10^7 nucleated cells/ml and 0.1 ml of the latter suspension added to 0.1 ml of the sensitized erythrocytes; thus giving an erythrocyte:nucleated cell ratio of 30:1.

The cell mixture was incubated in a water bath at 37°C for 60 minutes with gentle agitation every 2-3 minutes. Controls consisted of tanned unsensitized erythrocytes with lymph node cells from inoculated animals, and tanned sensitized erythrocytes with lymph node cells from control animals.

After incubation the number of RFC/1000 lymph node cells was calculated using improved Neubauer haemocytometers. A cell was only considered positive when 5 or more sheep erythrocytes were adhering to it.

Photomicroscopy: Photographs were taken on a Zeiss standard RA microscope with an Olympus PA35 camera attachment. Using Ilford FP4 the exposure was 1 second with an X40 oil objective.

RESULTS

Preinoculation and control RFC results: The background level of RFC amongst the 12 experimental animals ranged between 0.5 1.8 RFC/1000 lymph node cells (LNC). In the two control animals receiving Freund's complete adjuvant alone there was a marked increase in the size of the left prescapular lymph node. However, the RFC count never rose above 2.2 RFC/1000 LNC up to 63 dpi, the last day of sampling.

Similar low RFC values were obtained when tanned but unsensitized sheep erythrocytes were mixed with lymph node cells from immunized animals; however in a few samples taken between 18-32 dpi the RFC count rose to a maximum of 3.1 RFC/1000 LNC, but still much lower than the corresponding RFC count using sensitized erythrocytes.

Cattle inoculated with infective T. parva *stabilate:*
Clinical findings: Clinical details of the *T parva* infection in the 8 experimental cattle including temp. reactions and parasitaemia are shown in Table 1. A rise in rectal tempera-

ture to 103°F or above was regarded as significant; all animals showed a marked febrile response lasting from 6-17 days. Schizont infected lymphoid cells were detected in the lymph node biopsies of all eight animals, parasites first being seen after 8 dpi. Piroplasm infected erythrocytes were also found in all animals, the degree of peak parasitaemia varying between 0.25% to 58.0%.

In the group receiving a 1:10 dilution of *T. parva* stabilate 3 of 4 animals died, and in the group receiving 1:100 stabilate 1 of 4 died; typical ECF was diagnosed in all carcasses on post-mortem.

Table 1

Clinical Findings in Eight Cattle Inoculated with a 1:10 or 1:100 Dilution of Infective T. parva *Stabilate*

No.	Dilution of Stabilate	Days to Temp*	Duration of Febrile Response	Days to first Detectable Schizont	Days to first Detectable Piroplasm	Maximum % Parasitaemia of Erythrocytes	Days to Death
A32	1:10	9	15	9	14	26.7	24
A33	1:10	9	11	9	14	58.0	20
A34	1:10	8	8	8	19	0.25	REC**
A35	1:10	8	16	11	16	32.0	24
A42	1:100	11	17	11	19	17.0	REC
A43	1:100	11	10	13	20	1.5	REC
A44	1:100	14	6	14	19	1.5	REC
A45	1:100	13	9	11	17	31.6	28

* A significant increase in rectal temp. was taken as 103°F or above
** Animal recovered from clinical ECF

RFC response: The RFC response of the four cattle surviving clinical ECF is shown in Fig. 1., and of the four cattle dying of ECF in Fig. 2. All cattle showed a rise in the number of RFC over the background level, the initial increase being detected 6-8 dpi. Peak numbers of RFC were reached after 11-15 dpi, remaining at a high level for up to 27 dpi. As is shown in Figs. 1 and 2 there was a noticeable variation in the length of time that the high level of RFC was maintained. In animals A43, A42 and A34 the RFC count remained above 20 for up to 12 days before dropping to reach almost preinoculation levels by the 46-63 dpi; these three animals all recovered from clinical ECF.

With animal No. A44 the RFC response was of a lower magnitude but essentially similar to that of the other three animals recovering from ECF. This animal had the shortest febrile response and a noticeably mild clinical reaction.

In the four animals that died of ECF, although the number of RFC did plateau for 7-9 days, there was a marked drop in the number of RFC before death. This drop was especially noticeable in animal No. A45 where the final biopsy was taken two hours before death. This drop occurred at the time when a high level of RFC was being maintained in the animals eventually recovering from ECF.

Several of the early RFC were large irregularly shaped cells with only small numbers of adherent erythrocytes, examples being shown in Fig. 4a and 4b. More typical rosettes are shown in Fig. 4c. and 4d. Between 18-39 dpi several of the rosettes were much larger with several layers of adherent erythrocytes, examples are shown in Fig. 4e and 4f.

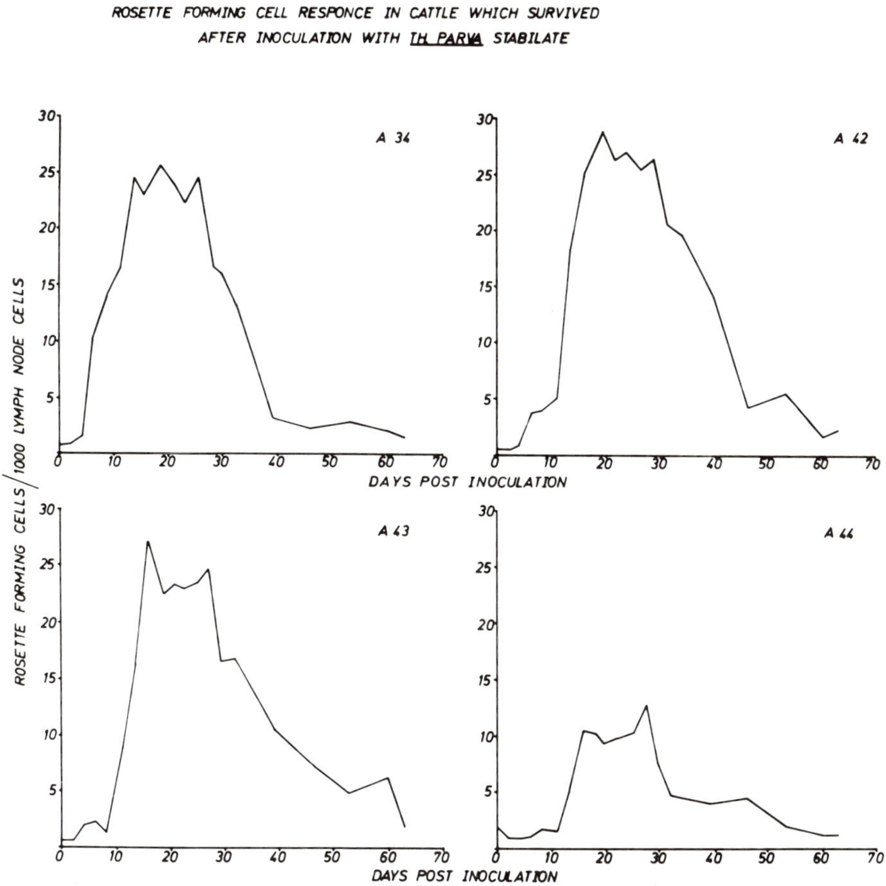

Fig. 1. The Rosette forming cell response in cattle which survived after inoculation with T. parva *stabilate.*

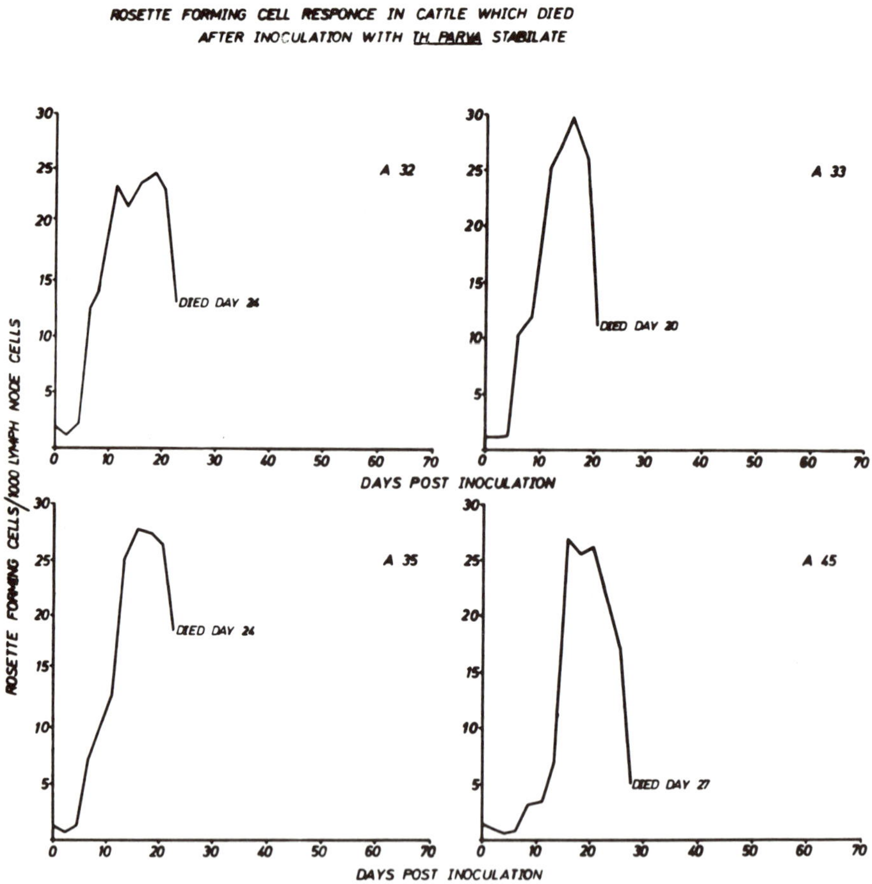

Fig. 2. The Rosette forming cell response in cattle which died after inoculation with T. parva *stabilate.*

RFC response in cattle inoculated with isolated T. parva *antigen:* A marked RFC response was observed in both animals inoculated with isolated *T. parva* piroplasm antigen. An increase was detected 4 dpi with a peak at 9 dpi, after which the numbers of RFC fell to reach approximately preinoculation levels by 32-35 dpi. This result, shown in detail in Fig. 3, was essentially similar in both experimental animals. The peak count was 28.1 RFC/1000 LNC. Many of the RFC between 9-16 dpi were large with multiple layers of adherent erythrocytes (Fig. 4f).

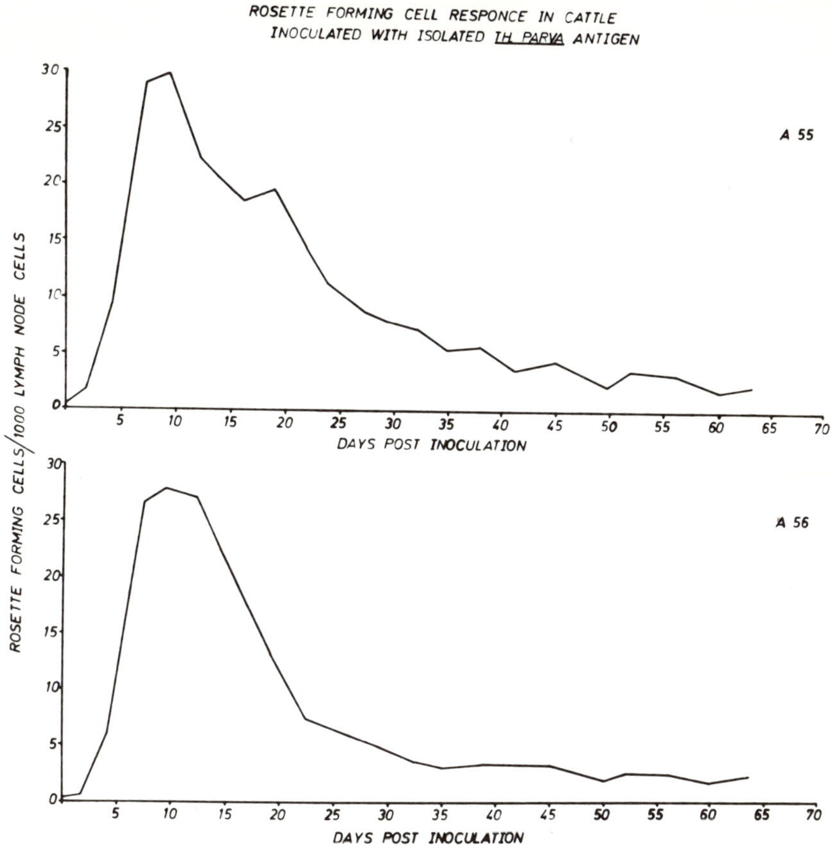

Fig. 3. The Rosette forming cell response in cattle inoculated with isolated T. parva *antigen.*

DISCUSSION

The above results indicate that the RFC technique is applicable in investigations of the cellular immune response in protozoal infections.

When cattle were inoculated with isolated *T. parva* antigen a rise in RFC was detected 4 dpi with a peak at 9 dpi followed by a fall to preinoculation levels by 32-35 dpi. These results are similar to the RFC response described by Cunningham, *et al.*, (1966) in the lymph nodes of sheep inoculated with dead *Salmonella muenchen*, and to the RFC response in rat popliteal lymph nodes after inoculation with sheep erythrocytes (Duffus and Allan, 1971).

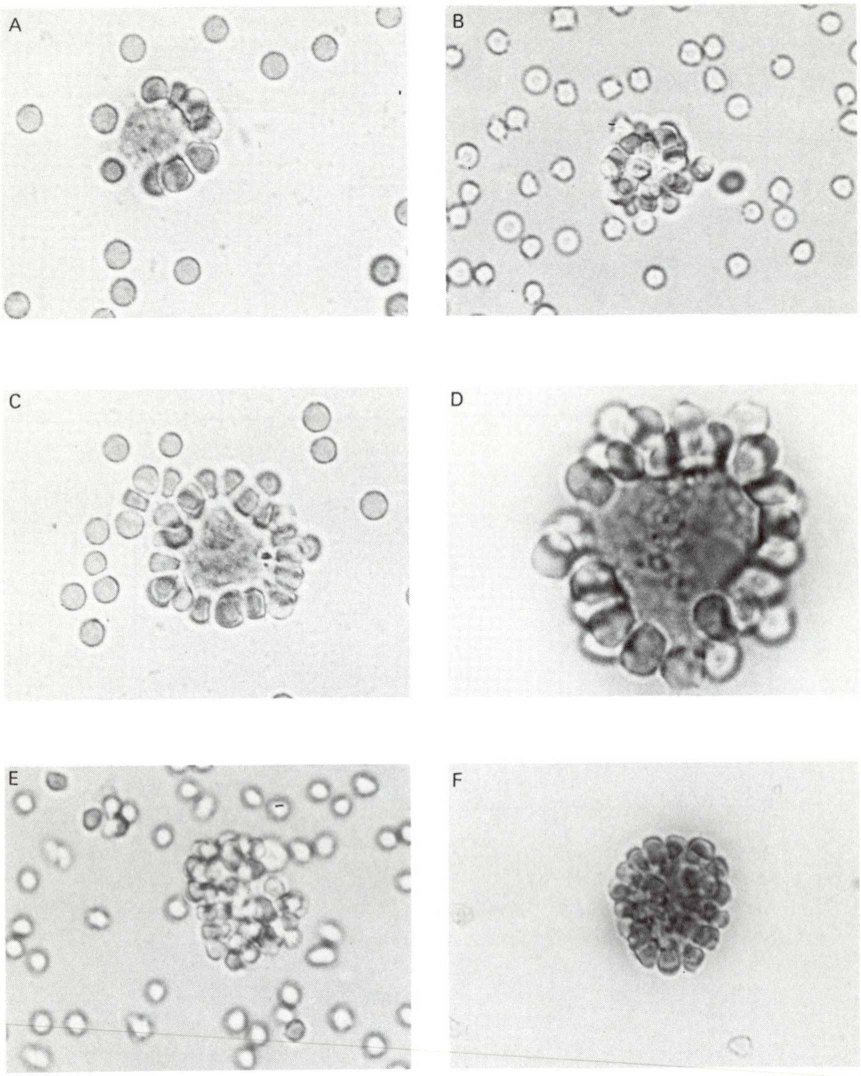

Fig. 4. Rosette formation by lymphoid cells of ECF infected animals at various days post inoculation. A, 11 days (x960); B, 13 days (x960); C, 13 days (x960); D, 20 days (x1500); E, 20 days (x480) F, 25 days (x480).

The RFC response when cattle were inoculated with virulent *T. parva* showed several differences. The initial increase in RFC was several days after the increase occurring when isolated antigen was the inoculum (6-13 dpi as compared to 4 dpi); a possible explanation could be the time taken for the parasite to multiply sufficiently within the host. Another noticeable difference was that instead of reaching a peak and falling, the number of RFC in the ECF infected cattle stabilized at a plateau for up to 12 days before dropping. The continual production and proliferation of protozoal antigen could be one explanation, as this plateau coincided with the multiplication of *T. parva*schizonts within the prescapular and other lymph glands.

However, in the four cattle dying of ECF although there was a similar plateau in the number of RFC, the latter showed a significant fall before death, emphasised in animal No. A45 where the RFC count had dropped to almost preinoculation levels, the samples being taken two hours before death. Part of the syndrome of terminal ECF is a marked destruction of both tissue lymphoid cells and blood leucocytes, which may well be involved in the explanation of this drop in RFC. However as the actual rosette count was per 1000 LNC and not therefore the total RFC population, there was probably a specific depletion in RFC. The significance of this depletion in terminal ECF should be investigated.

An interesting question arising from the results described in this paper is the nature of the lymphoblast cells containing *T. parva* schizonts, especially as the peak of RFC coincided with the multiplication of these infected lymphoblasts. Malmquist, *et al.,* (1970) and Moulten, *et al.,* (1971) have described the successful tissue culture isolation of *T parva* infected lymphoblasts. These latter cells exhibit a rapid multiplication rate in suspension culture, a situation rather like the hyperplasia of schizont infected lymphoblasts in animals with clinical ECF. Therefore, do these cells exhibit any type of immunoglobulin receptor, and can any specific antigen activity be demonstrated? Experiments to try and answer some of these questions are planned.

It has been increasingly suggested that cell mediated immunity (CMI) plays an important part in the immunity to protozoal diseases, this subject has been admirably reviewed by Soulsby (1970). Tremanti and Walton (1970) working with toxaplasmosis in guinea pigs demonstrated specific activity with both the macrophage migration inhibition and intradermal tests; and Yanovsky and Alboda (1972) have shown inhibition of leucocyte migration in *Trypanosoma cruzi* infections in mice. More recently, Buening (1973) has demonstrated CMI in anaplasmosis in calves, and using inhibition of leucocyte migration, Mohammed *et al.,* (1973) have also shown CMI in cattle after infection with *T parva.* As the RFC test can be used to study both bone-marrow derived and thymus derived lymphocytes (Bach and Dardenne, 1972a, 1972b; Kreeftenberg and Leerling, 1972), it may act as an indicator of the population of sensitized cells in studies on the cellular immune response, together with intradermal, leucocyte migration and serological tests.

The nature of the receptor site on RFC is still in doubt (Lay, *et al.*, 1971; Kreeftenberg and Leerling, 1972), some authors finding little if any inhibition of RFC by anti-immunoglobulins (Coombs, *et al.*, 1970) while others have stated that anti-immunoglobulins might have an inhibiting effect on rosette formation (Bach and Dormont, 1971). In our opinion, the experimental conditions of the rosette test, such as sedimentation, pH, erythrocyte source and temperature, can greatly alter the number of observed RFC (Duffus, unpublished data; Chaves and Arranhado, 1972; Kreeftenberg and Leerling, 1972).

In the experiments reported here, very little work was done on the morphology of the RFC. However, the large rosettes found later on in the response might be indicative of active antibody production by the central RFC, as has been suggested by Zaalberg, *et al.*, (1966) and Duffus and Allan (1971).

An interesting point was that we found very little increase in RFC when tanned unsensitized erythrocytes were the indicator cells; we also have serological data on ECF immune sera using the indirect haemagglutination test (Duffus and Wagner, 1973b) where there is similarly very little increase against control tanned unsensitized erythrocytes after infection. This is in contrast to results in trypanosomiosis where quite high titres of antibody against tanned unsensitized sheep erythrocytes have been shown in immune sera (Houba, personal communication).

ACKNOWLEDGEMENT

We would like to thank Dr. I. Muriithi, Director of Veterinary Services, Kabete, for permission to publish this papeer. We would also like to thank Charles Akwabi for excellent technical assistance and Norman Mitchell for the photomicroscopy.

REFERENCES

Bach, J.F. and Dardenne, M. (1972a). *Cellular Immunol. 3,* 1.
Bach, J.F. and Dardenne, M. (1972b). *Cellular Immunol. 3,* 11.
Bach, J.F. and Dormont, J. (1971). *Transplantation 11,* 96.
Buening, G.M. (1973). *Am. J. Vet. Res. 34,* 757.

Chaves, M.A. and Arranhado, E. (1972). *Lancet* No. 7740, 42.

Coombs, R.R., Gurner, B.W., Wilson, A.B., Holm, G. and Lindgren, B. (1970). *Int. Arch. Allery. Appl. Immunol. 39,* 280.

Cunningham, A.J., Smith, J.B. and Mercer, E.H. (1966). *J. exp. med. 124,* 701.

Duffus, W.P.H. and Allan, D. (1969). *Immunology 16,* 337.

Duffus, W.P.H. and Allan, D. (1971). *Immunology 20,* 345.

Duffus, W.P.H. and Wagner, G.G. (1973a). (Submitted for publication).

Duffus, W.P.H. and Wagner, G.G. (1973b). Submitted for publication).

Hulliger, L., Brown, C.G.D. and Wilde, J.K.H. (1965). *Abst. 2nd Internat. Conf. Protozool.* p. 37, London.

Kreeptenberg, J.G. and Leerling, M.F. (1972). *Transplantation 14,* 665.

Lay, W.H., Mendes, N.F., Bianco, C. and Nussenweig, V. (1971). *Nature 230,* 531.

Löhr, K.F. and Ross, J.P.J. (1969). *Res. Vet. Sci. 10,* 453.

Malmquist, W.A., Nyindo, M.B.A. and Brown, C.G.D. (1970). *Trop. Animal Hlth. Prod. 2,* 139.

Moulton, J.E., Krauss, H.H. and Malmquist, W.A. (1971). *Lab. Invest. 24,* 187.

Muhammed, S.I., Wagner, G.G. and Lauerman, L.H. (1973). (Submitted for publication).

Nota, N. R., Liacopoulos-Briot, M., Stiffel, C. and Biozzi, G. (1964). *C. R. Acad. Sci. 259,* 1277.

Purnell, R.E., Brown, C.G.D., Cunningham, M.P., Burridge, M.J. Kirimi, I.M. and Ledger, M.A. (1973). *Parasitology.* (In Press).

Soulsby, E.J.L. (1970). *J. Parasit. 56,* (Sect II) 534.

Tremanti, L. and Walton, B.C. (1970). *Am. J. Trop. Med. Hyg. 19,* 49.

Wagner, G.G., Duffus, W.P.H. and Burridge, M.J. (1973). (Submitted for publication).

Wagner, G.G., Duffus, W.P.H., Kimber, C.D. and Lule, M. (1973) (Submitted for publication).

Yanovsky, J.F. and Albado, E. (1972). *J. Immunol. 109,* 1159.

Zaalberg, O.B. (1964). *Nature 202,* 1231.

Zaalberg, O.B., Van Der Meul, V.A. and Van Twisk, J.M. (1966). *Nature 210,* 544.

Zaalberg, O.B., Van Der Meul, V.A. and Van Twisk, J.M. (1968). *J. Immunol. 100,* 451.

ANTI-LYMPHOCYTE ANTIBODY RESPONSE IN CATTLE INOCULATED WITH *THEILERIA PARVA* INFECTED LYMPHOBLASTOID CELL LINES

G.G. Wagner and W.P.H. Duffus

The U.S. Department of Agriculture Co-operative Research Project, at the East African Veterinary Research Organisation, Muguga, P.O. Box 32, Kikuyu; and the UNDP/FAO Special Fund Project (KEN 22), at the Veterinary Research Laboratory, P.O. Kabete, Kenya

INTRODUCTION

Theileria parva infections of cattle, known as East Coast Fever have never been shown to be secondarily transmitted to man. However, as a systemic protozoan infection, the theilerioses serve as an excellent model for the study of humoral and cellular factors in an immune response to similar intracellular infections.

The infection of cattle by *T. parva* is characterized by a febrile reaction, hyperplasia of lymph nodes, and the presence of two intracellular forms of the parasite: a schizont stage within lymphoid cells and a piroplasm stage within erythrocytes.

Recently, a continuous cell line of *T. parva* schizont-infected bovine lymphoblasts has been established (Malmquist *et al.*, 1970). These cultures are easily standarized and adaptable to bulk production, and they have provided a promising source of potentially immunogenic material. Thus far, 80% of the cattle that have received optimal doses of cell-culture material have been proved immune (Brown *et al.*, 1970).

Subsequent interest in these animals concerns not only the nature of the antibody response in those that are immune, but also the reasons for a lack of protective response in the other 20%.

Animals inoculated with a potentially immunogenic dose of *T. parva*-infected lymphoblasts receive not only the parasite, but also bovine lymphoid cells of possible foreign nature. Conceivably then, the introduction of these lymphoid cells might induce an anti-lymphocyte response either before or with the host's responses to the parasite. This report presents the results of experiments designed to determine whether such an anti-lymphocyte response might occur, and, if so, whether it could in any way influence the immune response to the parasite.

MATERIALS AND METHODS

Sera

Sera for the evaluation of anti-lymphocyte activity were collected at various intervals from cattle on experiment within the FAO Project at EAVRO. These sera were obtained primarily from animals that had been inoculated subcutaneously with 10^8 schizont-infected, cell-culture lymphoblasts, either from cattle (Malmquist *et al.*, 1970) or African Cape buffalo (Stagg *et al.*, 1974) as an immunogen. Sera were also collected from cattle undergoing experimental ECF and chemoprophylactic immunogenesis. In addition, sera were collected from a group of animals subcutaneously inoculated with 10^8 non-parasitized lymphoid cells previously obtained from the lymph nodes of a susceptible animal.

Negative control sera were obtained from ECF-susceptible cattle and were shown to be negative for ECF antibodies by the indirect fluorescent antibody (IFA) test (Burridge and Kimber, 1972). A positive control serum was obtained from an animal that was inoculated with 10^8 schizont-infected, cell-culture lymphoblasts. This animal was shown to be immune to homologous challenge with a tick stabilate (Lumsden and Hardy, 1964). A large bleeding for serum was obtained at the peak of specific IFA activity, approximately 30 days after challenge. This serum was also shown to contain a high level of ALA and was subsequently included in all tests as the positive control.

Cells

The cells used in the different assay procedures were from several sources. Lymphoblasts were maintained in cell culture as previously described (Malmquist *et al.*, 1970). Lymphocytes were harvested from various blood samples according to Aalund *et al.* (1970). Thymocytes were obtained from the thymus of 3-week-old calves presumed susceptible to ECF. Occasionally, the lymph nodes from the same calves were used as a source of lymphocytes.

Migration Tests

Lymphoblasts were harvested from cell cultures by centrifugation (250 g - 10 min) and washed several times in Hank's*

---

*Mention of a trade name proprietary product, or specific equipment does not constitute a guarantee or warrenty by the U.S. Department of Agriculture and does not imply its approval to the exclusion of other products that may be suitable.

balanced salt solution (BSS) containing antibody (penicillin 100 IU/ml, streptomycin 100 mcg/ml). The cell pellet was finally resuspended in Eagle's minimum essential medium (MEM) supplemented with 20% fetal calf serum (and antibiotics, as above) to give an approximate 10% cell suspension. Hematocrit tubes were filled with the cell suspension by capillarity, sealed at one end by melting the tips, and centrifuged at 250 g for 5 min. The tubes were cut at the cell-medium interface and the cut ends containing the cells placed in duplicate into Sykes-Moore Chambers (Bellco Glass Co., Vineland, N.J.). Chambers were filled with MEM supplemented with 10-15% fetal calf serum and 5-10% of the serum to be tested. Chambers were incubated at 37 C for 16-18 hr.

Lymphocytes for use in migration assays were harvested from peripheral blood samples as described by Aalund *et al.* (1970). After separation, the lymphocytes were washed in BSS and treated as above.

The area of migration was read with a low power inverted microscope with an ocular grid. The percentage of migration inhibition was calculated by comparing the migration area of cells in the presence of various test sera (average of 6 capillaries) with the migration area obtained by using a standard negative control serum. A result of less than 10% inhibition was not found to be significant by the student "t" test ($p < 0.05$). The standard, positive control serum was included in every test as a check on the reproducibility of the assay. This serum repeatedly gave 60-65% inhibition of either lymphoblasts or lymphocytes.

Fluorescent Antiglobulin Test

In this method, all sera to be tested were first precipitated with half-saturated ammonium sulfate solution. The globulin precipitates were washed several times by centrifugation (100 g - 20 min), redissolved in 0.1 m phosphate buffered 0.15 m saline (PBS) solution (pH 7.2), dialyzed exhaustively against PBS, and finally adjusted to a protein concentration of 20 mg/ml.

A single cell suspension of thymocytes was used for most tests although lymphoblasts and lymphocytes were also tested. The cells were washed several times in BSS by centrifugation (250 g - 10 min). The cell pellet was finally resuspended in MEM and adjusted to approximately 4×10^6 cells/ml.

Two-tenths-ml aliquots of various dilutions of the globulin fractions were added to equal volumes of the cell suspension. After 30-min incubation at room temperature, the mixtures were centrifuged (250 g - 2 min) and the cells washed twice with MEM. Finally, the cells were resuspended in 0.2

ml MEM containing 0.1 m sodium azide. Ten microliters of a rabbit antiserum, specific for bovine IgG and conjugated with fluorescein isothiocyanate, was then added, and this mixture was incubated a further 15 min at room temperature. The cells were again collected by centrifugation, washed twice, and finally resuspended in 0.2 ml MEM with 0.1 m sodium azide. Wet mounts of cell suspensions were prepared on microscope slides and observed with UV illumination. Cells that had reacted with sera containing antilymphocyte activity were brightly stained. Cells incubated with negative control sera were unstained. The same positive control serum was used as in the migration tests.

Additional Tests

All sera were tested for anti-*T. parva* schizont activity by the IFA technique (Burridge and Kimber, 1972). Several sera were tested for anti-Forssman activity in homolysin titrations (Mayer, 1964).

RESULTS

Five cattle were inoculated subcutaneously with 10^8 cell-culture lymphoblasts containing *T. parva* schizonts. Serum samples were obtained at 2 to 3-day intervals and tested for anti-lymphocyte activity against cell-culture lymphoblasts in the migration test. Significant ALA was detected as early as 5 days postinoculation (Fig. 1), reached a peak at 14 days, and declined to a plateau. A second group of two animals in this experiment were similarly inoculated subcutaneously with 10^8 non-infected lymphocytes obtained from the lymph nodes of a calf. This latter group (Fig. 1) also responded with ALA, but a significant response was not detected until 14-16 days postinoculation. Peak activity in this group was reached within the same period (i.e., 7 days) as the first but was of lesser magnitude and quickly declined.

Figure 2 shows the results with the sera from the same group of cattle as above, but tested in the fluorescent antiglobulin reaction. As with the migration inhibition assays, ALA was detected as early as day 5 postinoculation, reached a maximum level on day 25, and declined slowly. The responses of the animals that received the non-infected cells was also detected but was delayed and of lesser magnitude.

Circulating antibody as measured by the IFA test, and specific for *T. parva* schizonts, was detected 21 days postinoculation but only in sera from the group of cattle that received *T. parva*-infected lymphoblasts. This group was also immune on challenge with homologous infective material (tick stabilate).

Another group of 5 cattle was inoculated with 10^8 *T. lawrencei* schizont-infected lymphoblasts. These lymphoblasts had been established in cell culture from infected lymphocytes obtained from an African Cape buffalo. Sera from the cattle inoculated with these lymphoblasts were collected at 2- to 3-day intervals and tested by both migration inhibition and fluorescent antiglobulin techniques.

Table I shows migration inhibition results of several of the sera from each animal tested against *T. parva*-infected lymphoblasts. The data indicate a response similar to the group of cattle that received the *T. parva*-infected lymphoblasts in that the ALA rose to a peak by 14 days postinoculation, but tended to plateau at that level rather than decline as in the latter group (Fig. 1). The fluorescent antiglobulin assay indicated the same kinetics as the data in Table I. On challenge with *T. parva* tick stabilate, 2 of the 5 cattle succumbed with patent ECF (Table I). From the individual ALA results, the death of these animals could not have been predicted before challenge.

The IFA results using sera from this group did show a difference (Table I). The 3 cattle that were subsequently proved immune had significant anti-*T. lawrencei* schizont antibody 28 days after inoculation, whereas the 2 that succumbed did not.

Similar migration inhibition tests have been performed with non-parasitized lymphocytes obtained from either peripheral blood or lymph nodes of susceptible animals. As shown in Table II, the degree of inhibiiton with any particular serum was the same, regardless of the lymphocyte used as indicator. In addition, cells obtained from the thymus, lymph nodes, peripheral blood, kidney, and bone marrow of cattle have been examined by the fluorescent antiglobulin test. Positive results have been obtained only with cells of lymphoid origin.

Many sera have been tested by both techniques, including samples from animals undergoing experimental East Coast fever, from animals immunized by chemoprophylaxis, and from other cattle that have received cell-culture lymphoblasts as the immunogen. Only sera from animals in the latter category demonstrate anti-lymphocyte activity (Table II).

In a related series of experiments, we found that the anti-lymphocyte activity is not anti-Forssman in nature and that the fluorescent test works well when either rabbit anti-IgG or anti-bovine IgM conjugates are used.

TABLE I

Percentage of migration inhibition, IFA reaction and challenge response of animals receiving *T. lawrencei*-infected cell culture.

Animal No.	Migration inhibition (%)[a] Days Postinoculation 5	7	14	25	28	IFA titer[b]	Challenge response[c]
823	6	24	42	30	29	640	Immune
835	22	31	35	34	31	640	Immune
837	17	20	25	35	35	10,240	Immune
836	18	21	33	33	34	40	Susceptible
838	21	25	42	33	33	40	Susceptible

a Percentage of migration inhibition of lymphoblasts by serum, average of 6 capillaries.

b Serum collected at 28 dpi, tested against *T. lawrencei* schizont antigen. Titer expressed as reciprocal dilution.

c Each animal challenged with 1 ml subcutaneous inoculation of *T. parva* tick stabilate.

TABLE II

Peak percentage of migration inhibition by sera from several sources, tested against *T. parva*-infected lymphoblasts and normal lymphocytes.

Serum from animal inoculated with:	Days post-inoculation	Migration inhibition (%) Lymphoblasts	Lymphocytes
cc, *T. parva*[a]	14	49	46
cc, *T. lawrencei*[b]	14	42	ND
nor, Lymphocytes[c]	25	40	39
Stabilate, CP[d]	14	5	5
Stabilate, ECF[e]	29	0	2

a Animal received 10^8 bovine cell culture lymphoblasts infected with *T. parva*.

b Animal received 10^8 buffalo cell culture lymphoblasts infected with *T. lawrencei*.

c Animal received 10^8 lymphocytes obtained from the lymph nodes of a normal susceptible calf.

d Animal received *T. parva* tick stabilate plus chemoprophylaxis.

e Animal received a 1:10 dilution of *T. parva* tick stabilate, underwent East Coast fever and recovered.

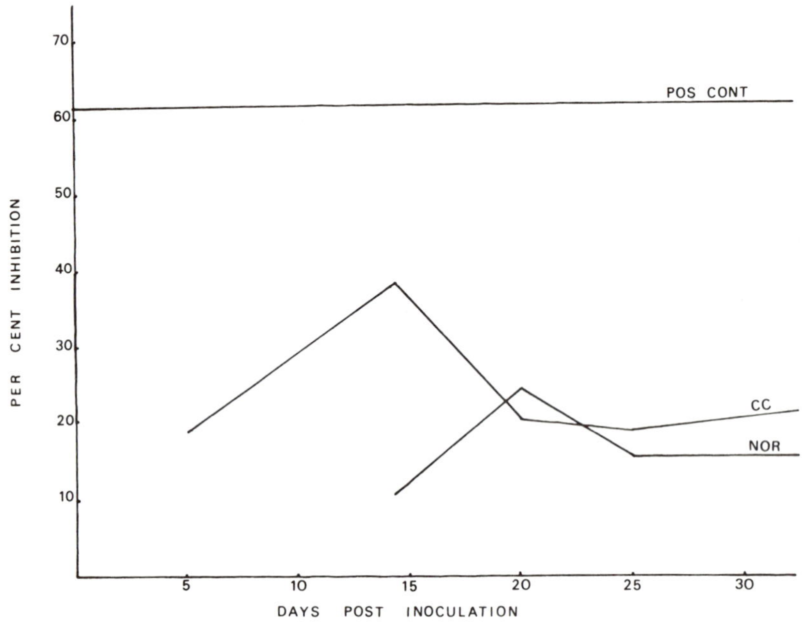

Fig. 1. Inhibition of migration of T. parva *schizont-infected lymphoblasts by serum from cattle inoculated with either* T. parva *schizont-infected lymphoblasts or non-infected lymphocytes from susceptible cattle.*

POS CONT *indicates inhibition by a standard positive control serum;* CC *indicates the mean observations of the sera from cattle inoculated with* T. parva *schizont-infected, cell-culture lymphoblasts;* NOR *indicates the mean observation of the sera from cattle inoculated with uninfected, "normal" lymphocytes.*

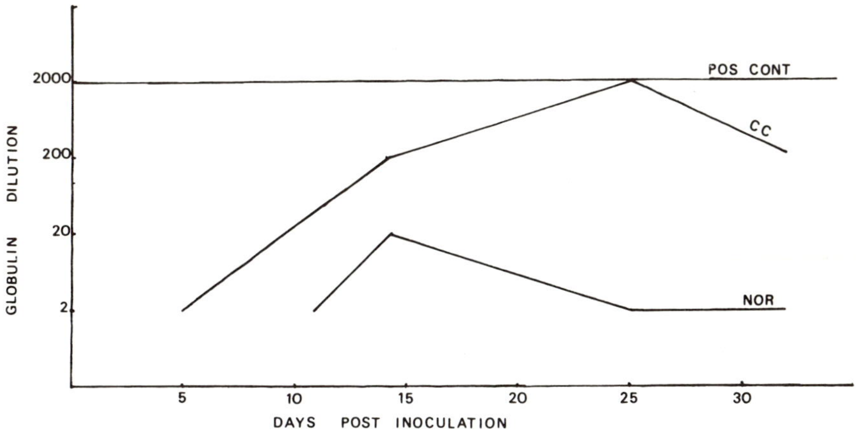

Fig. 2. Fluorescent antiglobulin reaction of bovine thymocytes with serum from cattle inoculated with either T. parva *schizont-infected lymphoblasts or non-infected lymphoblasts or non-infected lymphocytes from susceptible cattle.*

POS CONT *indicates inhibition by a standard positive control serum;* CC *indicates the mean observation of the sera from cattle inoculated with* T. parva *schizont-infected, cell-culture lymphoblasts;* NOR *indicates the mean observations of the sera from cattle inoculated with uninfected, "normal" lymphocytes.*

DISCUSSION

The results of the experiments reported indicate that when cattle are inoculated with cell-culture lymphoblasts infected with either *T. parva* or *T. lawrencei* schizonts, an anti-lymphocyte response is initiated, apparently unrelated to the specific antibody response to the parasite itself. This response, as manifested in these experiments, does not appear to either interfere or enhance the development of subsequent immunity to challenge with the homologous parasite.

One point of interest was the comparison of the kinetics of the anti-lymphocyte response in sera from cattle inoculated with parasitized cells with those inoculated with non-parasitized cells. In the former group, the responses not only was detected earlier, but also was of greater magnitude. Although the antigenic character of the lymphoblasts, which are considered to be a "transformed" cell type (Malmquist *et al.*, 1970), can only be speculation at present, these cells are apparently more "foreign" than the "normal". Perhaps in the process of transformation, a major antigenic determinant is exposed. This determinant may be relatively inaccessible on the "normal" cell. Perhaps also the transformed cells are a particular cell type; for instance, either "T" (thymus-derived) or "B" (bone marrow-derived). The percentage of the same cell type (although similar numbers of cells were inoculated) in a preparation of cells from the lymph nodes of a "normal" animal might be low and thus account for the delay in the response.

The latter possibility might be examined by inoculating only thymocytes or perhaps by inoculating other "transformed" lymphoblasts, for example, lymphocytes stimualted by either phytohemagglutinin or bacterial lipopolysaccharide.

Another point of interest was the finding that no ALA was detected in sera from cattle undergoing experimental ECF (even acute prefatal cases) or during chemoprophylaxis-induced recoveries. Although schizont-infected cells are considered to be "transformed" *in vivo* (Malmquist *et al.*, 1970), there might not be enough antigen to induce ALA. Also, cattle undergoing ECF are possibly not immunocompetent to an unrelated antigenic stimulus.

A final point of interest concerns the ALA induced by the *T. lawrencei* infected buffalo lymphoblasts. The kinetics of the ALA response of the group of cattle inoculated with these cells was very similar to the response of the cattle inoculated with the *T. parva* infected bovine lymphoblasts. The data suggest that the antigen responsible for the induction of ALA is similar for both cells.

The answer to the question of why 20% of cattle inoculated with parasitized lymphoblasts do not become immune remains unanswered. Possibly the activity detected in these experiments has some other property that has not been ascertained but that can influence the response. An answer may await elucidation of the histocompatibility system operable in the bovine.

We need to reiterate that *T. parva* and East Coast fever are being used in these experiments as a model for other intracellular parasitic diseases of zoonotic importance. As cell cultures of these other disease agents are developed, with the idea of using such cultures as vaccine material, the possibility of a concurrent anti-cell response must also be kept in mind.

ACKNOWLEDGMENTS

We wish to acknowledge the invaluable assistance of M. Cunningham and members of the UNDP/FAO Immunological Research on Tickborne Cattle Diseases and Tick Control Project (AFR REG 77) at EAVRO. Special thanks are due to D. Brown, M. Burridge, J. Crowford, C. Kimber and G. Chege.

REFERENCES

Aalund, O., Hoerlein, A.B. and Adler, H.C. (1970). *Acta Vet. Scand.*, *11*, 331.

Brown, C.G.D., Malmquist, W.A., Cunningham, M.P., Radley, D.E. and Burridge, M.J. (1970). *Proceedings of the Second Int. Cong. Parasit.* (Part 4). Washington,D.C., 6-12 September

Burridge, M.J. and Kimber, C.D. (1972). *Res. Vet. Sci. 13*, 451.

Lumsden, W.H.R. and Hardy, G.J.C. (1965). *Nature*, *205*, 1032.

Malmquist, W.A., Nyindo, M.B.A. and Brown, C.G.D. (1970). *Trop. Animal Hlth. Prod.*, *2*, 139.

Mayer, M.M. (1964). *In* Experimental Immunochemistry (S.A. Kabat and M.M. Mayer, eds.). pp. 133-240. Charles H. Thomas, Springfield, Illinois.

Stagg, D.A., Brown, C.G.D., Crawford, J.G., Kanhai, G.K. and Young, A.S. (1974). *Res. Vet. Sci.* (In press)

PARASITOLOGICAL AND ZOONOTIC FINDINGS IN SOUTH AMERICAN MONKEYS*

J.M. Bafort and P. Kageruka

Department of Malariology and Department of Veterinary Medicine, Institute of Tropical Medicine, Antwerpen, Belgium.

INTRODUCTION

Chagas' disease is an important disease in humans in the Americas. More than 100 animal species have been found to harbour the etiological agent, *Trypanosoma (Schizotrypanum) cruzi* Chagas, 1909 (Hoare, 1972). The natural infection exists in some new world monkeys, as has been demonstrated by several authors (Pifano, 1961; Deane and Damasceno, 1961; Ayala, 1961; Garnham and Gonzalez - Magaburu, 1962; Dunn *et al.*, 1963; Marinkelle, 1964; Bullock *et al.*, 1967 and 1969; Albuquerque, 1969). Nevertheless, hiterto, *Aotus trivirgatus*, the owl monkey, has not been included as an animal reservoir of Chagas' disease.

Since the demonstration of the receptivity of *Aotus trivirgatus* to human plasmodiums by Porter and Young (1966), and Geiman and Meagher (1967), this new experimental malaria model is widely used in laboratories throughout the world. The monkey also serves as a laboratory host for Chagas disease, but before any experimental use is made of the monkeys, it is necessary to ascertain whether natural infections occur. Such infections could possibly interfere with the results of experiments and could be transmissible to human beings.

This paper reports the discovery of *Aotus* as a new host for Chagas' disease and presents data on the susceptibility of laboratory animals to *T. (Schizotrypanum) cruzi (Aotus* strain).

AOTUS TRIVIRGATUS: *A NEW HOST FOR* TRYPANOSOMA CRUZI

Isolation of T. cruzi

During investigations of *Plasmodium vivax* infection in owl monkeys (Bafort and Kageruka, 1972), three trypanosome species, *T. cruzi*, *T. rangeli*-like and *Megatrypanum* sp. were found in seven of the monkeys. The *T. rangeli*-like and *Megatrypanum* sp. were readily demonstrated by the usual microsco-

*This study was supported in part by the World Health Organization, Geneva, and in part by N.F.W.O., Brussels, Belgium.

pic techniques and the *T. rangeli*-like organism has been obtained on artificial media (Fig. 3). However, despite numerous microscopical investigations [direct smear, thick smear, and the concentration method of (Bennett, 1962)], splenectomy and administration of an immunodepressant (Betametasone(R), Glaxo), *T. cruzi* could not be demonstrated in the peripheral blood of the monkeys. The natural infection of *Aotus* was demonstrated xenodiagnosis and isodiagnosis, immunoelectrophoretic study confirmed *T. cruzi* infection and the immunofluorecent test revealed antibodies of Chagas' disease in the monkeys.

Xenodiagnosis, using *Triatoma infestans*, showed that 6 out of 7 bugs, fed at different times on a naturally infected owl monkey, were positive. Microscopical examination of the intestinal contents of the bugs, cyclical transmission of the infection to *Aotus trivirgatus* and subcutaneous inoculation of *Chinchilla lanigera* with ground up bugs confirmed the presence of *T. cruzi*.

Experimental infections

An *Aotus* monkey, previously been shown to be negative by xenodiagnosis and serological techniques, was cyclically infected with a bug fed on a naturally infected monkey. The monkey developed subclinical infection. Trypanosomes were found in peripheral blood from the 33rd day after feeding until the 125th day. Parasitaemia was low and fluctuating, and the animal survived the infection. Chinchillas infected subcutaneously with a suspension of homogenized infected bugs showed a high degree of parasitaemia and acute infection. Peripheral blood was positive for *T. cruzi* on the 13th day until death on the 28th day (Fig. 1).

Several species of laboratory rodents, including *Chinchilla lanigera*, were used for the isodiagnosis test. Transmission by the intraperitoneal inoculation of blood (0,2 to 0,5 ml) from naturally infected monkey was successful only with *Chinchilla lanigera*. Mice, (GIF/TB), young Wistar rats, guinea pigs and rabbits were insucceptible as assessed by parasitological, histological and immunological critera.

The chinchillas developed an acute infection, leading to death in 30 days. At necropsy, typical lesions of Chagas' disease; e.g. cardiac hypertrophy and exudative myocarditis were present. Hydrothorax ascites, splenomegaly and decoloured liver were also present and numerous trypanosomes could be found in direct smears from all the organs. Histological examinations revealed pseudocysts of amastigotes in cardiac muscle, and in other tissues such as the striated muscles, the gut wall and the lymph nodes (Fig. 2).

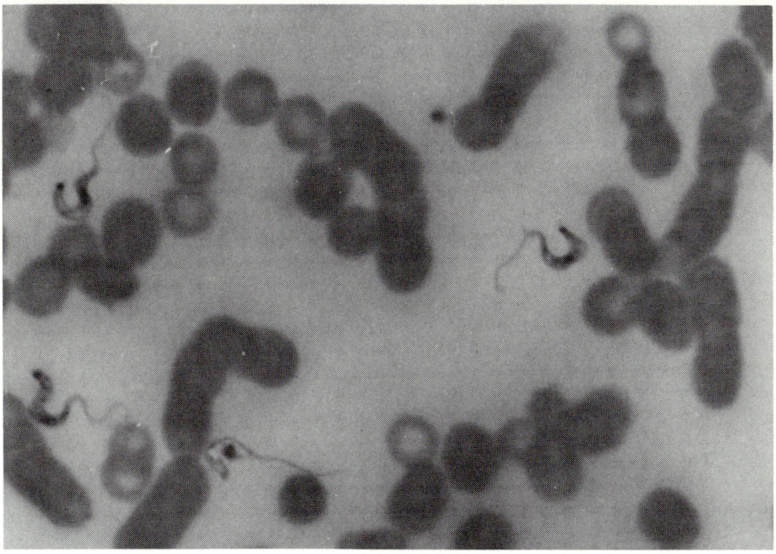

Fig. 1. T. cruzi *in the blood of chinchilla (X1000).*

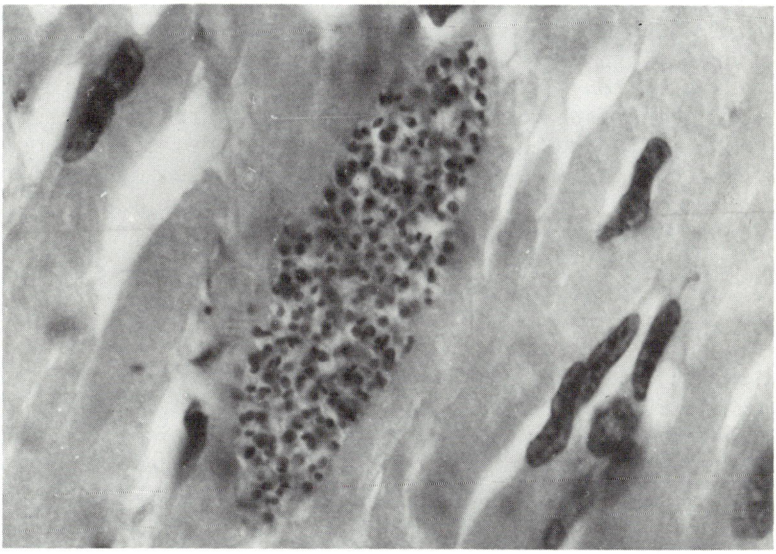

Fig. 2. Pseudocysts of T. cruzi *in the heart muscle of a chinchilla (X750).*

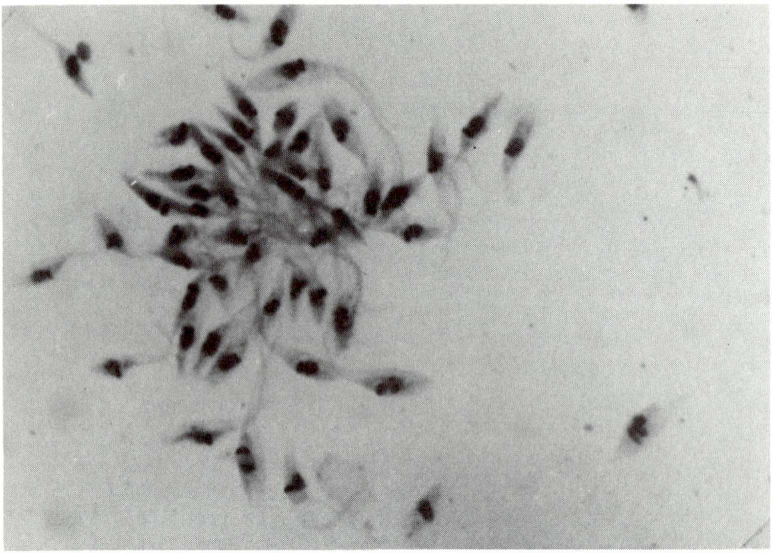

Fig. 3. Culture forms of T. cruzi (Aotus *strain) (X1000).*

Immunofluorescent tests on sera using *T. cruzi* culture antigen, gave positive reactions. Immunoelectrophoresis revealed the precipitin arc (arc No. V) which is considered by Afchain and Capron (1969) to be specific for *T. cruzi*. In addition, comparison of the *T. cruzi (Aotus* strain) antigen with that of *T. cruzi* (Tehventepec) by immunoelectrophoresis indicated that the antigens of the strains were identical.

SUSCEPTIBILITY OF LABORATORY ANIMALS TO T. CRUZI (AOTUS *STRAIN) INFECTION.*

In the initial studies the number of trypanosomes in the inocula was too low and the parasites were not detectable by microscopical examination in any animal. Subsequently, a larger number of parasites was used for inoculation; being obtained from blood taken from a chinchilla during the acute parasitaemic stage of infection. A variety of laboratory animals, GIF/TB mice, normal and splenectomized NMRI mice, young Wistar rats, guinea pigs, rabbits, and Syrian gold hamsters were used. Rabbits were inoculated intraperitoneally with 0,2 ml of chinchilla blood and the other species received 0,1 ml. by the same route.

Mice

In GIF/TB mice, trypanosomes could be detected in the ascitic fluid for 7 days after inoculation. The blood of these animals showed trypanosomes after the 13th day but parasitaemia was low and irregular. All the animals survived for at least 100 days after infection.

Non-splenectomized NMRI mice showed trypanosomes in the blood between the 15th and the 33rd day after infection. Half of the mice died during the first 40 days while the others survived beyond 60 days. Splenectomized NMRI mice behaved similarly to the non-splenectomized mice. One mouse died on the 25th day; the blood of four out of five became negative on the 38th day and all survived.

Rats

Young Wistar rats showed a few trypanosomes in the blood on the 9th day after the inoculation. After one month parasitaemia was very high, but it became negative after two months. A few pseudocysts were found in cardiac muscle.

Guinea pigs

Guinea pigs became positive 10 days after infection. The number of trypanosomes in the blood gradually increased until the 36th day, when the animals were sacrificed. Histological section of cardiac muscle showed the presence of a few pseudocysts.

Rabbits

Rabbits showed a moderate parasitaemia from the 13th to the 30th day, thereafter they became negative.

Hamsters

Hamsters did not develop a parasitaemia. A few parasites were observed in the ascitic fluid on the 6th day after the inoculation and they persisted here until the 30th day. All the animals survived the infection.

Chinchillas

Chinchillas infected with chinchilla derived material developed acute infections. Cardiac lesions and pseudocysts in the cardiac muscle and in other tissues were detected. Trypanosomes appear in ascites fluid before they are detectable in the peripheral blood. This confirms similar findings of Le Ray, (1967).

Triatoma bugs fed on chinchillas during the peak of parasitaemia failed to become infected.

SUMMARY AND CONCLUSIONS

Aotus trivirgatus was found to be infected with *Trypanosoma (Schizotrypanum) cruzi*. The morphology of the organism corresponded to the classic description of the parasite; the measurement of the blood forms was 23,65 μ (range 17,55 - 29,74 μ); cultures were readily obtained and pseudocysts were produced in tissues. The identity of the parasite was confirmed by immunoelectrophoresis and immunofluorescent tests.

Infection with *T. cruzi* in owl monkeys was inapparent. However, the inoculation of blood into susceptible laboratory animals, xenodiagnosis, culture in artificial media and immunological tests revealed its presence.

Of the laboratory animals tested, *Chinchilla lanigera* (Chinchilla) was the most sensitive to the infection. It developed an acute parasitaemia, detectable by microscopic examination. The infection induces some of the typical lesions of Chagas Disease in this host. These observations suggest the use of the chinchilla as an experimental model for Chagas' disease. Since the geographical distribution of the chinchilla coincides with that of Chagas' disease, the role of the chinchilla as an animal reservoir of *T. cruzi* should be investigated.

Since the spider monkey (*A. trivirgatus*) may be a reservoir host for *T. cruzi*, the increased direct importation of it into North America and Europe for experimental studies of malaria, may pose hazards to human health. Hence, isodiagnosis and xenodiagnosis on imported *A. trivirgatus* and indeed on other genera of monkeys such as *Ateles, Saimiri, Alouatta, Lagothrix* and *Saguinus*, some of which are known to be reservoirs of *T. cruzi*, is recommended.

ACKNOWLEDGEMENTS

The authors thank Mr. Van den Bergh, Director, Royal Zoological Society, Antwerp, for providing the chinchillas. The facilities provided by the Departments of Protozoology and of Serology, and the help received from Mr. D. Afchain, S.I.B.P. of the Faculty of Medicine, Lille, is gratefully acknowledged.

REFERENCES

Afchain, D. and Capron, A. (1969). *C. R. Acad. Sc. Paris, 269*, 272.

Albuquerque, R.D.R. and Barretto, M.P. (1969). *Rev. Inst. Med. Trop. S.Paolo, 11*, 115.

Albuquerque, R.D.R. and Barretto, M.P. (1969). *Rev. Inst.*

Med. Trop. S.Paolo, 11, 394.
Ayala, F.M. (1961). *Rev. Brasil. Malariol. 13,* 99.
Bafort, J.M. and Kageruka, P. (1972). *Ann. Soc. Belge Med. Trop. 52,* 235.
Bennett, G.F. (1962). *Canad. J. Zool. 40,* 124.
Bullock, B.C., Lehner, N.D.M. and Clarkson, T.B. (1969). *Primates in Med.,* Karger, New York, *2,* 62.
Bullock, B.C., Wolff, R.H. and Clarkson, T.B. (1967). *J. Amer. Vet. Med. Ass. 151,* 920.
Deane, L.M. and Damasceno, R.M.G. (1961). *Rev. Inst. Med. Trop. S.Paolo, 3,* 61.
Dunn, F.L., Lambrecht, F.L. and du Plessis, R. (1963). *Amer. J. Trop. Med. Hyg. 12,* 524.
Garnham, P.C.C. and Gonzalez-Magaburu, L. (1962). *Rev. Inst. Med. Trop. S.Paolo, 4,* 79.
Geiman, Q.M. and Meagher, M. (1967). *Nature, 215,* 437.
Hoare, C.A. (1972). *The trypanosomes of Mammals.* Blackwell, Oxford.
Marinkelle, C.J. (1966). *Trans Roy. Soc. Trop. Med. Hyg. 60,* 109.
Marinkelle, C.J. (1964). *Mem. III. Congr. Latino Amer. Microb.,* Bogota, Columbia.
Pifano, F.C., Guerrero, L., Martin, G.G., Vasquez, A.D. and Maekelt, A. (1961). *Rev. Venez. San. Assist. Soc. 26,* 7.
Woo, P.T.K., (1969). *Can. J. Zool. 47,* 921.

CURRENT STATUS OF VACCINATION AGAINST CHAGAS' DISEASE: USE OF IRRADIATED PARASITES

William L. Hanson, Julia J. Chien, Willie L. Chapman, Jr.*, and Edward L. Roberson

Departments of Parasitology and * Medicine and Surgery, College of Veterinary Medicine, University of Georgia, Athens, Georgia

INTRODUCTION

The development of effective immunizing agents for use against *Trypanosoma cruzi* infections in man and animals has been the objective of numerous investigations. A variety of antigens prepared from the epimastigote stage of *T. cruzi* has been tested in laboratory animals for their potential as vaccines. These preparations include formalin-killed epimastigotes (Hauschka *et al.*, 1950) and epimastigotes subjected to pressure, ultrasonication, lyophilization, or shaking with glass beads (Goble *et al.*, 1964; Menezes, 1965; Garcia, 1967; Gonzalez-Cappa *et al.*, 1968; Hanson, unpublished). While some limited success has been achieved with certain of these preparations, none have been satisfactory.

The most successful vaccination attempts have been those in which so-called avirulent strains of *T. cruzi* have been used (c.f. Menezes, 1970, 1971; Kagan and Norman, 1961; Seah and Marsden, 1969). While animals which have undergone a primary infection with one of these strains of *T. cruzi* are resistant to challenge with highly virulent strains of the parasite, some severe limitations should be considered (see Goble, 1970). One of the primary limitations of this procedure is the fact that it is impossible to predict the virulence for man of these so-called avirulent strains of *T. cruzi*. Furthermore, little information is available regarding the possible role of these relatively avirulent strains of the parasite in the production of chronic Chagas' disease in man. Until this information is available, the use of these strains of *T. cruzi* for immunization of man involves considerable risk.

Since antigens prepared previously from the epimastigote stage of *T. cruzi* generally have not been satisfactory for use as vaccines against *T. cruzi*, it appeared reasonable that antigens prepared from those stages of the parasite which predominate in the vertebrate host (i.e. trypomastigotes and amastigotes) should be more effective. This communication presents some results of studies in our laboratory using irradiated trypomastigotes and amastigotes of *T. cruzi* to stimulate immunity to acute Chagas' disease in mice. The success in immunizing animals with various other species of parasites subjected to irradiation (Jarrett *et al.*, 1957; Miller, 1971; Duxbury *et al.*, 1972) suggested that this approach with the American trypanosomes might be worthwhile.

MATERIALS AND METHODS

Animals

Female CF_1 albino outbred mice (Carworth Farms, Portage, Michigan, U.S.A.), 18-25 grams, served as experimental animals in all the immunization attempts. Female C_3H brown inbred mice (Flow Laboratories, Dublin, Virginia, U.S.A.) served as donors of infected and normal blood for the experiments in which irradiated infected blood was used. C_3H mice also were used in studies requiring a highly susceptible host for the detection of small numbers of virulent *T. cruzi* in mouse blood and in suspensions of irradiated parasites.

Maintenance and production of parasites

A Brazil strain of *T. cruzi* was used in these studies and is maintained in our laboratory in four-week old CF_1 mice by intraperitoneal (IP) injection of infective whole blood every 17-21 days.

Trypomastigotes and amastigotes subjected to irradiation and subsequently used for immunization of animals were obtained from infected C_3H mice or were mass produced in vero (African green monkey kidney) cell cultures according to the method of Hanson (unpublished). Regarding the former, C_3H mice were inoculated with 50,000 *T. cruzi* in mouse blood via the intraperitoneal route. The mice were exsanguinated on day 18 post-infection, which is the time of maximum parasitemia (approximately 5.0×10^6 trypomastigotes per ml blood), and whole infected blood was subsequently subjected to the desired level of gamma irradiation. Parasites grown in cell culture (consisting generally of 50-70% trypomastigotes and 30-50% amastigotes) were collected from the liquid medium from roller cultures by centrifugation at 10,000 X G for 15 minutes in a RC2-B Sorvall refrigerated centrifuge at 4°C. The parasites were washed one time by centrifugation in cold Lockes' solution and resuspended in this solution to the desired concentration in preparation for irradiation.

Irradiation of T. cruzi, *immunization and challenge of mice, and quantitation of parasitemia*

T. cruzi from cell culture was suspended in Lockes' solution to a concentration of 40-50 X 10^6 trypomastigotes per ml and exposed to 30, 60, 75, 85, 90, 100, 125, 150, 175, 200 or 300 KR of irradiation from CO_{60} in a Gammacell 200 Irradiator. Mouse blood containing 0.5-7.5 X 10^6 parasites per ml was subjected to 150 KR irradiation as described above for the cell culture parasites.

To immunize mice with irradiated *T. cruzi* from cell culture, groups of mice were given three weekly intraperitoneal injections of 0.2 ml aliquots of suspensions of parasites containing 8-10 X 10^6 trypomastigotes which had been exposed to each level of irradiation. For immunization of mice with irradiated infected blood, groups of mice were given 2, 3, 4, or 5 weekly intraperitoneal inoculations of 0.1 ml blood containing 0.1 to 1.0 X 10^6 parasites. Some control groups received vero cells only, uninfected mouse blood, or Lockes' solution which had been handled in a manner identical to that of parasites from cell culture or infected blood. Other control groups received nothing.

Seven days after the last immunizing injection of irradiated cell culture pasasites and 20 days after the last immunizing injection of irradiated infected blood, all immunized mice along with appropriate controls were challenged with 5 X 10^4 virulent *T. cruzi* in mouse blood and the parasitemia and mortality subsequently recorded.

Parasitemia counts were made with the quantitative thick smear procedure (Roberson, *et al.*, 1973).

Cell culture and mouse inoculation procedures for detection of small numbers of T. cruzi

The viability and virulence of the irradiated parasites were tested by inoculation into vero cell culture (this procedure is capable of detecting a single viable organism in an inoculum; see "Results" section), or by inoculation into C_3H inbred mice (this procedure also is capable of detecting a single viable organism in an inoculum; see "Results" section), or both.

The evaluation of these two procedures for the testing for the presence of viable or virulent parasites in an inoculum or in mouse blood was done as described below. *T. cruzi* grown in vero cell cultures were harvested by centrifugation, suspended in 5 ml cell culture medium, and the parasites counted by quantitative fresh preparations (Roberson *et al.*, 1973). Tenfold dilutions of parasites ranging from 100,000 to 10 organisms per ml were prepared in cell culture medium and 0.1 ml aliquots of each dilution (numbers of organisms per aliquot ranging from 10,000-1 per aliquot) were added to each of five vero cell monolayers in 250 ml Falcon flasks prepared as described by Hanson (unpublished). A drop of culture medium was removed from each flask at weekly intervals following inoculation with parasites and examined for the presence of *T. cruzi*. Flasks not found positive for parasites after one month were discarded and recorded as negative.

Blood containing trypomastigotes of *T. cruzi* was obtained by cardiac puncture from a mouse 18 days after experimental infection. The number of parasites was determined by the quantitative fresh count procedure (Roberson *et al.*, 1973). Tenfold dilutions of parasites ranging from 100,000 to 10 organisms per ml were prepared in Hanks' balanced salt solution (BSS) and 0.1 ml aliquots of each dilution (range of 10,000 to 1 parasites per aliquot) were inoculated either into each of five vero cell monolayers or into groups of 10 C_3H mice via the intraperitoneal route. The presence and numbers of parasites in the cultures were determined as described above and presence and numbers in the blood of the mice were determined subsequently from quantitative thick smears prepared at two to seven-day intervals during the period of 7-47 days following injection. If parasites were not observed in the blood during this time, the mice were considered negative for *T. cruzi*.

Indirect fluorescent antibody and agglutination procedures

To obtain sera for serological tests, blood was collected from groups of mice which were either untreated, immunized, immunized and challenged, or challenged only. Indirect fluorescent antibody (IFA) and/or agglutination (Agg) studies were conducted according to the procedure of Logan and Hanson (1973) and Vattuone and Yanovsky (1971).

RESULTS AND DISCUSSION

Detection of small numbers of viable T. cruzi *in blood and other fluids*

When designing experiments to investigate immunization of animals against *T. cruzi*, at least two important problems should be considered. First, it is necessary to devote some attention to the desired morphological stage of the parasite to be used as the antigen. Second, because of the extreme virulence of this parasite for man and animals, the antigens used in immunization should be free of virulent parasites which might produce eventual disease in the immunized animal. Regarding the stage of *T. cruzi* to be used, it was reasoned that those stages which occur in the mammalian host (i.e. trypomastigotes and amastigotes) should be the most desirable as antigens in vaccination attempts. In our experience these states can be grown consistently only in cell culture. Thus a cell culture procedure for mass production of these stages was developed as described above. Regarding assurance that vaccines contained no virulent parasites, considerable effort was devoted to developing dependable procedures for the detection of low numbers of *T. cruzi*.

Preliminary observations indicated that vero cell cultures were efficient in detecting small numbers of *T. cruzi* in various fluids. C_3H inbred mice had also been observed to be exceptionally susceptible to *T. cruzi* and all animals injected with small numbers of parasites developed severe acute Chagas' disease which was accompanied by heavy parasitemia and 100% mortality. Results of experiments designed to evaluate these two procedures for efficacy in the detection of small numbers of viable or virulent *T. cruzi* indicated that both procedures were quite sensitive in the detection of small numbers of *T. cruzi* in fluids.

All of five vero cell cultures inoculated with either 10,000, 1,000, or 100 parasites from mouse blood or from cell cultures were observed to develop increasing numbers of *T. cruzi* in the medium by two to three weeks (Table 1). Five of five flasks inoculated with 10 parasites from cell culture and four of five flasks inoculated with 10 parasites from mouse blood became positive. Even inocula containing theoretically only a single parasite from mouse blood or from cell culture were infective respectively for three of five and two of five vero cell cultures.

All of 10 mice in each group inoculated with either 10,000, 1,000, 100, or 10 parasites from mouse blood developed fulminating infections of acute Chagas' disease and died (Table 2). Six of 10 mice inoculated with a single trypomastigote .to *T. cruzi* also developed heavy parasitemias and died by 43 days post-inoculation.

The preceding results indicate that both the vero cell culture procedure and C_3H mouse inoculation procedure are reliable methods for the detection of a single viable or virulent parasite in the blood of animals or in other types of suspensions of *T. cruzi*. One or both of these procedures were used subsequently in determining the presence of living, virulent organisms in irradiated vaccines or in the blood of vaccinated mice.

Immunization of mice with irradiated T. cruzi

A number of experiments were performed to determine the level of irradiation necessary for attenuation of *T. cruzi* to

Table 1

Efficacy of vero cell cultures in the detection of Trypanosoma cruzi *in blood or other fluids*

Source and Number of Parasites Inoculated into Cell Culture	Number of Positive Cell Cultures/Total Number of Cell Cultures
Blood	
10,000	5/5
1,000	5/5
100	5/5
10	4/5
1	3/5
Cell Culture	
10,000	5/5
1,000	5/5
100	5/5
10	5/5
1	2/5

Table 2

Efficacy of C_3H brown inbred mice in the detection of Trypanosoma cruzi *in blood or other fluids*

No. of Organisms Injected	Positive Mice/Total No. Injected	No. of Mice that Died No. Mice Positive
10,000	10/10	10/10
1,000	10/10	10/10
100	10/10	10/10
10	10/10	10/10
1	6/10	6/10

an extent that no virulent organisms remained. Suspensions of cell culture parasites subjected to 30, 60, 75, 85, 90, 100 or 125 KR gamma irradiation were found to be capable of producing infections in cell cultures or in the vaccinated CF_1 mice themselves (Table 3). On the other hand, suspensions of *T. cruzi* subjected to 150, 200, or 300 KR gamma irradiation were not observed to contain parasites capable of infecting cell cultures, C_3H mice, or the vaccinated animals (Table 3). It was concluded from these studies that exposure to at least 150 KR gamma irradiation is necessary to attenuate the Brazil strain of *T. cruzi* used in these experiments to an extent that the parasites are incapable of producing prolonged infection in cell culture, C_3H mice, and, thus, in vaccinated animals under the conditions of these experiments.

Table 3

Relation of the level of gamma irradiation administered to Trypanosoma cruzi *from cell culture to the infectivity of the parasites*

Level of gamma Irradiation Administered (Kr)	Infectivity Demonstrated By:		
	Cell Culture Technique	Injection into C_3H Mice	Injection into CF_1 Mice
30	+	ND*	+
60	+	ND	+
75	+	ND	+
85	+	ND	+
90	+	ND	+
100	+	ND	+
125	+	ND	+
150	-	-	-
175	-	-	-
200	-	-	-
300	-	-	-

*Not Done

Based on these observations, 150 KR gamma irradiation was used to attenuate *T. cruzi* in blood and 150, 200, or 300 KR were used to attenuate cell culture parasites in subsequent experiments. In a preliminary experiment designed to determine if irradiated *T. cruzi* stimulated any increased resistance to challenge with *T. cruzi*, each of four groups of CF_1 mice were injected with either 2, 3, 4, or 5 weekly doses of the irridiated infected C_3H blood. Inoculation of aliquots of irradiated blood into C_3H mice indicated the absence of virulent organisms in each of the four preparations of immunizing material. In addition, examination of the blood of each of the CF_1 mice at 20 days following the last immunizing injection revealed no parasites. Thus, on the 20th day following the last immunizing injection, immunized and control mice were challenged with virulent *T. cruzi*. Protection against challenge with virulent *T. cruzi* was evident in the mice which were immunized with irradiated infected blood (whether given 2, 3, 4, or 5 injections) as judged by significantly lower parasitemias in these mice as compared to that of untreated controls ($p<.005$, t test) or controls immunized with irradiated but uninfected blood ($p<.025$ to .05 during the week of peak parasitemia, Fig. 1). As the number of immunizing injections increased, the degree of protection increased. For example, when two injections of irradiated infected blood were given, the maximum average parasitemia of the challenged immunized mice was 0.75×10^6 trypomastigotes/ml and when three injections were given it was 0.5×10^6 trypomastigotes/ml. Maximum protection was observed in mice receiving five injections of irradiated infected blood in which the maximum mean parasitemia was 0.2×10^6 trypomastigotes/ml blood. It may be possible to completely prevent the development of a parasitemia in challenged mice if the number of immunizing doses is increased above five or if the numbers of parasites in each immunizing injection is increased. These possibilities are being investigated further.

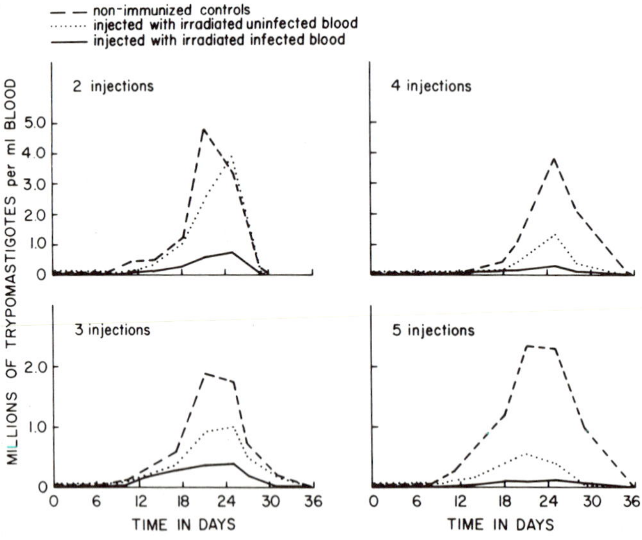

Fig. 1. Effect of immunization with T. cruzi *in C_3H mouse blood exposed to 150 KR gamma irradiation on parasitemia in CF_1 mice challenged with 50,000 trypomastigotes in mouse blood.*

No mortality occurred among mice immunized with irradiated infected blood while 9 to 20% mortality was recorded among control groups.

It is of interest to note that mice receiving irradiated uninfected mouse blood were afforded some protection against *T. cruzi* as evidenced by lower mean parasitemias and reduced mortality (Fig. 1). The degree of protection appeared to increase concomitantly with the number of injections. For example, mice immunized with five injections of irradiated uninfected blood were observed to have maximum mean parasitemia of approximately 0.5×10^6 trypomastigotes per ml blood as compared to 2.3×10^6 per ml in the untreated controls ($p<.005$) on the same day. Further, mortality in the former was only about one-half as great in the mice receiving irradiated uninfected blood as compared to untreated controls. The reason for this protection is not understood at present but it is possible that it is related to non-specific phagocytic enhancement or enhancement of the ability of the macrophages to destroy parasites picked up by macrophages. Taliaferro and Pizzi (1955) have suggested that phagocytic activity is a factor in arresting acute infections of Chagas' disease and that phagocytes of immune animals are more efficient in the destruction of parasites which have been ingested by macrophages. In these experiments, C_3H mice were used as donors of infected blood for irradiation since high numbers of trypomastigotes can be obtained from this strain of mouse. Uninfected control blood was also obtained from C_3H mice and subsequently irradiated. CF_1 mice (used for previous immunological studies in our laboratory) were used as recipients of irradiated infected or uninfected blood in the present immunization experiments. Perhaps the C_3H blood was sufficiently incompatible in CF_1 mice to result in enhancement of nonspecific phagocytosis and a consequent reduction in the numbers of virulent parasites upon challenge.

While injections of irradiated uninfected blood resulted in some increased resistance to challenge in mice, a significantly greater protection ($p<.05$) was afforded those mice which were injected with irradiated infected blood as compared with that of the former group. We attribute the greater degree of protection in the latter group to the presence of the parasite in the immunizing material.

Since the use of irradiated infected blood in the previous experiments was complicated by the presence of relatively large amounts of contaminative red blood cells, it is obvious that a cleaner preparation of parasites was necessary for additional experiments. Trypomastigotes and amastigotes relatively free of contaminative cells or other substances can be produced in cell culture. Experiments were then carried out to determine the efficacy of *T. cruzi* grown in cell culture and exposed to 150 KR gamma irradiation to induce immunity in recipient mice. Mice which were given three weekly IP injections of cell culture forms of *T. cruzi* irradiated with 150 KR developed significantly lower mean parasitemia when challenged with virulent *T. cruzi* seven days after the last immunizing injection than that observed in untreated control mice or control mice which were injected with vero cells only (Fig. 2). No significant difference was observed between the mean parasitemias of the two control groups. However, the mean parasitemia of the group immunized with irradiated *T. cruzi* was significantly lower than that of the other two on days 19, 21, and 24 ($p<0.005$ to <0.05). For example mean parasitemia of 10 immunized mice increased to maximum numbers of only about 500,000 on day 24 while control mice receiving vero cells were observed to have mean parasitemias of approximately 3.25×10^6 per ml on the same day.

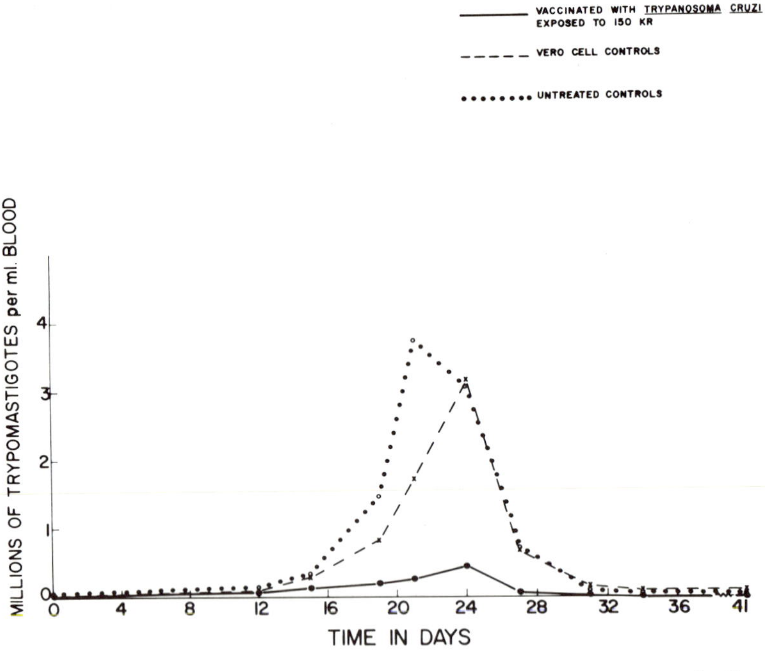

Fig. 2. Effect of immunization with Trypanosoma cruzi *from cell culture exposed to 150 KR gamma irradiation on parasitemia in mice challanged with 50,000 trypomastigotes in mouse blood.*

The question subsequently arose regarding the relationship of the ability of the parasites to stimulate protective immunity in mice to the level of irradiation administered to *T. cruzi* grown in cell culture. Levels of 200 and 300 KR were used to attenuate separate suspensions of *T. cruzi*. Following three immunizing injections and challenge, mice receiving parasites exposed to 200 or 300 KR irradition were noted to have significantly lower mean parasitemias ($p<0.005$ to 0.05 on days 19, 21, 23, and 25) than untreated control mice or those receiving vero cells only (Fig. 3). Since no significant difference was observed between the mean parasitemias of the latter two groups on any day examined, these data were combined (Fig. 3). No significant differences were observed between the mean parasitemias of mice immunized with parasites exposed to 200 or 300 KR and these mice developed resistance to challenge which appeared to be equivalent to that seen in mice receiving parasites subjected to 150 KR.

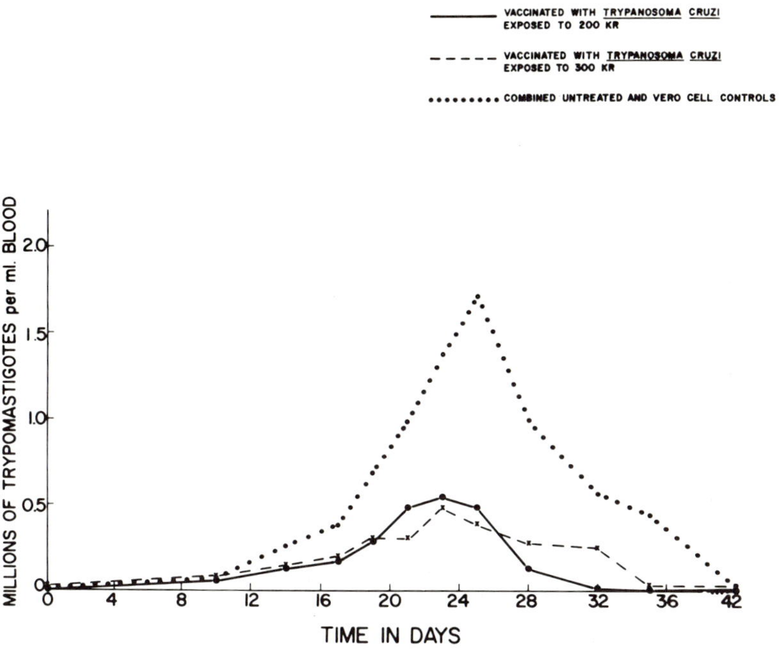

Fig. 3. Effect of immunization with Trypanosoma cruzi *from cell culture exposed to 200 or 300 KR gamma irradiation on parasitemia in mice challenged with 50,000 trypomastigotes in mouse blood.*

A total of 40 mice in three separate experiments have been immunized with *T. cruzi* grown in vero cell culture and exposed to 150, 175, 200, or 300 KR gamma irradiation while a total of 50 mice served as either untreated controls or controls inoculated with vero cells only. Fourteen of the 50 control mice died following challenge with 50,000 trypomastigotes from mouse blood while only one of the 40 mice immunized with irradiated parasites died following challenge.

IFA and Agg studies of sera from immunized and control mice indicated that immunized mice developed measurable antibody titers detectable by both of these procedures (Table 4). Slightly higher IFA and Agg titers were found in sera from challenge immunized mice (three-week infection) then were seen in non-immunized controls with infections of the same duration.

These studies indicated that inoculation of mice with *T. cruzi* subjected to gamma irradiation resulted in a significant protective immune response which was accompanied by an antibody response and that immunization enabled the mice to produce a more rapid antibody response when challenged with virulent parasites.

Although the degree of protection in this work was not as great as that observed by Duxbury *et al.*, (1972) with *T. rhodesiense*, it appears from these experiments that trypomastigotes and amastigotes of *T. cruzi* subjected to 150-300 KR gamma irradiation offer significant promise for immunization of animals against Chagas' disease. Additional work is underway to study the relation of the number of parasites in the immunizing injection and the number of immunizing injections given to the ability to stimulate protective immunity. It is anticipated that some improvement in the degree of protection can be realized from additional work. While we cannot be sure that the fluorescent antibody and the agglutination procedures used in this work measure protective antibody, the data suggest that vaccination possibly stimulates a protective antibody response. Passive transfer experiments using serum from immunized animals are planned in an effort to elucidate this further.

SUMMARY

Groups of CF_1 mice received either 2, 3, 4, or 5 weekly immunizing injections of gamma irradiated (150 KR) infected mouse blood containing trypomastigotes of *T. cruzi* and were challenged 20 days following the last immunizing injection. Other CF_1 mice received three weekly immunizing injections of gamma irradiated (150, 200, or 300 KR) of trypomastigotes and amastigotes of *T. cruzi* grown in cell culture and were chal-

Table 4

Serology of CF_1 *mice (either immunized with gamma irradiated* T. cruzi *or non-immunized) as determined by the indirect fluorescent antibody (IFA) procedure (using cell culture parasites as antigen) or by the agglutination (Agg.) procedure (using trypsinized epimastigotes of* T. cruzi *as antigen).*

Immunization: Dosage of Gamma Irradiation for *T. cruzi* or vero Cells; 3 weekly Injections	Challenge: 50,000 *T. cruzi* Yes or No	Time of Serum collection: After Last Immunizing Dose (PI) or Post-Challenge (PC)	(No. Serum Samples) and Reciprocal of Highest Dilution Obtained on 1/2 the No. of Serum Samples	
			IFA	Agg.
150 KR *T. cruzi*	No	1 wk PI	(4) 16	
200 KR *T. cruzi*	No	1 wk PI		(5) 8
300 KR *T. cruzi*	No	1 wk PI		(3) 8
150 KR Vero Cells only	No	1 wk PI	(4) 0	(3) 0
Untreated	No	-		(3) 0
150 KR *T. cruzi*	Yes	4 wk PI, 3 wk PC	(4) 64	
200 KR *T. cruzi*	Yes	4 wk PI, 3 wk PC		(5) 256
300 KR *T. cruzi*	Yes	4 wk PI, 3 wk PC		(3) 128
200 KR Vero Cells only	Yes	4 wk PI, 3 wk PC		(3) 32
Untreated	Yes	3 wk PC	(4) 16	(4) 64
Untreated	Yes	6 wk PC	(2)1024	(9) 512

lenged one week following the third immunizing injection. Both of the above groups were significantly protected upon challenge with 50,000 virulent blood forms of *T. cruzi* as evidenced by lower parasitemia and mortality in the immunized mice as compared to that in controls.

The viability and virulence of the irradiated parasites were tested by inoculation into vero cell culture (this procedure was found to be capable of detecting a single viable organism in an inoculum), or by inoculation into C_3H inbred mice (this procedure also was found to be capable of detecting a single viable organism in an inoculum), or both. While parasites exposed to the above levels of irradiation stimulated protective immunity in inoculated mice, they were apparently completely attenuated since none of the immunizing material exposed to 150, 200, or 300 KR produced detectable infections in vero cell cultures. Gamma irradiation of *T. cruzi* from cell culture at levels below 150 KR (i.e., at 30, 60, 75, 85, 90, 100, or 125 KR) failed to attenuate the parasites as judged by the development of parasites in vero cell cultures and/or in C_3H mice inoculated with parasites exposed to these lower levels of irradiation.

These studies indicate that the possibility of immunizing animals and possibly man with irradiated *T. cruzi* grown in cell culture holds considerable promise.

ACKNOWLEDGEMENTS

This work was supported in part by Contract # DADA 17-69-C-9167 from the U.S. Army Medical Research and Development Command. We wish to thank Mrs. Allene Ranew and Mrs. Ginny Waits for their technical work in these experiments.

REFERENCES

Duxbury, R.E., Sadun, E.H., and Anderson, J.S. (1972). *Am. J. Trop. Med. Hyg. 21*, 885.

Garcia, A. (1967). *Primer Congreso Lationamericano de Parasitologia*, Santiago de Chile, Resumenes, p. 35.

Goble, F.C. (1970). *In: Immunity to Parasitic Animals*, (G.J. Jackson, R. Herman and I. Singer, Eds.), Vol. II, Appleton-Century-Crofts, N.Y., N.Y. 597.

Goble, F.C., Boyd, J.L., Grimm-Wehner, M. and Konrath, M. (1964). *J. Parasit. 50*, (Suppl.) 19.

Gonzalez Cappa, S.M., Schmunis, G.A., Traversa, O.C., Yanovsky J.F., and Parodi, A.S. (1968). *Am. J. Trop. Med. Hyg. 17*, 709.

Hausckha, T.S., Goodwin, M.G., Palmquist, J. and Brown, E.

(1950). *Am. J. Trop. Med. 30,* 1.
Jarrett, W.F.H., Jennings, F.W., McIntyre, W.I.M., Mulligan, W., and Urquhart, G.M. (1957). *Vet. Rec. 63,* 1329.
Kagan, I.G. and Norman, L. (1961). *J. Infect. Dis. 108,* 213.
Logan, L.L. and Hanson, W.L. (1973). Submitted to *Exptl. Parasit.*
Menezes, H. (1965). *Revta. Bras. Med. 22,* 536.
Menezes, H. (1970). *Revta. Soc. Bras. Med. Trop. 4,* 1.
Menezes, H. (1971). *Revta. Soc. Bras. Med. Trop. 5,* 1.
Miller, T.A. (1971). *Adv. Parasit. 9,* 153.
Roberson, E.L., Hanson, W.L. and Chapman, Jr., W.L. (1973). *Exptl. Parasit. 34,* 168.
Seah, S. and Marsden, P.D. (1969). *Ann. Trop. Med. Parasit. 63,* 211.
Taliaferro, W.H. and Pizzi, T. (1955). *J. Infect. Dis. 96,* 199.
Vattuone, N.Y. and Yanovsky, J.F. (1971). *Exptl. Parasit. 30,* 349.

IMMUNOSUPPRESSION IN TRYPANOSOMIASIS

P. K. Murray, F. W. Jennings, Max Murray and G. M. Urquhart

Glasgow University Veterinary School, Bearsden, Glasgow, Scotland

INTRODUCTION

There is a current awareness that a variety of infectious agents can exert at least some of their pathogenicity through a suppressive effect on the hosts' immune defences in that it may enhance their susceptibility to secondary infections. Such immunosuppressive events have been shown to occur in diseases as widely disparate as viral infections (McGregor, 1972), mycoplasmosis (Kakalamanis *et al.*, 1972), bacterial infections (Rees and Waters, 1972), helminth infections (Faubert and Tanner, 1971) and in a variety of protozoal infections (Clinton *et al.*, 1969; Strickland *et al.*, 1973).

Although circumstantial evidence of immunosuppression, e.g., the association of severe secondary streptococcal infection and sleeping sickness, has existed for many years, the real importance of this phenomenon in the epidemiology of disease has only recently been recognized. In 1962 McGregor and Barr working in areas of endemic malaria in The Gambia, found that the responsiveness of children to immunisation with tetanus toxoid was significantly reduced and suggested that there was a "possibility that malaria may interfere with the antibody response to specific vaccines". These observations were confirmed and extended by Greenwood *et al.* (1972) who also showed that the suppression which occurred in human malaria was selective in that certain cellular immune responses remained normal. Perhaps the immunosuppression associated with malaria may be said to have one beneficial effect as it has been suggested that the conspicuous absence of autoimmune disease in Nigerians is related to the occurrence of malaria (Greenwood, 1968), and this has been substantiated by experimental evidence obtained in laboratory animals (Greenwood and Voller, 1970; Greenwood and Greenwood, 1971).

Infection of laboratory rodents with malaria parasites have provided useful models for studying the mechanisms of immunosuppression. Using such a system, various workers have shown a marked reduction in the responsiveness of infected mice to heterologous erythrocytes (Sengers *et al.*, 1971; Barker and Powers, 1971; Greenwood *et al.*,1971a). A more extensive investigation into the mechanisms of this immunosuppression has been conducted by Greenwood *et al.* (1971a). By studying the humoral and cellular responses of mice infected with the non-pathogenic *Plasmodium berghei yoelii* to a variety of antigens it was suggested that the immunological defect might be due to a disturbance of macrophage function. Further investigation into the role of the mononuclear phagocytic system of infected mice. (Greenwood *et al.*, 1971b) provided no further evidence of abnormality in this cell population but did indicate that there was a defect in the transport of antigen-antibody complexes by lymphocytes into germinal centres of the spleens of these infected mice. However the macrophage was again incriminated as being the defective component in the immune response by Loose *et al.* (1973) who concluded that there was a failure of "macrophage antigen processing" in mice infected with *P. berghei yoelii*. It can be seen from such reports that the nature of the immunosuppression is still poorly understood and that opinions as to the underlying cause vary considerably.

The earliest experimental evidence that immunosuppression was a feature of trypanosomiasis was reported by Goodwin (1970) and Goodwin *et al.* (1972). Sheep erythrocytes were used as an antigen in these studies in *Trypanosoma brucei* infected rabbits and mice and it was found that after infection the haemagglutinin response was significantly reduced. Since then, investigations have been directed towards characterising the immunological defect induced by trypanosome infections by using a broadly similar approach to those conducted in malaria and the results of such investigations by ourselves and others are presented and discussed in this paper.

Pathology of the immune system in rodents infected with T. brucei

In rats and mice infected with *T. brucei*, generalised lymph node enlargement, marked splenomegaly (Fig. 1) and hepatomegaly are the most obvious post-mortem findings (Hu, 1931; Losos and Ikede, 1972; Murray *et al.*, 1974a,b). Such changes develop soon after inoculation, persist throughout the infection and are attributable mainly to an expanded mononuclear phagocytic system and to massive plasma cell hyperplasia.

The number of cells in the mononuclear pahgocytic system of the liver, lymph nodes (Fig. 2), spleen, bone marrow and also of non-fixed macrophages in all tissues is markedly increased. These cells appear active and have abundant vacuolated cytoplasm often containing debris, possibly ingested trypanosomes and in the spleen they are frequently packed with red blood cells.

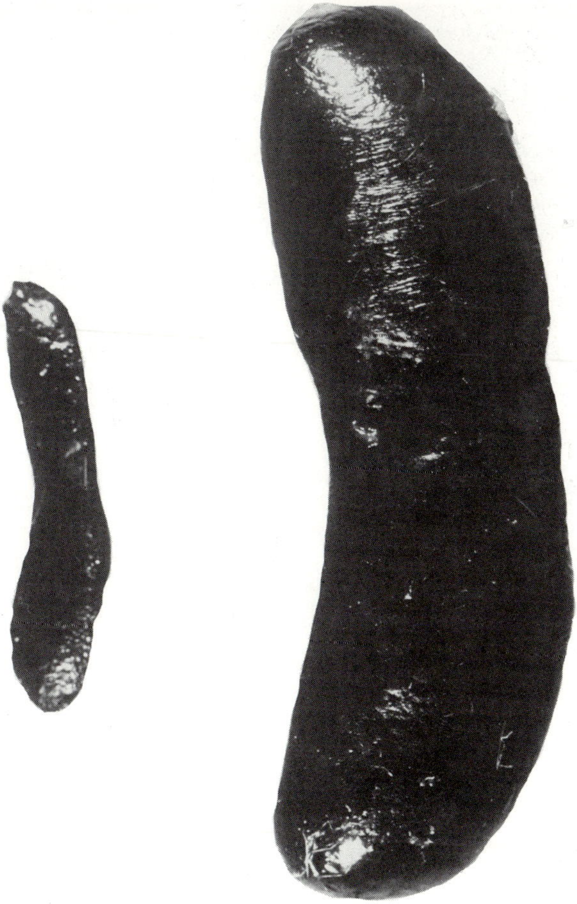

Fig. 1. Splenomegaly in mouse infected with Trypanosoma brucei.

Within a few days of infection, the medullary cords and juxtamedullary area of lymph nodes become populated by large lymphoid cells, many of which are found in mitosis, and then by plasma cell hyperplasia (Figs. 3 and 4). A similar series of events occur in the spleen where, by 14 to 21 days, the plasma cells occupy most of the white pulp and much of the red pulp (Fig. 5).

Early in the course of infection, foci of cellular lysis with depletion of plasma cells are present in lymph nodes and these are usually in association with aggregations of trypanosomes. In mice, later in infection, an occasional extensively depleted lymph node may be found but in general the plasma

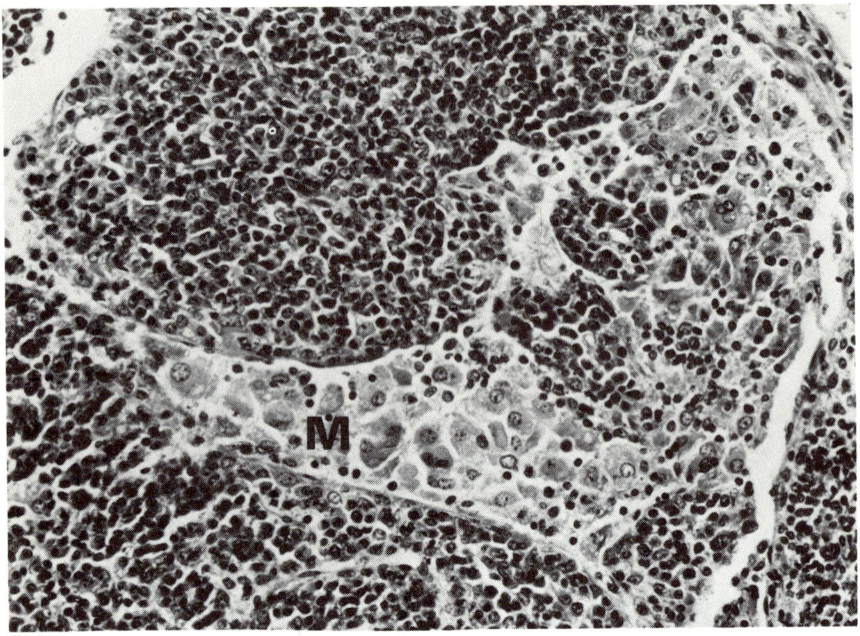

Fig. 2. Medulla of mouse lymph node **21** *days after infection with* Trypanosoma brucei. *Medullary sinus is packed with macrophages (M). Haematoxylin and Eosin x300 (by courtesy of the Editor of* Immunology*).*

cell hyperplasia persists for the duration of the infection, around 70 days (Murray *et al.*, 1974b). In rats, however, between 5 and 8 weeks of infection, severe cellular depletion occurs in the lymph nodes and spleen (Figs. 5 and 6) (Murray *et al.*, 1974a). Whether this change is due directly to trypanosomes or some form of immunological exhaustion is unknown.

Soon after infection, marked changes are found in the thymus. The cortex becomes narrow and irregular and numerous macrophages are present in the cortex and medulla where large lymphoid cells and plasma cells are also seen (Fig. 7). These changes are not progressive however, and the thymus is never ablated.

Thus extensive morphological alterations occur in all components of the immune system, i.e., the macrophage, B cells and T. cells; there is an expansion and increase in activity of the mononuclear phagocytic system, massive plasma cell hyperplasia, followed at least in the rat by depletion, and marked changes in the T lymphocyte components with replacement of the thymus-dependent areas of the lymph nodes and spleen by plasma cells and alterations in the thymus as

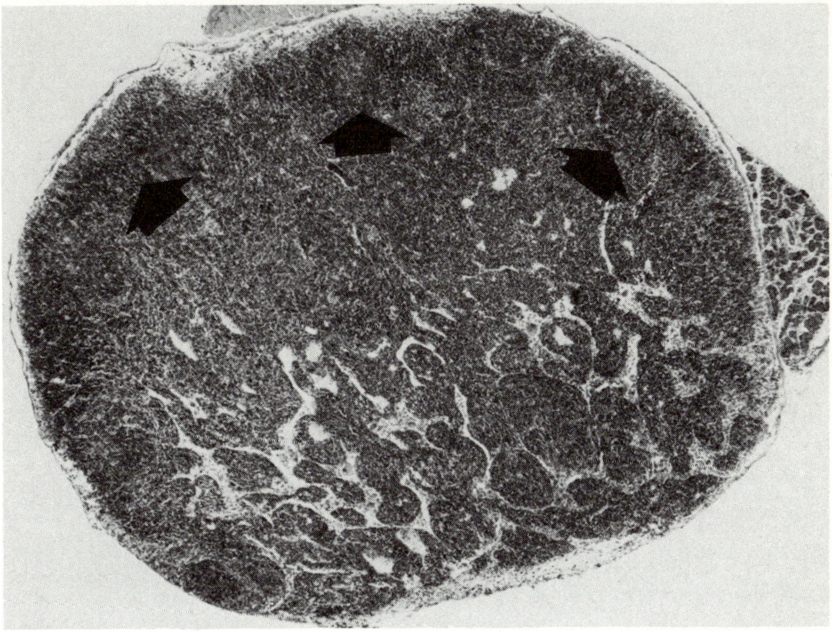

Fig. 3. Lymph node of mouse 21 days after infection with T. brucei. *The medullary cords are packed with plasma cells which are replacing the paracortical area and encroaching on the cortex. The outline of the cortex is outlined with arrows. Haematoxylin and Eosin. x45*

described above.

The role of the mononuclear phagocytic system in immunosuppression.

One aspect of the immunological response in malaria-infected mice which appeared to be at fault was the processing of antigen by macrophages and the histological evidence of an expanded and active macrophage system (Fig. 2) in *T. brucei* infected mice by following the circulating clearance and organ distribution of sheep erythrocytes (SRBC) labelled with the isotope sodium Cr^{51} chromate (Murray *et al.*, 1974c). Such investigations showed that one hour after intravenous injection of various doses of Cr^{51} SRBC the activity which remained in the circulation of infected mice was half that of the normal control mice. Since the rate of disappearance of particulate material from the blood has been widely used as a measure of the activity of the mononuclear phagocytic system, this increased blood clearance of Cr^{51} SRBC in in-

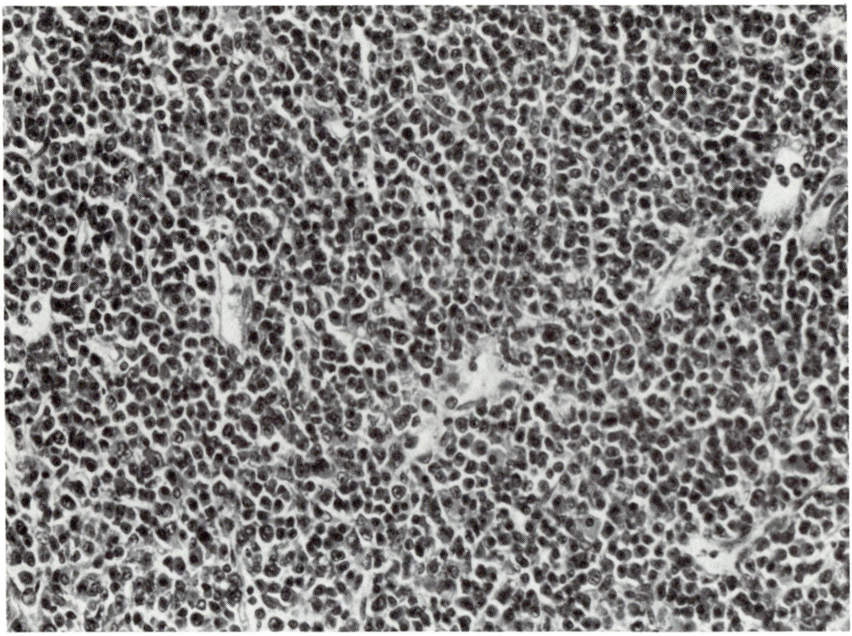

Fig. 4. Lymph node medulla from same mouse showing massive plasma cell response. Haematoxylin and Eosin. x 300.

fected mice indicating that its phagocytic potential was increased. With the highest dose level used (2.0 x 10^9 SRBC) the livers of infected mice showed an enhanced uptake. Confirmatory evidence of this increased potential for hepatic phagocytosis was obtained by injecting infected mice with coloidal carbon before the Cr^{51}SRBC. It was found that the miced coped readily with both these particulate materials without causing a characteristic redistribution of SRBC to the spleen as happens in normal mice after liver blockade with carbon (Souhami, 1972). It appears from such results that hepatic mononuclear phagocytic system of infected mice has an enhanced ability for phagocytosis and that this aspect of macrophage function at least is not suspect. Paradoxically, the very efficiency of the hepatic phagocytic system may be responsible, if only partially, for immunosuppression by effectively reducing the localisation of antigen in the spleen below the level necessary to stimulate an immune response. Although we have found that the numbers of SRBC reaching the spleens are no less in infected mice than in their normal counterparts, it should be realised that splenomegaly (Fig. 1) is a marked feature of murine trypanosomiasis (the spleen may weigh up to 30 times normal weight) and there may well be

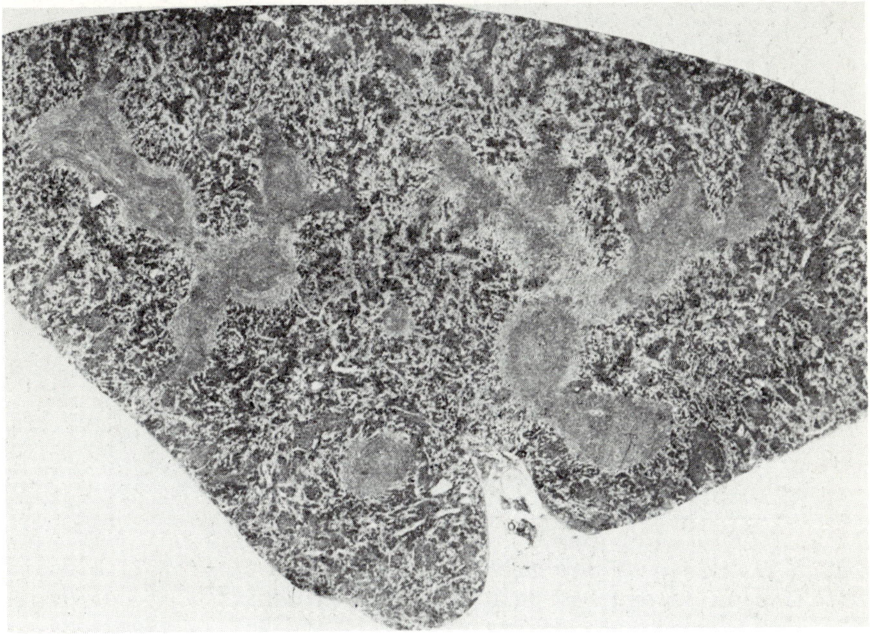

Fig. 5. Spleen of rat with a 4 week infection of T. brucei. *The white pulp and red pulp contain numerous plasma cells and there is marked extramedullary erythropoiesis. Haematoxylin and Eosin. x 10*

a relative deficiency of splenic antigen. In this respect attempts to increase the splenic localisation of SRBC by increasing the injected dose above 2.0×10^9 SRBC have resulted in the death of the infected mice.

In addition to having a scavenging function, the macrophage is considered to play an integral part in certain immune responses by processing antigen and presenting it in an immunogenic configuration on its plasma membrane to immunologically competent lymphocytes (Unanue and Cerottini, 1970; Sohnle and Sussdorf, 1972; Gottlieb and Waldman, 1972). We have found by means of cell transfer experiments that glass adherent peritoneal exudate cells derived from *T. brucei*-infected mice could transfer immunogenic information to normal recipient mice (Murray *et al.*, 1974c). Thus, while the macrophages of infected mice appeared competent in their ability to process antigen in the requisite manner, it should be noted that they were transferred from an infected to a normal environment; it is possible that had they been defective such an environmental alteration may have allowed a

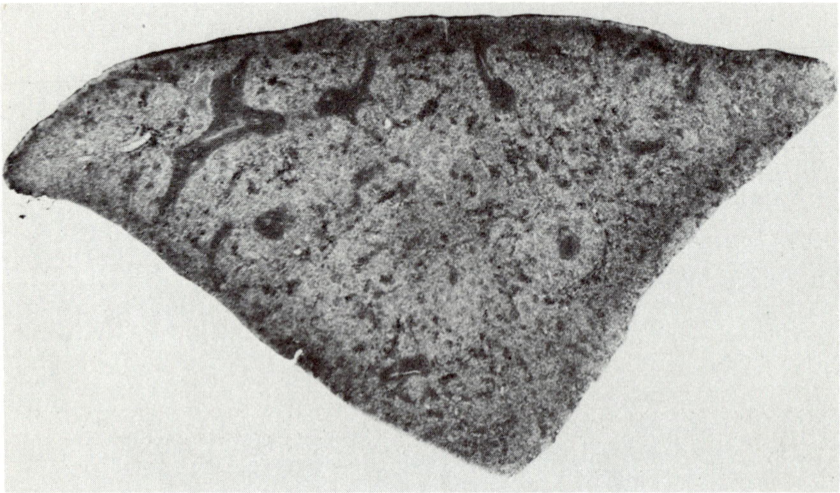

Fig. 6. Spleen of rat with an 8 week infection of T. brucei. *Both the white and red pulp are largely depleted of cells. (By courtesy of the Editor of* Res. Vet. Sci.*). Hematoxylin and Eosin. x 15.*

return to normal function. Despite this reservation these findings tend to indicate that this aspect of macrophage activity is unimpaired and taken with the observations on the phagocytic ability of the mononuclear phagocytic system, suggest that the integrity of this cell population remains intact in *T. brucei* infections mice.

Humoral responsiveness in T. brucei *infected mice.*

Responses to SRBC

Much of the work conducted so far on immunosuppression has involved the use of SRBC as antigen. The kinetics of the antibody response to SRBC in mice is well documented and the co-operative cellular events in the immunological response to this antigen have been reported in depth. Goodwin *et al.* (1972) showed that rabbits and mice infected with *T. brucei* have a profoundly depressed haemagglutinin response to SRBC and this was later confirmed in mice by Murray *et al.* (1974c); with their strain of *T. brucei* suppression occurred within 1 week of infection and persisted throughout the course of the disease. Apart from the non-specific participation of an adherent cell population (Mosier, 1967) the production of IgG antibody to SRBC in mice depends on the specific inter-

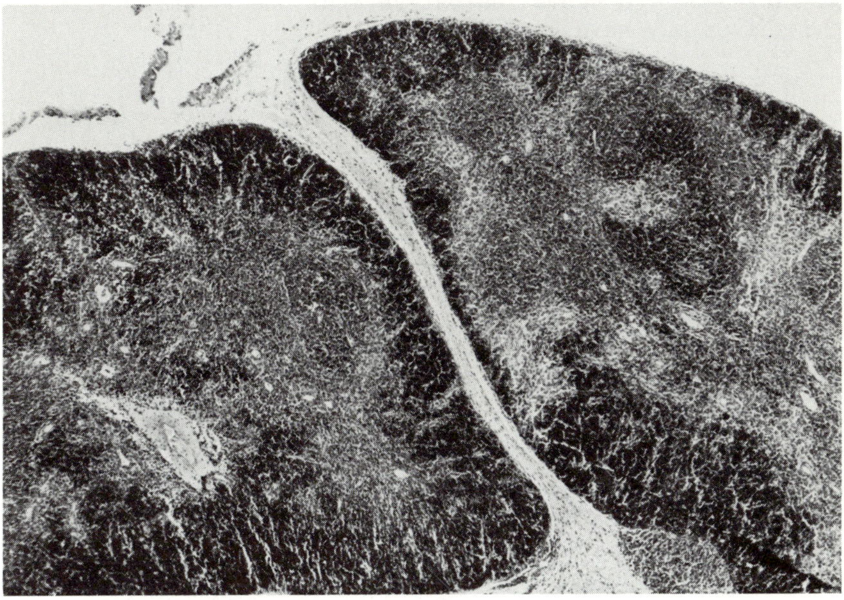

Fig. 7. Thymus of mouse 21 days after infection with T. brucei. *The thymus cortex is narrow and irregular while the medulla contains numerous macrophages, large lymphoid cells and plasma cells as well as small lymphocytes. (By courtesy of the Editor of* Immunology*). Hematoxylin and Eosin. x 45*

action of thymus-derived (T) lymphocytes and bursa-equivalent (B) lymphocytes (Playfair, 1971). Similarly, much of the IgM response to SRBC requires such co-operation. However, it has been demonstrated that a proportion of the anti-SRBC IgM response can be accomplished by B cells alone (Playfair and Purves, 1971; Pantelouris and Flisch, 1972). Three weeks after infection with *T. brucei* Murray *et al.* (1974d) showed that there was a complete suppression of both IgM and IgG responses to sheep erythrocytes using a technique of localised haemolysis in gel (Dresser and Wortis, 1973). These results are in agreement with those of Freeman *et al.* (1974) who found that by 10 days of infection, "numbers of both IgM and IgG producing cells are down to below 2% of normal value". This absence of IgM response at 3 weeks is remarkable in that it occurs during a phase of marked plasma cell proliferation in the lymphoid tissues of these mice (Figs. 3,4 and 5) and the presence of such large numbers of immunoglobulin-producing B cells together with a complete failure in cellular production of anti-SRBC IgG seems indicative that the B lymphocytes themselves may have become defective.

Responses to lipopolysaccharide (LPS)

The functional capacity of the B lymphocytes during immunosuppression have been further investigated by using lipopolysaccharide derived from the bacteria *E. coli* 0111; B4 as an antigen. It is widely accepted that LPS is an antigen which selectively stimulates B cells (Andersson and Blomgren, 1971; Gery *et al.*, 1972; Manning *et al.*, 1972), and although the macrophage may play a significant co-operative role in the *in vitro* response to LPS (Bona *et al.*, 1973) its degree of involvement *in vivo* is less clearly defined (Baker and Landy, 1967).

T. brucei infected mice show a marked depression in the antibody response to LPS (as judged by passive haemagglutinin and PFC assays) when studied during the proliferative plasma cell phase of the disease 3 weeks after infection. This inability to produce anti-LPS antibody complements the finding that these mice also fail to produce any anti-SRBC IgM and again points to a possible failure in B lymphocytes as being the underlying cause of immunosuppression. However, the results do not exclude a faulty macrophage participation in the response to LPS although, as mentioned above, there is no evidence of abnormality in macrophage-antigen processing in *T. brucei* infections.

T cell responsiveness of T. brucei *infected mice.*

The above conclusion does not, of course, preclude the co-existence of a defective T cell population particularly since marked histological changes are found in the thymus and thymus dependent areas of the immune system of both mice and rats infected with *T. brucei* (see earlier). However, Urquhart *et al.* (1973) showed that, after a *T. brucei* infection of 3 weeks duration, mice were able to mount a significant delayed type response (DTH) to the skin-sensitising agent oxazolone as measured by the increased thickness of their ears 24 hours after a challenge application of this chemical (Asherson and Ptak, 1968). In these mice there was also histological evidence of extensive infiltration of mononuclear cells into the epidermis of the sensitised ears and the thymus-dependent paracortical areas in the draining lymph nodes were expanded. This response of mice to oxazolone is dependent on the active participation of sensitised T lymphocytes (DeSousa and Parrott, 1969) and can therefore be considered as a measure of T cell responsiveness. These results in *T. brucei*-infected mice suggest that at least one aspect of the T cell function, i.e., the ability to mount a delayed-type response is intact.

Subsequent investigations into the role of the T cell utilised the more sensitive technique of incorporation of isotopically labelled deoxyuridine (I^{125} UdR) into DNA of newly formed cells (Pritchard and Micklem, 1972). Davies *et al.* (1969) have shown that the increased I^{125} UdR incorporation a few days after sensitisation with oxazolone is specifically associated with proliferation of thymus-derived cells in the paracortical areas of the lymph nodes. Thus the cellular reactivity of T cells of *T. brucei* infected mice may be accurately assessed on the basis of I^{125} UdR incorporation in the regional lymph nodes following exposure to oxazolone (Jennings *et al.*, 1974; Murray *et al.*, 1974d). The results showed that in a 3 week infection there was significantly increased T cell division in the draining nodes of mice 3 days after sensitisation with oxazolone.

Thus neither the delayed-type hypersensitivity reaction nor the primary responsiveness of T cells to oxazolone were significantly depressed by a 3 week *T. brucei* infection suggesting that the immunosuppressive effect is unlikely to be present in this cell population at least during this phase of the disease.

In contrast, however, is the finding that mice infected for longer period, i.e., 5 to 6 weeks, failed completely to respond to oxazolone sensitisation. This suggests that T cell failure may ultimately occur, probably in the terminal stages of the disease, and indicates that immunological unresponsiveness in murine trypanosomiasis may be attributable to more than one factor depending on the duration of infection. Interestingly, no new morphological changes were found to account for this depression in contrast to the marked cellular depletion of the immune system which occurs in rats at this time (Fig. 6) (Murray *et al.*, 1974a,b).

The effects of T. brucei *infection on* Nippostrongylus brasiliensis *infection.*

Many of the conclusions on the aetiology of immunosuppression have been derived from analysis of the responses of animals to certain defined antigens. Although these findings have given important clues as to the immunological nature of the defect, the effects of immunosuppression on the occurrence and significance of concurrent disease in the infected host has been less well documented. In this respect the model system of *N. brasiliensis* in the rat has proved valuable in assessing the interaction between helminth disease and trypanosomiasis.

In the normal course of events, rats with a single infection of *N. brasiliensis* undergo what has been called a "self cure" in that 10 to 16 days after the infection the adult worms in the small intestine are expelled by a process which is known to be immunolgoical (see review Murray, 1972). The effect of *T. brucei* on this helminth infection is therefore readily assessed in terms of the numbers of *N. brasiliensis* remaining in the intestine after the period when immune expulsion is normally completed. Initial experiments showed that *T. brucei* infection could abrogate the primary response of rats to *N. brasiliensis* and that an infective dose of *N. brasiliensis* which was normally tolerated could, in the presence of the trypanosome infection, be lethal (Urquhart *et al.*, 1973). More recent investigations have demonstrated that if rats are allowed to undergo initial infection of *N. brasiliensis* and are subsequently infected with *T. brucei* after the phase of immune expulsion they lose their ability to expel a challenge infection of *N. brasiliensis* (personal observation). These results show that the suppression of the immune responses associated with murine trypanosomiasis not only affects the development of the primary response but also prevents the expression of a secondary response.

Recovery of the immune response after trypanocidal therapy.

The possible importance of immunosuppression in the field has already been mentioned and preliminary findings indicate that the experimental *T. congolense* infection can actively suppress the responses of Zebu cattle to immunisation with a polyvalent clostridial vaccine* (Holmes *et al.*, 1974). In view of these findings the efficacy of trypanocidal drug treatment, not only in curing trypanosome infection, but also in allowing a return to normal immunological function is likely to be a consideration of importance. The effect of curative treatment on immunological recovery has not yet been investigated in bovine trypanosomiasis although experimental evidence in *T. brucei* infection in mice indicates that treatment with diminazine aceturate** very quickly restores their responsiveness to certain antigens. Murray *et al.* (1974d) showed that immunisation of mice with SRBC as soon as 3 days after their *T. brucei* infection had been terminated by trypanocidal therapy resulted in a normal haemagglutinin response.

The ability of mice infected for 36 days, i.e., at a time when reactivity to oxazolone is absent, to recover their

* Tribovax - Wellcome Research Laboratories, Beckenham.
** Berenil - Farbwerke-Hoechst, Frankfurt.

responsiveness to an application of oxazolone was also investigated using the technique of assessing the incorporation I^{125} UdR in their lymph nodes 3 days after sensitization. T cell reactivity in the nodes of these treated mice was restored and as might be anticipated it appeared at an even earlier stage than the serological response to SRBC. These findings gained support from experimental results presented by Freeman *et al.* (1974) who found that the plaque-forming cell response to SRBC returned to normal when *T. brucei* infected mice were treated with berenil on the same day as they were immunised with SRBC.

The effect of trypanocidal therapy on the recovery of the immune responses has also been demonstrated with *N. brasiliensis* infection. As mentioned previously, rats which have undergone immune expulsion and were subsequently infected with trypanosomes, failed to exhibit any immunity to challenge with *N. brasiliensis*. When, however, the trypanosome infection was treated, the rats were able to mount a full secondary response which was indistinguishable from that of uninfected, immune control rats. One important conclusion of this experiment was that immunolgoical memory was not destroyed by a subsequent trypanosome infection, being merely suppressed to re-emerge unscathed after treatment.

It would thus appear that immunosuppression caused by trypanosome infection, although profound, is reversible in that the death of these organisms leads to a rapid and complete return to normal immunological function.

DISCUSSION

In many parts of the world and in particular Africa, trypanosomiasis causes economic loss on a huge scale. The findings discussed here indicate that immunosuppression is another aspect of trypanosomiasis which might be found to contribute to these serious economic effects through interference with immunisation and predisposing to other infections. If only for these reasons, the phenomenon is one worthy of investigation and clarification. However, it is also apparent that the underlying causes of immunosuppression in this disease and others impinge on the very nature of the immunological response and as such may be found to be useful tools in the investigation of immune mechanisms.

Interpretation of experimental findings in terms of current immunological concepts is difficult in view of the complexity of this subject at present. It is apparent from such considerations that there are a wide variety of possible levels of failure in the immunological response. Immunosuppression may occur during the inductive phase of the immune response and involve macrophages or alternatively it may be the result of an acquired fault in either the T or B lymphocyte populations or indeed in any of their various sub-populations. Interference in the proper function of these cell types may also occur in an indirect fashion, e.g., through an upset in the normal regulatory functions of the immune response or by a deficiency of any of the specific factors necessary for this process.

Any interpretation of the immunological changes which occur in trypanosomiasis must take into account the marked and severe changes in the immune system. During the initial phases of the disease the lymph nodes and spleen become packed with plasma cells and macrophages and histologically the picture is one of proliferation. The effect of this is a complete disruption of normal lymph node and splenic structure with replacement of the paracortical T-dependent areas by plasma cells. Despite this there is complete absence of antibody production to SRBC throughout this phase. Concurrently, the trypanosomes in the circulation are found to undergo a cyclic variation in numbers, generally attributed to the production by the host of a series of specific anti-trypanosome variant antibodies (Gray, 1970). Apparently on the one hand there is a failure of specific antibody production to any antigenic stimuli encountered after *T. brucei* infection while on the other there is an apparent continuous responsiveness to new antigenic variants of trypanosomes. These observations indicate the anomaly of the phenomenon of immunosuppression in this disease.

The macrophage population in *T. brucei* infected mice appears to be functional particularly with regard to its phagocytic capabilities, but as pointed out earlier such an enhancement in the activity of Kuppfer cells can lead to a relative reduction of antigen in the spleen, the main source of antibody production to circulating antigen. In transfer experiments the immunogenic capabilities of macrophages containing SRBC derived from infected mice have been demonstrated to be normal. However, it is possible that, if the suppression was caused by some extra-cellular substance which acted at the level of macrophage-antigen processing, then this might be removed on transfer of the macrophages to a normal environment. The presence of suppressive factors might be confirmed if serum from infected mice or dead trypanosomes could be shown to affect macrophage-antigen processing either *in vivo* or *in vitro*.

Feldman (1973) proposes that the site of antigenic competition is at the surface of the macrophage and, if so, it is possible that the large amount of trypanosome antigen which is present during infection gives rise to competition with other antigens at these sites. Unfortunately the rapid return to competence after trypanocidal therapy provides no clear answer to this hypothesis.

Thymus-derived lymphocytes fulfil a variety of functions in the immune response. It is hypothesised that they are the initial cell to interact with antigen as a consequence of which they produce carrier-specific factors which can coat macrophages (Taussig and Lackmann, 1972). These macrophages are then able to fix the antigen on their surfaces and so facilitate its presentation to the antibody-producing B cell line. This "co-operative role" of T cells in *T. brucei* infection can only be investigated by careful reconstitution experiments and there are no reports to date that such experiments have been conducted. However, two aspects of T cell function were investigated *in vivo*. Firstly, proliferation of T cells in response to oxazolone stimulation, and secondly their ability to mount a characteristic DTH reaction in the ears of infected mice. In both respects the T cells in infected mice were found to mount a significant response although perhaps slightly less than that occurring in normal mice. The evidence at present therefore suggests that the T cells are responsive and indicates that the area of fault may lie in the B cells or in the co-operative event itself.

B lymphocytes are the progenitors of plasma cells and in trypanosomiasis the marked plasma cell proliferation in the spleen and lymph nodes together with the high level of circulating IgM give the impression of vigorous B cell responses. However, much of this IgM is thought to be "non-specific", i.e., not directed against trypanosome antigens; for example it contains a wide variety of auto-antibodies (McKenzie *et al.*, 1972). We have also shown that there is a complete failure of specific response to LPS and SRBC. These findings suggested another possible cause of immunosuppression namely that an apparent aspecific activation of B cells might occur due to the production by the trypanosome of a mitogenic factor (Urquhart *et al.*, 1973). Certain plant mitogens, e.g., pokeweek mitogen, produce plasma cell proliferation not unlike that of *T. brucei* infections (Jorgenson *et al.*, 1972). Recent evidence shows that another mitogen Concanavalin A can also cause immunosuppression by activating a population of T suppressor cells (Rich and Pierce, 1972).

In attempting to determine the validity of either of these two theories as the cause of immunosuppression, i.e., antigenic competition by trypanosome variant antigens, or the production by the trypanosomes of a mitogen-like substance which aspecifically activates the B cells, it might be useful to establish the specificity to trypanosome antigens of the excessive amount of immunoglobulin produced in this disease, and secondly in *in vitro* studies in lymphocyte cultures, to find if trypanosomes or their products are in fact mitogenic or immunosuppressive.

In conclusion, it would appear that in laboratory mice *T. brucei* infection causes a severe impairment in responsiveness to certain other antigens and investigations suggest that this may be due to an acquired fault in the B lymphocyte population, perhaps through the agency of a mitogenic factor. The results of experiments on the restoration of immune responses after chemotherapy indicate that the strategic use of trypanocidal drug may be important in areas of endemic trypanosomiasis. If these results can be further extrapolated to the field situation, then immunological memory, temporarily held in abeyance by the trypanosome infection, can be restored after treatment. In general terms, immunosuppression is a phenomenon of major interest and possibly one of great consequence in the pathogenicity of protozoal disease in the tropics.

ACKNOWLEDGEMENTS

We would like to thank the Wellcome Trust and The Rockefeller Foundation for the financial support which made this work possible.

REFERENCES

Andersson, B. and Blomgren, H. (1971). *Cell. Immunol.*, *2*, 411.

Asherson, G.L. and Ptak, W. (1968). *Immunology*, *15*, 405.

Baker, P.J. and Landy, M. (1967). *J. Immunol.*, *99*, 687.

Barker, L.R. and Powers, K.G. (1971). *Am. J. Trop. Med. Hyg.*, *20*, 389.

Bona, C., Robineaux, R., Anteunis, A.A. and Astesano, A. (1973). *Immunology*, *24*, 831.

Clinton, B.A., Stauber, L.A. and Palczuk, N.C. (1969). *Expt. Parasit.*, *25*, 171.

Davies, A.J.S., Carter, R.L., Leuchars, Elizabeth and Wallis, Valerie (1969). *Immunology*, *17*, 111.

DeSousa, Maria A.B. and Parrott, Delphine, M.V. (1969). *J. Exp. Med.*, *130*, 671.

Dresser, D.W. and Wortis, H.H. (1973). *Handbook of Experimental Immunology*. Ed. D.M. Weir, Blackwell Scientific Publ., Oxford

Faubert, G. and Tanner, C.E. (1971). *Expt. Parasit.*, *30*, 120.
Freeman, J.C., Hudson, K.M. and Byner, Carole (1974). 14th Seminar in Trypanosomiasis Research. *Trans. Roy. Soc. Trop. Med. Hyg.* (In press)
Gery, I., Kruger, J. and Spiesel, S.Z. (1972) *J. Immunol.*, *108*, 1088.
Goodwin, L.G. (1970). *Trans. Roy. Soc. Trop. Med. Hyg.*, *67*, 797.
Goodwin, L.G., Green, D.G., Guy, M.W. and Voller, A. (1972). *Br. J. Exp. Path.*, *53*, 40.
Gottlieb, A.A. and Waldman, S.R. (1972). In "*Macrophages and Cellular Immunity*". Eds. A. Laskin and H. Lechevalier, Butterworths, London.
Gray, A.R. (1970). In: "*The African Trypanosomiasis*", p. 113. Ed. H. W. Mulligan. George Allen and Unwin, London.
Greenwood, B.M. (1968). *Lancet*, *2*, 380.
Greenwood, B.M. and Voller, A. (1970). *Clin. Exp. Immunol.*, *7*, 793.
Greenwood, B.M. and Greenwood, Alice M. (1971). *Trans. Roy. Soc. Trop. Med. Hyg.*, *65*, 581.
Greenwood, B.M., Playfair, J.H.L. and Torrigiani, G. (1971a). *Clin. Exp. Immunol.*, *8*, 467.
Greenwood, B.M., Brown, J.C., DeJesus, D.G. and Holborow, E.J. (1971b). *Clin. Exp. Immunol.*, *9*, 345.
Greenwood, B.M., Bradley-Moore, Alice M., Palit, A. and Bryceson, A.D.M. (1972). *Lancet*, *1*, 169.
Holmes *et al.* (1974). Personal communication.
Hu, C.H. (1931). *Nat. Med. J. China*, *17*, 435.
Jennings, F.W., Murray, P.K., Murray, Max and Urquhart, G.M. (1974). *Trans. Roy. Soc. Trop. Med. Hyg.* In *Proceedings of 14th Seminar on Trypanosomiasis* (In press).
Jorgenson, H.P., Jensen, M.K. and Olsen, J.R. (1972). *Acta Path. Microbiol. Scand.*, *80*, 367.
Kakalamis, Evangelia and Pavlatos,Mary (1972). *Immunology*, *22*, 695.
Loose, L.A., Cook, J.A., DiLuzio, N.R. (1973). *Proc. Helm. Soc. Wash.*, *39* Special Issue, 484.
Losos, G.J. and Ikede, B.O. (1972). *Vet. Path.* (Suppl)., *9*.
Manning, Judith K., Reed, N.D. and Jutila, J.W. (1972). *J. Immunol.*, *108*, 1470.
McGregor, I.A. (1972). *Br. Med. Bull.*, *28*, 22.
McKenzie, A.R., Boreham, P.F. and Facer, Christine (1972). *Trans. Roy. Soc. Trop. Med. Hyg.*, *66*, 344.
Mosier, D.E. (1967). *Science*, *158*, 1573.
Murray, Max (1972). In "*Immunity to Animal Parasites*". Ed. E. J. L. Soulsby. Academic Press, New York and London.
Murray, Max, Murray, P.K., Jennings, F.W., Fisher, E.W. and

Urquhart, G.H. (1974a). *Res. Vet. Sci., 16*. (In Press)
Murray, Max, Murray, P.K., Jennings, F.W. and Urquhart, G.M. (1974b). (In press)
Murray, P.K., Jennings, F.W., Murray, Max and Urquhart, G.M. (1974c). (In press).
Murray, P.K., Jennings, F.W., Murray, Max and Urquhart, G.M. (1974d). (In press).
Pantelouris, E.M. and Flisch, P.A. (1972). *Immunology, 22,* 159.
Playfair, J.H.L. (1971). *Clin. Exp. Immunol., 8,* 839.
Playfair, J.H.L. and Purves, Elizabeth C. (1971). *Immunology, 21,* 113.
Pritchard, Helen and Micklem, H.S. (1972). *Clin. Exp. Immunol., 10,* 151.
Rees, R.J.W., and Waters, M.F.R. (1972). *Br. Med. Bull., 28,* 16.
Rich, R.R. and Pierce, C.W. (1972). *J. Exp. Med., 137,* 649.
Sengers, R.C.A., Jerusalem, C.R. and Doesburg, W.H. (1971). *Expt. Parasit., 30,* 41.
Sohnle, P.G. and Sussdorf, D.H. (1972). *Immunology, 23,* 361.
Souhami, R.L. (1972). *Immunology, 22,* 685.
Strickland, G.T., Pettitt, L.E. and Voller, A. (1973). *Am. J. Trop. Med. Hyg., 22,* 452.
Taussig, M.J. and Lachmann, P.J. (1972). *Immunology, 22,* 185.
Unanue, E.R. and Cerottini, J.C. (1970). *J. Exp. Med., 131,* 711.
Urquhart, G.M., Murray, M., Murray, P.K., Jennings, F.W. and Bate, Elma (1973). *Trans. Roy. Soc. Trop. Med. Hyg., 67,* 528.

ZOONOTIC CESTODES

J. A. Euzeby

Ecole Nationale Veterinaire, Lyon, France

INTRODUCTION

Definition

Metacestodiasis is defined as parasitism by the larval stages of cestodes (=metacestodes) of normal intermediate hosts for the cestode or of hosts which are incidentally interposed in the life cycle. Man may act as either. Human metacestodiasis may result from metacestodes, the definitive host of which is man (e.g., cysticercosis cellulosae and, much less frequently, cysticercosis bovis) or from metacestodes which their adult forms in animals. The latter only are true zoonotic metacestodiases and they only will be dealt with in this review.

The metacestodes of zoonotic origin are classified in Table 1. Some of these metacestodes may produce daughter-forms. This often occurs in *Coenurus* and chiefly in *Echinococcus*. It is of great importance in the latter and very severe forms of diseases may be associated with this process. Plerocercoids sometimes proliferate too, but without generating active forms, and without producing serious pathological consequences. Solid metacestodes seldom are enclosed in a tissue reaction, while vesicular larvae usually are. The envelope so formed around the larva is called the adventica; however, no adventica develops around the larvae of one species of *Echinococcus (E. multilocularis)* and the pathogenicity of this larval stage is greater because of this.

The general life-cycles of zoonotic metacestodes and corresponding cestodes are summarized in Table 2.

In the Diphyllobothriidae life-cycle the plerocercoid-infected 2nd intermediate host may not be eaten by the normal definitive host but by an accidental host. In that case, the plerocercoid larva usually encysts in the accidental host, awaiting for the latter to be eaten by the normal host. This re-encystation process is the paratenic process or parateny. It may occur in man, who can be infected either as a normal intermediate or as a paratenic host.

In most cases, metacestodes in man are lost for the life-cycle of the parasite, man not normally being eaten by carni-

TABLE I

The important metacestodes of zoonotic origin in man.

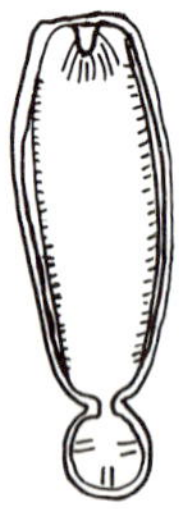

a) Procercoïd = 1st stage larva of Diphyllobothriidae. Two parts ; the posterior one carries embryonic hooks (= cercomere) while the anterior one does not bear a fully developped scolex. Develops in Copepod Crustacea (1st intermediate hosts). Unable to infect vertebrates.

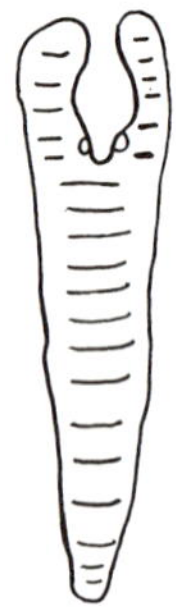

b) Plerocercoid = 2nd stage larva of Diphyllobothriidae. No more cercomere nor embryonic hooks, but a fully developped scolex at the anterior end. Originates from procercoïd and is formed in lower aquatic vertebrates (Fish, Amphibian) (2nd intermediate hosts) eating procercoïd-infected copepods.

1. SOLID LARVAE. ADULT CESTODES = PSEUDOPHYLLIDEA

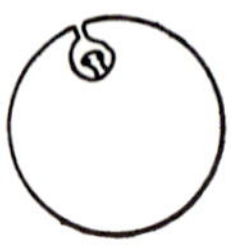

a) Cysticercus : Volume : from pea to nut. One cephalic invagination bearing one scolex. No daughter - vesicles. Adult worm = Taenia.

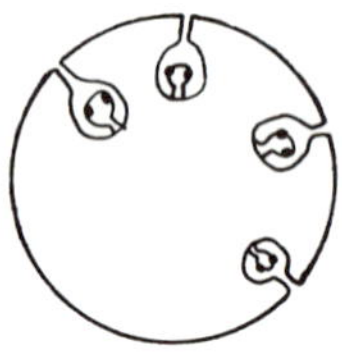

b) Coenurus : Volume : from cherry to egg. Several cephalic invaginations, each bearing one scolex. May form exogenous or endogenous daughter-vesicles. Adult worm = Multiceps.

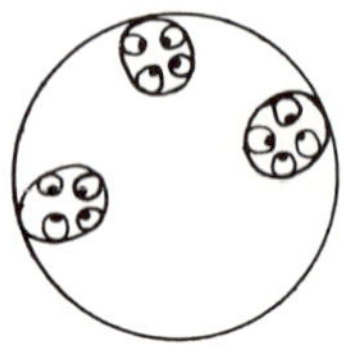

c) Echinococcus : Volume : from cherry to orange. Several cephalic invaginations, each containing several scoleces (= protoscoleces) (*). Exogenous and endogenous daughter-vesicles very frequent. Adult worm = Echinococcus.

2. VESICULAR LARVAE. ADULT WORMS = CYCLOPHYLLIDEA

(*) Sometimes protoscoleces do not develop and the larva remains sterile for not being able to give birth to an adult worm in the definitive host.

TABLE II

General life cycles of zoonotic metacestodes

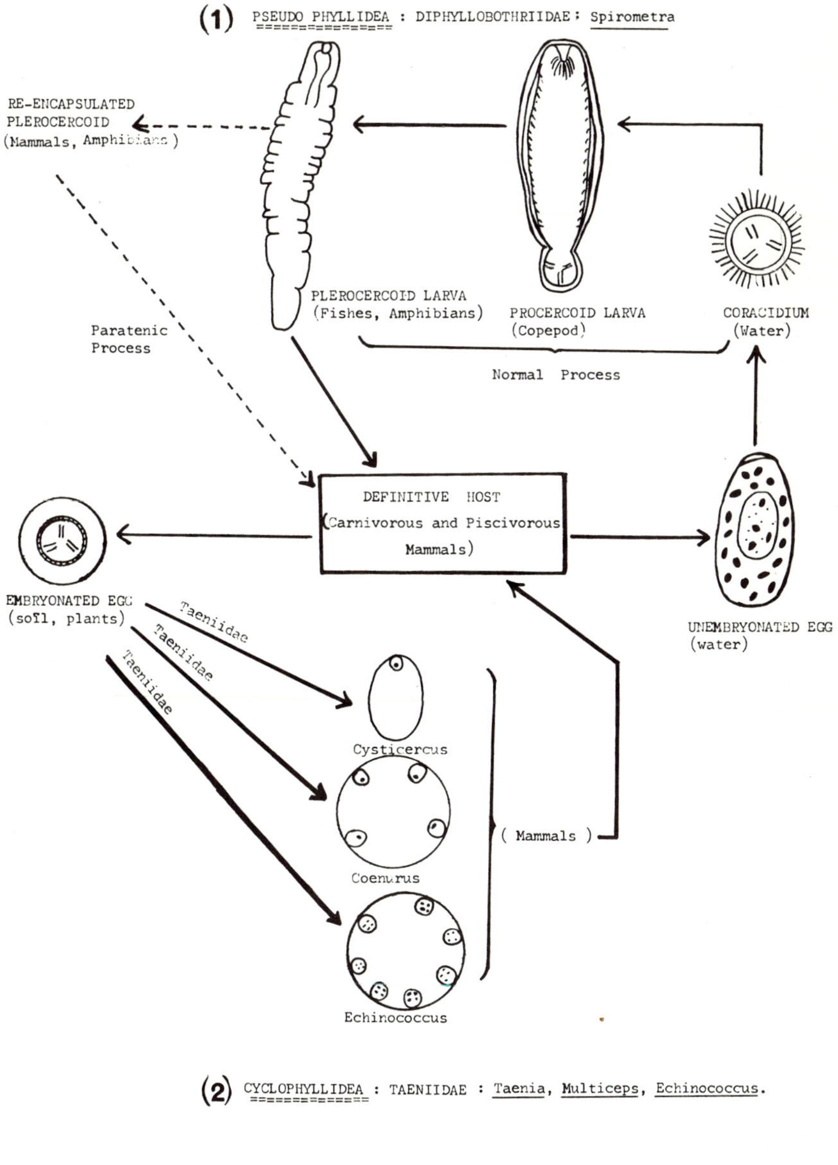

vores. Under special circumstances, however (e.g., the special customs of certain central African tribes, where human corpses are offered to hyenas) the life cycles may be completed.

ZOONOTIC METACESTODES AND THEIR LIFE-CYCLES

Plerocercoids

In this view, the only plerocercoids considered as agents of zoonotic metacestodiasis belong to the genus *Spirometra* and are usually known as Spargana*. Many species of Spargana have been reported, but most of them are not valid and should be synonymized. Three are of medical importance (These may be synonymous).

Spirometra mansoni Joyeux and Houdemer, 1927, is widely spread in the Far East. The adult worm lives in the cat and dog and up to 95% of cats and 20% of dogs may be infected (Brumpt, 1949). Plerocercoids may be found in several vertebrates except fishes, and their normal hosts are adult amphibians. According to Galliard (1946) tadpoles can be infected but their infection disappears at the time of metamorphosis into the adult animal. Plerocercoids are observed in reptiles (various snakes), birds and small mammals (rodents, insectivor) in which infection comes from the paratenic process. Human sparganosis is also a paratenic process, infection being acquired from frogs, snakes and rodents.

Spirometra erinacei europaei (Rudolph, 1891). This worm, in spite of its specific name, seems to be quite ubiquitous.

It occurs, under several names, in Europe: Italy (Bianchi, 1964), USSR (Sokolova *et al.*, 1961); Africa: Kenya (Sambon, 1907; Cox, 1965; Nelson *et al.*, 1965), Uganda (Jones, 1962), Ruanda-Urundi (Fain and Piraux, 1959); various Central African Countries (de Meillon and Leech, 1943), Liberia (Brujning, 1960); Western Portuguese Africa (Alves *et al.*, 1954); Madagascar (Byggoo *et al.*, 1961); North America: various parts

* The genus *Diphyllobothrium* only infects man as an adult worm. The genus *Sparganum* was erected by Diesing (1854) to include all unidentified plerocercoid larvae. Later, this was reserved for *Spirometra* plerocercoids. This may still lead to confusion and it would be better to name a plerocercoid according to the specific binome of the corresponding adult worm.

of the U.S., Florida (Stiles, 1908), Shortt and Lewis, 1964), Texas (Moore, 1915; Read, 1952), Mississippi (Brooks *et al.*, 1960), Alabama (Gleason, 1960), Virginia (Wirth and Farrow, 1961), New York (Mueller, 1963a), Arkansas (Cross, 1963), Louisiana (Corkum, 1966), several other Southern States (Schwartzwelder *et al.*, 1964); South America: Venezuela (Garcia, 1961), Ecuador (Leon, 1972), Uruguay and Columbia (Faust, 1970) and in the West Indies (Faust, 1970) and Australia (Sandars, 1959).

The definitive hosts of *S. erinacei* are chiefly Felidae, either domestic cats or wild cats and leopards (*Felis pardalis*, etc. ...) and even man (Faust *et al.*, 1929)*. Plerocercoids infect amphibians and re-encystment occurs (parateny) in snakes and small mammals (rodents, hedgehogs) and in man. Sometimes large mammals such as pigs, *Phacochoerus* spp, antelopes and zebras may be infected (Bearup, 1953; Rukavina, 1957; Dinnik, 1969) in a paratenic manner, and such forms can induce further parateny in man.

Spirometra mansonoides has been stated to be the chief agent of human sparganosis in the U.S.A., where experimental human infections have been established by Mueller and Coulston (1941). The definitive hosts of the worm are Canidae (dog, fox), Mustelidae (Otter) and, chiefly, Felidae (domestic and wild cat, lynx). Plerocercoids develop in tadpoles, but such infection is lost at the time of metamorphosis. Parateny occurs in snakes and mammals. The following mammals have been reported to be infected: Rats, *Procyonidae*; Raccoon, *Procyon lotor* (Harkema and Miller, 1964); dogs, "foxes", including the grey fox, *Urocyon cinereo-argentus* (McIntosh, 1937); and the oppossum, *Didelphys virginica* (Corkum, 1966). The domestic pig can be infected experimentally. On the other hand, *Sparganum mansonoides* has never been found in adult amphibians.

The specific identity of the above three parasites is not wholly agreed upon. *S. mansonoides* is identified as *S. erinacei europaei* by Iwata (1936) and Ryzenkho (1971). More recently, Iwata (1972) has identified *S. mansoni* as *S. erinacei*, and according to such views, the latter would be the only species of plerocercoid which causes human spargansis.

---

* The worm recorded from man was named *S. houghtoni*. It fell into synonmy with *S. erinacei europaei*. The main other synonyms of this worm are *decipiens*, *raillieti*, *okumurai*, etc. ...

Iwata, (1972) believes *Sparganum proliferum* Ijma 1905, to be a degenerative form of *Sparganum erinacei* from lesions caused by this parasite.

Finally, the Central-African *Spirometra, S. pretoriensis,* Baer, 1924 must be considered. The adults of this infect Canidae such as *Lycaon pictus* and *Otocyon megalotis* (Fain *et al.,* 1959), but chiefly Hyenidae (Nelson *et al.,* 1965). In the districts where this species occurs, man appears to be the only host for the plerocercoids; if so he would be the true intermediary host of the parasite. Infections of hyenas may occur when they devour human corpses which are offered to them, according to local custom.

Cysticercus

Since *C. cellulosae* and *C. bovis* are not considered to be of true zoonotic origin the only zoonotic cysticerci so far reported from man are:

C. ovis: this was found in a human spinal cord in a sheep breeding area in USSR (Madyarov *et al.,* quoted by Abdulaze and Sadykov, 1971).

C. crassiceps: this budding cysticercus normally infects rodents (Sciuridae, Cricetidae) and is the larval form of *Taenia crassiceps,* of dogs and foxes. It was recently observed in the eye of a 17 year old girl in Canada (Anon, 1972).

Coenurus

In man the following coenurus larvae have been reported:

C. cerebralis: This is the larval stage of *Multiceps multiceps,* the adult of which lives in the small intestine of domestic and wild Canidae. This cestode is common in temperate countries but does not exist in tropical areas (Nelson *et al.,* 1965). The larval stage occurs in the central nervous system of herbivorous animals, chiefly ruminants. It does not produce daughter-vesicles. The Leporidae are not receptive to infection (Bondareva, 1953, 1958). Man may be infected and about 25 cases have been reported, either in the central nervous system or in the eye (Baylis, 1932; Clapham, 1941; Roger, 1942; Buckley, 1947; Cruz, 1948; Johnstone, 1950; Becker and Jacobson, 1951; Ranque and Nicolle, 1955; Watson, 1955; Caballero and Caballero, 1956; Boase, 1956; Bertrand and Callot, 1956; Wainwright, 1957; Epstein, 1959; Correa, 1962; Sadikov, 1965; Hermos, 1970; Deiana, 1971).

C. seralis: this is the larval stage of *Multiceps serialis*, the adult of which infects domestic and wild canidae. The parasite is well known in temperate countries but does not occur in tropical Africa. The coenurus can generate daughter-vesicles which develop in connective tissue of Leporidae. Man may be infected too, either in the connective tissue or in the central nervous system (Bonnal *et al.*, 1933; Brumpt *et al.*, 1934; Harant and Midrouille, 1949; Rodriguez-Gallego, 1957). *C. serialis* differs from *C. cerebralis* in some morphological features but chiefly by biological features (e.g. daughter-vesicles and infectivity for leporidae). These differences are evidence against the hypothesis of Dollfus (1959) that *M. multiceps* and *M. serialis* are identical.

C. brauni: this is the larval stage of *M. brauni*, the adult of which develops in dogs and jackals (Fain, 1952, 1958). The parasite is widespread in tropical Africa (Central and East) and also in South Africa, where, as in other temperate countries, *C. cerebralis* and *C. serialis* also exist (Ortlepp, 1938). The coenurus infects wild rodents such as gerbillidae (from which it was first reported by von Linston, 1902). Muridae (*Rattus rattus, Lemnicosmys barbarus, Otomys irroratus, O. angomiensis, Dendromys pumilio lineatus*) palacidae (*Tachyoryctes ruandae*); Hystricidae (the porcupine *Hystrix galatea*, Nelson *et al.*, 1956) and from monkeys (*Cercopithecus natis dogetti*, Fain, 1952, 1958; Nelson *et al.*, 1965). Neither the leporids nor the insectovors serve as hosts (Fain, 1952) but mice can be infected experimentally (Fain, 1956). About 25 cases of human coenuriasis brauni have been observed in Central Africa (Taramelli and Dubois, 1939; Fain, 1956; Raper and Dockeray, 1956; Vanderick *et al.*, 1964; Templeton, 1968) and this coenurus is the only one found in tropical Africa. It develops in connective tissue of its hosts and also in splanchnic cavities such as the lungs, brain and eyes. The chief difference between *C. brauni* and *C. serialis*, besides some morphological features, is the biological characteristic that wild Muridae are the main hosts while the leporids are not receptive.

Other coenurid forms include *C. glomeratus* (Railliet and Henry, 1915), which Turner (1959) reported from man in Nigeria. Its description is somewhat imprecise (Railliet and Henry, 1919), and it may be an incompletely developed form of *C. brauni*. A cornurus extracted from a Texas woman by Orihel *et al.*, (1970) was not identified. Recently Wilson *et al.*, (1972) have found a coenurus in man in Ghana, the morphological features of which are intermediate between those of *C. brauni*, *C. serialis* and *C. cerebralis*.

Echinococcus

Three main species and their subspecies must be considered. As adults they occur in the small intestine of canidae and felidae.

E. granulosus: This is very widespread and adults only mature in canidae. The vesicular larvae (hydatids) develop in herbivorous and omnivorous mammals such as ruminants, horses and pigs. They are the cause of hydatid disease or hydatidosis in man. Four subspecies have been recognized (Cameron, 1960; Sweatman and Williams, 1963; Williams and Sweatman, 1963).

E. g. granulosus: The ovigerous adult of this subspecies infects chiefly *Canis* species (dog, wolf, lycaon, dingo) and sometimes also foxes (*Vulpes vulpes*) (Cameron, 1926; Deiana, 1962; Malczewski, 1963; and Lubke, 1968). A parasite, maturing in foxes, named as *E. cameroni* by Ortlepp (1934) was identified as *E. granulosus* by Rausch (1953). The report of mature *E. granulosus* in a simocyonine dog, *Cuon primaerus* in South Viet-Nam (Le Van Hoa, 1967) may require re-evaluation in view of the discovery of a new species, *E. vogeli,* in another simocyonine, *Speothus venaticus* in Ecuador (Raush and Bernstein, 1972).

Hydatid larvae develop in ungulates and man (Deve, 1946, 1949) which are hosts with a long potential life span. Larval development is very slow, protoscolices being formed after 7-8 months or even after one year. Sometimes they are not formed at all (sterile hydatids). Development to the fertile stage occurs most satisfactorily in sheep. Neither rodents nor lagomorphs (Leporidae) are spontaneously receptive, or only exceptionally so (Sulimov, 1965). However, in Argentina, Schantz *et al.*, (1972) have reported a natural *Echinococcus* life cycle between the red fox (*Ducicyon culpaeus*) and the european hare (*Lepus europaeus*) and the features of the parasite correspond to those of *E. g. granulosus* (see also remarks on *E. patagonicus,* below). All organs and tissues, even bones of a host, may be infected, but the chief locations are the liver and the lungs.

Echinococcus granulosus granulosus is known all over the world. It occurs chiefly in South America, the Near and Middle East, Australia and New Zealand, where it is very widespread. In other countries, it occurs in small endemic foci.

E. g. canadensis: The mature adult forms of this subspecies infect dog and wolf and never the fox (Cameron, 1960); hydatids only infect Cervidae (Reindeer) and neither the bovine nor the pig can be infected (Cameron, 1960). Man can also be infected and hepatic hydatids occur in man. In animals the main location of hydatids is the lung.

The geographical distribution of *E. g. canadensis* is Northern Canada.

E. g. borealis: This differs from *E. g. canadensis* in that the adult worms infect foxes, dogs and wolves and the hydatid will infect sheep experimentally. Infection of man may also occur and the elective location is the lungs. The geographical distribution is Northern Canada.

E. g. equinus: As an adult worm this subspecies infects dogs and foxes. Hydatids develop in equines (horses and asses) and the parasite occurs mainly in Belgium, Northern France, Great Britain and Ireland. It is characterized by the frequency of fertile hydatids and by its elective location in liver. Receptivity of man for the hydatids is questionable since in Britain and Ireland where up to 61% and 30% of horses (Dixon, 1973) are infected respectively hydatidosis of man is no more than in other western European countries.

E. multilocularis: The adult ovigerous worms live in Canidae and Felidae and larvae develop mainly in microtine rodents of the following genera: *Microtus, Clethrionomys* and, less frequently, *Lemmus, Ondatra* and *Elobius*. Gerbillidae, Cricetidae, Dipodidae and Muridae may also be affected, while only one species of lagomorph (*Onchoterra daurica,* Lagomyidea) has been found infected. Besides rodents, the insectivors *Sorex jacksoni* and *S. tundrensis* may act as intermediate hosts (Rausch, 1967). The receptivity of the microtidae and of the domestic mouse is of interest from the epidemiological viewpoint, since these intermediate hosts have a short life span (Rausch, 1967) and larvae develop in them very quickly, in 2 to 3 months (Rausch, 1968). On the other hand, ungulates such as sheep, cattle and pigs are never infected and reports of such infections result from the confusion of certain developmental forms of *E. granulosus* with larval stages of *E. multilocularis*. However, man may be infected with the larval stage of this parasite. The larval form is not a voluminous hydatid, rather it produces many external daughter and granddaughter vesicles which spread into the parenchyma of the liver, the main location of the larvae (Fig. 1).

Echinococcus multilocularis has a wide geographical distribution and has been reported from all continents. The important foci occur in North American, Asia (Siberia, Japan) and Central Europe. However, its distribution is extended when it is searched for: for example, in France it has been found nearly every time it has been searched for (Euzeby, 1960, 1968; Coudert *et al.,* 1970; Romano, 1970).

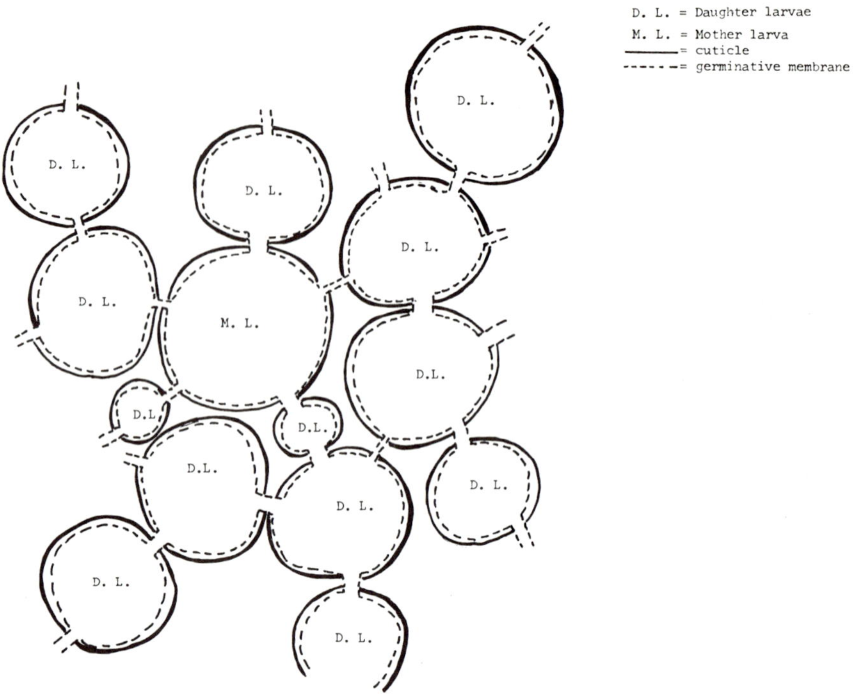

Fig. 1. Mode of replication in multilocular hydatidosis.

Two sub-species of *E. multilocularis* have been recognized *viz.*

E. m. multilocularis: This sub-species occurs in Europe and the temperate countries of Asia and North America, the definitive hosts of which are foxes (*Vulpes vulpes*), dogs and domestic cats. The larvae develop chiefly in *Microtus* spp and, incidentally, in the mouse.

E. m. sibiricensis: This sub-species occurs in arctic areas, infecting, as the adult, chiefly polar foxes (*Alopex lagopus*) and, as the larva, several species of Microtidae. The sub-species *E. m. kazakhensis* Schultz 1962 and *E. m. veterinorum* (Rudolphi, 1810) are not valid. The first one seems to be a nomen nudum; as to the second, Abdulaze (1964) thinks it is only a modified form of *E. granulosus*.

E. oligarthrus: This species is somewhat intermediary between *E. granulosus* and *E. multilocularis*. The adult worms only infect Felidae. In natural conditions, the parasite is found in wild species such as *Felis concolor* (Puma), *Panthera onca* (jaguar) and *Felis (Herpailurus) eyra* (Jaguarandi) while the domestic cat can be infected in the laboratory, the dog cannot. Larvae are found in a Dasyproctidae, *Dasyprocta agouti* (Agouti), in a marsupial, *Didelphis marsupialis* (oppossum) and in a rodent Echimyidae, *Prochimys guyanensis* (spinose rat) (Thatcher, 1972). Ruminants cannot be infected. Man is probably infected by *E. oligarthrus*, since in countries such as Panama, where *E. oligarthrus* is the only known *Echinococcus* species, human hydatid disease exists (Thatcher and Sousa, 1966; Thatcher, 1972). In all intermediate hosts, the striated muscles, including the myocardium, are the predeliction sites for the larvae. However, in man the parasite also infects the liver. Larvae appear as small vesicles (1-5 mm) often divided by septa, so as to give the appearance of a multilocular vesicle.

E. patagonicus: This species was described by Szidat (1960, 1963) from the patagonian area of Argentina. This author considers that the larval stage may infect man. The validity of *E. patagonicus* is not wholly agreed upon since the adult form only has been described, in *Ducicyon culpaeus* (Patagon fox). According to Rausch (1968) it is a *species inquirenda*. *Echinococcus patagonicus* may be identical to the form reported by Schantz *et al.* (1972) which occurs in *D. culpaeus* and hares and which they state is a form of *E. g. granulosus*.

CLINICAL AND ANATOMICAL FEATURES OF ZOONOTIC METACESTODIASIS IN MAN

The following is a brief review of the diseases caused by zoonotic metacestodes.

Sparganosis

Spargana infections may be external, affecting the connective tissue of the skin, vagina, eyelids, etc., and also the sub-conjuntival area of the eyes. The organism causes oedema, pruritis and nodules that may become abcesses. Sometimes, an immediate cutaneous hypersensitivity reaction may occur (Mueller and Coulston, 1941).

The internal, or visceral form of sparganosis may affect the wall of the small intestine, mesentery, urethra and pulmonary artery. These lesions may resemble those of carci nomas (Kiremerwa *et al.*, 1956). In addition, larvae may be found in the lymph nodes, especially the inguinal nodes, and genital oedema and even elephantiasis may result from such infections. A larva migrans syndrome may result from cutaneous or mucosa infections by plerocercoids, but encephalitic sparganosis, as reported by Faust (1970) is quite rare. Parasite induced weight gain, as reported in mice, rats and hamsters (Mueller, 1963a, 1965, 1972) has not been observed in man.

Cysticercosis

Zoonotic cysticercosis in man is represented by *C. ovis*, which affects the spinal cord and *C. crassiceps* which affects the eye causing endophthalmy.

Coenurosis

Three forms of coenurosis are recognized. These are:

A nervous syndrome which has been reported only from temperate countries and, so far, never from tropical Africa. It is mainly due to *C. cerebralis* but sometimes also to *C. serialis*. A coenurus induced nervous syndrome may be observed in areas where ovine coenurosis is unknown but where *C. serialis* in Leporidae is frequent (Hermos, 1970). The most typical form is a posterior-fossa syndrome, resulting from the presence of a coenurus in the sub-arachnoid space. Coenuri may localize in the brain or the spinal cord and in such cases the clinical manifestations are dependent on the location of the larval stage.

An ocular syndrome is less common than the nervous one. It is well known in tropical Africa and in temperate areas and two forms have been described: an endophthalmic syndrome chiefly of the vitreous chamber and due either to *C. cerebralis* or to *C. brauni*; and a syndrome associated with the subconjunctival location of coenuri, either *C. serialis* or *C. brauni*, and which may be associated with displacement of the eyeball.

A soft tissue involvement is more frequent in tropical Africa (*C. brauni*) than in temperate countries (*C. serialis*). The infection occurs chiefly in the subcutaneous and the intramuscular connective tissue, but it may also occur in the orbital cavity. Clinical signs vary with the location of the parasite, but the most frequent form consists of pseudo-tumoral soft, mobile, painless pseudo-lipomatous nodules.

Echinococcosis

Two types are recognized, *viz:*

a. Hydatid disease due to *E. granulosus* and its sub-species and which is characterised by well defined hydatid cysts surrounded by an adventia reaction. This form mainly affects the liver, with the lungs as the second most common site of infection. This form of hydatid disease is world wide in distribution. In Northern countries the lungs are preferentially affected, but hydatid cysts may be found in every part of the body, including the bones. The disease may be complicated by abscess formation or by rupture of the cyst when secondary cyst formation may result.

b. Alveolar disease, due to *E. multilocularis*, and which is characterised by the formation of liver pseudo-carcinomatous lesions. This is associated with discontinuities of the cuticular layer of the vesicular larvae of this parasite which allow hydatid fluid and germinative membranes to escape from the mother vesicle. The germinative membrane then migrates in the liver parenchyma necrotised by the hydatid fluid and generates daughter vesicles, which then produce grand-daughter vesicles. No adventia tissue reaction occurs to limit the extension of the process.

The larval stage of *oligarthrus* causes polycystic lesions in the liver intermediate between a typical hydatid cyst and alveolar lesions but well contained by an adventia reaction.

To summarize, the zoonotic metacestodiases consist of the following entities:

Subcutaneous - sparganosis, coenurosis serialis and brauni
Muscular - coenuriasis serialis and brauni
Ocular - sparganosis, coenuriasis cerebralis and brauni
visceral - hepatic; hydatidosis granulosus and alveolar echinococcosis
-pulmonary; hydatidosis granulosus, canadensis and borealis
-intestinal; sparganosis
Nervous - coenuriasis cerebralis, hydatidosis granulosus, sparganosis and less frequently submucosal and ganglion forms.

AETIOLOGY OF ZOONOTIC METACESTODOSIS

Reservoir of parasites

Table III emphasizes the canidae and felidae species that are definitive hosts of cestodes, the reservoirs of human zoonotic metacestodosis and the various species that, acting as intermediary hosts, allow the completion of life cycles (Table III).

Means of infection

Three infection modes are recognized (Fig. 2):

a. Direct infection: This requires that the eggs of adult cestodes are immediately infective for man; only Taeniidae eggs are such. Infection occurs by direct contact with wild Canidae and Felidae. Man may acquire eggs from his hands which have been contaminated, for example, by being licked by dogs and cats which have contaminated their tongues by licking an egg contaminated, pruritic, anal region, by stroking dogs and cats whose fur is contaminated by eggs in the grooming process or by skinning wild fur bearing animals for the pelt, a process which is sometimes done using the teeth. Similarly, veterinarians and laboratory technicians may become infected when they conduct autopsy, fecal or obstetrical examinations.

b. *Semi-direct.* This is possible from domestic cats and dogs infected with taeniid cestodes. It occurs most usually when domestic pets contaminate food utensils, such as dishes, with eggs carried on their tongues.

c. *Indirect infection.* This occurs through indirect contact with the animal reservoir. It is possible with the taeniid cestodes of domestic and wild Canidae and Felidae and is the only means of infection with the Diphyllobothriidae (*Spirometra*) the eggs of which cannot infect man directly. Indirect may occur by the following routes:

i. *Ingestion of contaminated food and water*

Contamination of vegetables occurs with taeniid eggs. For example short stemmed raw-eaten vegetables and fruits may be spoiled by eggs originating from disintegrated proglottids. This may occur in all forms of coenurosis and echinococcosis but is the most frequent means of infection in alveolar echinococcosis. Thus wild strawberries, gooseberries, bilberries, etc, may be spoiled with eggs from foxes harbouring *E. multilocularis*. The sterilization of raw vegetables and fruits has been impossible hitherto, but recently Williams *et al.* (1973) have indicated that eggs exposed to an 11% aqueous solution of "Bunamidine" for one hour will be killed.

Infection through contaminated meat is restricted to plerocercoids of *Spirometra*. Such larvae, when ingested by man, re-encyst in him as part of the paratenic process, and cause sparganosis. Man can be infected through eating the raw meat of snakes, frogs, rats, raccoons, oppossums and sometimes pork in which, through a previous paratenic process, encysted plerocercoids occur. Even the handling of infected flesh, followed by licking of the spoiled fingers may cause infection. Such contaminated meat can infect man only if it is eaten raw or very lightly cooked since boiling or frying kill the plerocercoids. While deep-freezing or salt curing

TABLE III: *Animal reservoirs of zoonotic metacestodes.* (Intermediate hosts in brackets)

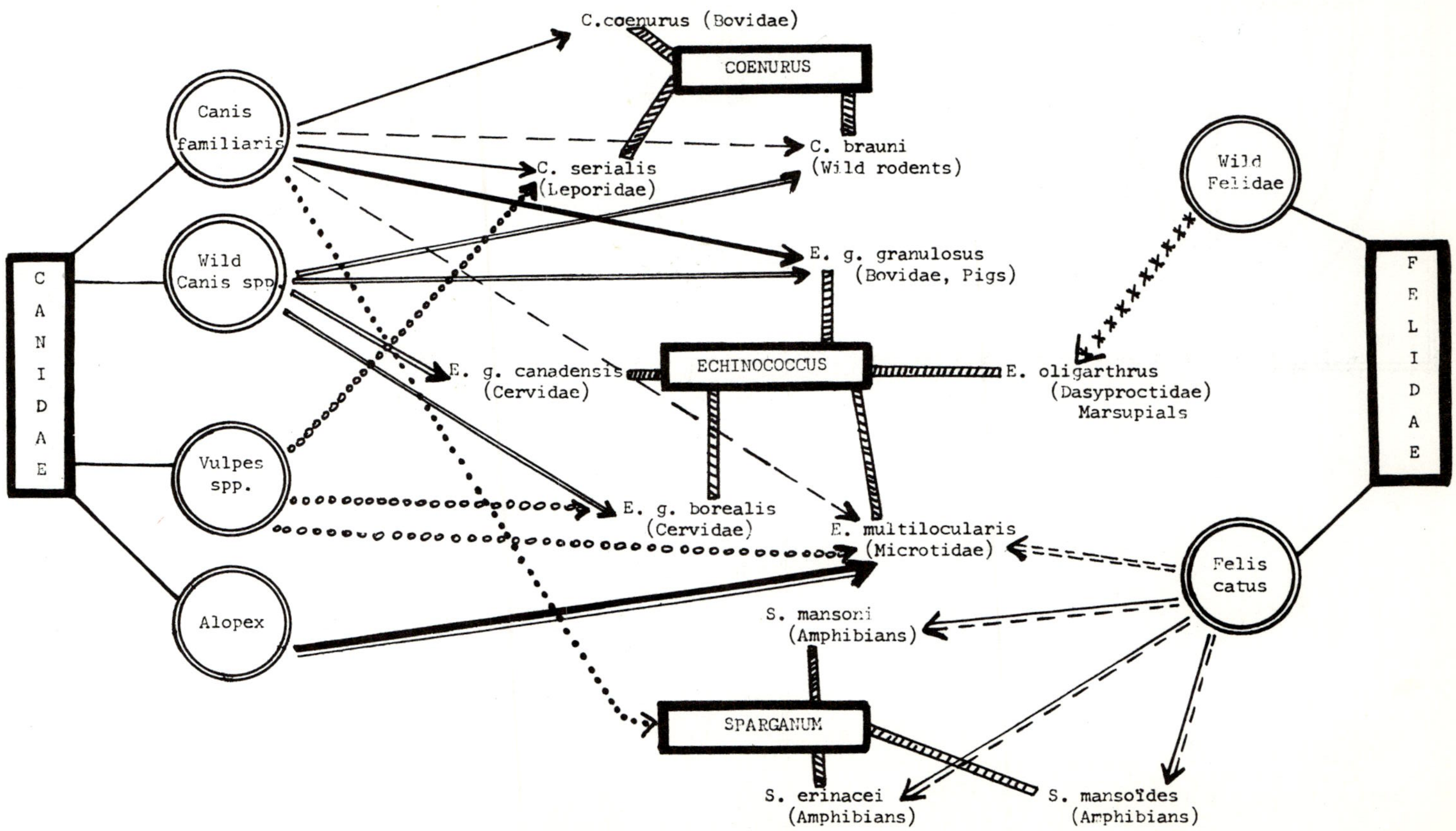

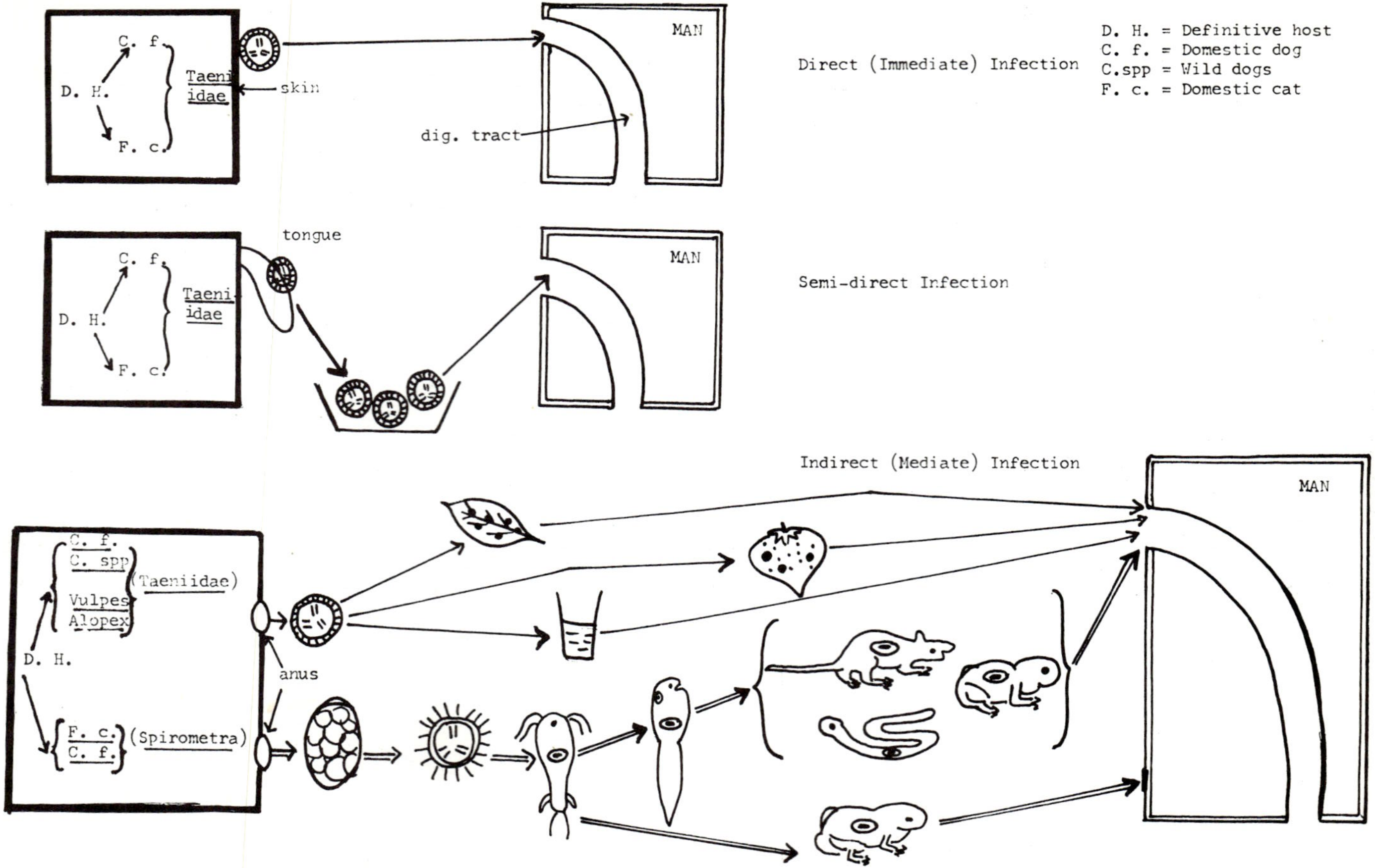
D. H.
C. f.
F. c.
Taeni idae
skin
MAN
dig. tract
Direct (Immediate) Infection
D. H. = Definitive host
C. f. = Domestic dog
C.spp = Wild dogs
F. c. = Domestic cat
tongue
Semi-direct Infection
Indirect (Mediate) Infection
C. f.
C. spp
Vulpes
Alopex
(Taeniidae)
(Spirometra)
anus

(dry or brine) of infected meat will kill the plerocercoids, smoking of meat will not do so.

Drinking water also can be a source of taeniid eggs and, possibly also plerocercoid infected tadpoles. However, the possibility of acquiring sparanosis by drinking water containing procercoid-infected copepods **is** dubuis since the administration of such copepods to pigs does not result in sparganosis (Corkum, 1966).

ii. Parenteral infection

The hypothesis proposed by Templeton (1971) that taeniid embryos may penetrate the human skin can be dismissed since it is difficult to envisage how the embryos could be activated to hatch outside the digestive tract in such circumstances. While procercoid larvae liberated from dead copepods cannot penetrate the skin (Mueller, 1964) plerocercoid larvae can penetrate into the subcutaneous or submucosal tissues (vagina, eyelids, ocular conjonctiva) when infected frog-flesh is applied as a topical remedy to the skin or mucosae. This is a common practice in some parts of the Far East.

EPIDEMIOLOGY

Geographical distribution of the zoonotic metacestodes

These diseases are world-wide in distribution, but their prevalence is not uniform and the majority are somewhat localized to certain geographic areas.

Thus, sparganosis occurs chiefly in South-East Asia and is much less frequent in Europe and America. This is attributable to the custom of Asian people of eating raw flesh of various plerocercoid-infected animals, and using frog-flesh as topical application for curing external diseases.

Coenurosis is more frequently reported from tropical Africa than from temperate countries (32 cases against 18) (Templeton, 1968). In temperate countries coenurosis is more frequent in South Africa than in France Great Britain or the U.S.A. (in that order). The distribution of coenurosis due to *M. brauni*, in which the larval stage occurs in wild African mammals, is less well established than that for *M. multiceps* or *M. serialis*. It is of note that cerebral coenurosis due to *M. cerebralis* is unknown in tropical Africa.

Hydatidosis occurs chiefly in South America, mediterranean and Middle-eastern countries, New Zealand and Australia, but foci are knwon in almost every country (e.g. 5,3 p. 100,000

Fig. 2. Infection routes to man by the zoonotic metacestodes

in Marseilles area, Quilici *et al.*, 1972; 9 p. 100,000 in Corsica, Panorazi, 1971; 2.4 to 7.5 in West and South-West France, Bailenger, 1957, 1960). Hydatidosis is closely linked with sheep raising, but not in an absolute quantitative manner. For example, even with a relatively small ovine population, human hydatidosis may be important if the infection rate of sheep is high. Thus in Corsica 46% of the 170,000 sheep carry hydatid cysts (Panorazi, 1971). On the other hand the type of sheep husbandry also may influence the incidence of human hydatidosis. (See below)

Alveolar echinococcosis occurs in West-Central Europe and Arctic countries, and it is unknown in America below the latitude of North Dakota. Its absence in Iceland, Greenland, Australia, New Zealand and South Africa, where hydatid disease is common, is striking.

Local distribution in a definite area may occur. Thus while hydatidosis is usually extensively distributed in endemic countries, it occurs in small foci outside these areas, these foci being centered on domestic dog-sheep relations. The distribution of the other metacestodoses is usually focal and depends upon the life cycle of the parasite. Thus sparganosis only occurs in watery areas and tropical African coenurosis (*C. brauni*), and alveolar echinococcosis occur in foci where their intermediary hosts (wild rodents) have their biotypes.

Seasonal distribution

Zoonotic metacestodoses of man, because of the long developmental periods involved are uniformly spread all over the year. However, infection may take place only in particular seasons. In animals, homologous metacestodes sometimes have a seasonal incidence, according to the time of the year when the reservoirs are mostly infected. Thus farm-dogs appear to be chiefly parasitised by *E. g. granulosus* in winter, so that for example, pig-hydatidosis is maximal in August (Lubke, 1972). As further examples, foxes, in Alaska, are infected by *E. m. sibiricensis* only in autumn (Fay *et al.*, 1964) while in Europe, maximal infection by *E. m. multilocularis* occurs in spring (Kurashvili, 1964; Coudert *et al.*, 1970). In temperate areas, *Spirometra* eggs can only develop at +8 to +10° C so that sparganosis probably has a seasonal incidence, though this has still to be determined.

Epidemiological types of zoonotic metacestodes

Zoonotic metacestodosis are endemic in various countries because the life-cycles of the parasites take place in definitive and intermediate hosts living in the country.

Three kinds of epidemiological cycles are known, *viz:*

i. rural type: This is the most frequent and is concerned with domestic dogs and cats and intermediate hosts which are usually domestic animals. Man is infected, directly or indirectly, from dogs and cats in villages or on farms. This cycle chiefly occurs with hydatidosis and coenurosis cerebralis and serialis.

ii. sylvatic type: This cycle is completed through wild Canidae and Felidae and their wild prey (wild rodents). This is the most frequent type for multilocular echinococcosis and man is indirectly infected by the alveolar form of this disease, from wild Canidae and Felidae. The same is true for most cases of coenurosis brauni.

iii. urban type: This cycle is completed through the domestic cat and mice. It has been recognized for some time for alveolar echinococcosis (Vogel, 1960) and has recently been re-emphasised by Leiby and Kritsky (1972).

However, variations can occur with these epidemiological types of infection. For example hydatidosis and coenurosis cerebralis and serialis may occur as sylvatic types at the periphery of forest areas. In such situations the life cycles of the parasites are completed in wild ungulates (hydatidosis, coenurosis cerebralis) or Leporidae (coenurosis serialis) and wild dogs and foxes that indirectly infect man and his domestic animals. Apparently, this type of cycle does not occur in Kenya, since the wild ungulates do not harbour hydatid cysts (Nelson *et al.*, 1963).

Hydatidosis may also have an urban cycle, even in large cities, especially when sanitary regulations are relaxed or ignored. For example, cases of hydatidosis due to such circumstances are reported from Wales (Cook, 1963) and New Zealand (Sweatman and Williams, 1962). Sometimes small foci occur when, in North Africa, a few sheep are kept for "mechoui" and at slaughter, the entrails are given to domestic dogs (Quilici *et al.*, 1972).

Alveolar echinococcosis may become rural,when the life cycle is completed through farm-dogs or cats and Microtidae and Muridae (*Apodemus agrarius, Mus musculus*).

Epidemiology in relation to habits, customs and occupations

Habits, customs and occupations may influence the prevalence of metacestode infections in certain groups. The increased risk of infection with echinococcus has been noted above for veterinarians and laboratory technicians handling dogs and cats, performing autopsies or conducting fecal examinations. The practices of using the flesh of frogs as an anti-phlogistic therapy and the consumption of the meat of of frogs, snakes etc. in a raw state greatly influence the prevalence of sparganosis. Hydatid infection of shoe-makers in the Middle East is attributable to the practice of softening leather by the use of a liquid suspension of dog faeces (Schwabe and Daoud, 1961). In some parts of the world the carcases of dead ruminants are not buried or are insufficiently buried, allowing scavengers such as dogs, jackals, etc. to become infected with *E. granulosus*. The unique example of human corpses being offered to hyenas has been referred to previously: this practice facilitates the spread of coenurosis brauni and sparganosis pretoriensis.

Religious practices may limit the prevalence of zoonotic metacestodes, an example of which is the distribution of hydatidosis in North East Iran where close contact with dogs is not allowed.

CONTROL

Control of metacestode infection consists of interrupting the life cycles of the parasites concerned. This is illustrated in Fig. 3.

Prevention of infection of definitive hosts (Fig. 3, I)

This is a most important measure since it results, ultimately, in the elimination of reservoirs for the infection. When domestic dogs are concerned in the epidemiology of metacestode infection, the most effective measures consist of effective meat inspection with immediate destruction of infected organs (Pampiglione, 1965), careful supervision of abattoirs to prevent the entry of dogs, the capture and destruction of stray dogs, the effective disposal of carcases of dead ruminants and the practice of sheep husbandry without dogs. Such measures, which can lead to the elimination of taeniid infections have been recognized for many years, but nevertheless have required re-emphasis by Murray (1971). However, the prevention of infections with *Spirometra* spp. is very difficult since it is not possible to eliminate the sources of infection such as pools and the intermediate hosts therein.

Novel approaches to control include vaccination against *E. granulosus* (Turner *et al.*, 1933, 1936; Forsek and Rukavina, 1959; Perez-Fontana, 1961; Gemmel, 1962; Movsesijan, 1967; Movesijan *et al.*, 1968, 1970). Gemmel (1962) found that extracts of adult worms injected subcutaneously would produce enhanced resistance to adult parasites and similar results were obtained by movsesijan *et al.* (1968)using x-irradiated protoscolices given by the oral route. However,

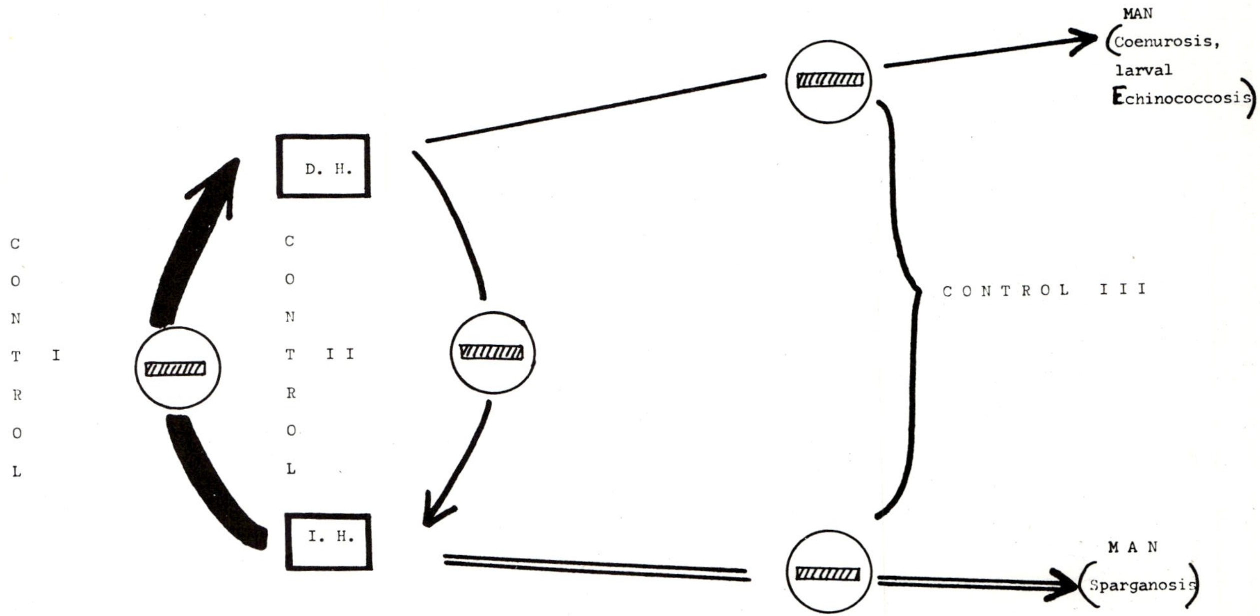

Fig. 3. *Outline of control for the zoonotic metacestodes of man.*

a commercial vaccine is not available at the present time.

The prevention of infection in wild carnivores is difficult and would require the slaughter of such hosts. This is impossible for aesthetic and ecological reasons.

Prevention of infection of intermediate hosts (Fig. 3, II)

In rural and urban epidemiological cycles the most satisfactory control consists of treating dogs and cats with an effective taeniacidal drug. Systematic and regular administration should be practiced on all animals in endemic areas or foci and the drug should be given at intervals, depending on the prepatent period of the worm (6-8 weeks for *E. granulosus*, 5-6 weeks for *Multiceps spp.*, 4 weeks for *E. multilocularis*, 3-5 weeks for *Spirometra)*.

The most satisfactory drugs are those which expel immature and ovigerous strobila quickly. This permits the segments to be collected and destroyed. Since there is no drug which is ovicidal, the use of drugs which expel mature cestodes may not produce the necessary interruption of the developmental cycle. A slow acting taeniicide may be dangerous because it does not prevent dispersion of eggs from the expelled proglotids. Such is the case with "Bunamidine" (N-N di *N* butyl 4 hexoly, 1 naphtamidine hydrochloride) when it is used for mature ovigerous worms. It is active against immature worms (Guilhon *et al.*, 1967; McCristell, 1967; Gemmel, 1968c; Williams and Trejos (1970) but it is necessary either to dose animals twice for 2 consecutive days with 25 mg/kg (which is tedious) or once with 200 mg/kg (which is near the toxic dose and is not always 100% effective).

Arecoline bromide is, in our opinion, better. At 3-4 mg/kg, with only one dosing, it causes expulsion of cestodes within one hour. Thus, by keeping dogs indoors for 3-4 hours it is easy to collect all worms and infected faeces from treated animals and to destroy them.

Immunization of cattle, sheep and pigs against larval taeniids has been considered (Deve, 1927, 1933, 1934; Turner *et al.*, 1936) and has been investigated recently (Ferro, 1953; Moya and Blood, 1964; and Gemmel, 1968). Promising results were obtained by Gemmel (1968) by the intramuscular inoculation of hatched activated embryos into sheep.

In addition to therapy and immunization, improved sanitation will assist in the prevention of infection of intermediate hosts. However, with contaminated areas there is no chemical agent which will kill eggs on pastures and thus not possible to prevent dogs and cats from defecating in pools or ponds. In the sylvatic cycles the eradication of wild Canidae and Felidae is impossible but selective control measures against these animals might be useful. More success could be achieved by the elimination of the use of dogs in sheep husbandry.

INDIVIDUAL PROPHYLAXIS IN MAN

Even though the control measures referred to above are widely practiced, the risk of human infection still exists. It is still necessary to recommend precautions to avoid direct and indirect infection. Thus, close contact with pets should be avoided, protective clothing should be worn when canine and feline autopsies are performed or when faecal samples are examined and such material should be sterilized by heat (Gemmel, 1968b). Some chemical agents can destroy taeniid eggs for example, 10% formalin with 2% sodium hydroxyde or 0.5% toxychloramide sodium (Gall and Wikerhauser, 1970) but they do so only after 1 hour's contact.

Indirect infections can be prevented by avoiding eating raw or under-cooked flesh of potentially infected animals, by avoiding irrational treatments such as the application of frog flesh to the skin or the mucosae (Sparganosis) and by avoiding drinking suspected contaminated water or raw fruit and vegetables, that cnanot properly be sterilised.

REFERENCES

Abdulaze, K.A. and Sadykov, V.M. (1971). *In Pathology of Parasitic Diseases.* (Ed. S.M. Faafar). Purdue University Studies, Lafayette, p. 275.
Anon. (1972). *J. Amer. Med. Assoc., 222,* 891.
Alves, W.D., Gelfand, M. and Weinberg, R. (1954). *Trans. Roy. Soc. Trop. Med. Hyg., 48,* 87.
Baer, J.G. (1924). *Rev. Suisse Zool., 31,* 529.
Bailenger, J. (1957). *Rev. Hyg. Med. Soc., 5,* 707.
Bailenger, J. (1960). *Arch. Intern. Hidat., 19,* 158.
Baylis, H.A. (1932). *Trans. Roy. Soc. Trop. Med. Hyg., 25,* 275.
Bearup, A.J. (1953). *Aust. Vet. J., 29,* 217.
Becker, B.J.F. and Jackobson, S. (1951). *Lancet, 2,* 198.
Bertrand, I. and Callot, J. (1956). *Presse Med., 64,* 333.
Bianchi, L. (1964). *Proc. 1st Intl. Congr. Paras. Rome, 2,* 820.
Boase, A.J. (1956). *Brit. J. Ophth., 40,* 183.
Bonnal, G., Joyeux, C. and Bosch, P. (1933). *Bull. Soc. Path. Exot., 26,* 1060.
Bondareva, V.I. (1953). *Akad. Nauk. Kazakhs. U.S.S.R.*, 66.
Bondareva, V.I. (1958). *Kazakhs. Gozudarstv. Izdatelsts.,*

p. 100.
Brooks, T.J.J., Hutchison, W.F., Safley, T.F. and Ross, T.G. (1960). *Amer. J. Trop. Med. Hyg.*, *9*, 192.
Brujning, C.F. (1960). *Trop. Geogr. Med.*, *12*, 356.
Brumpt, E., Duvoir, M.E. and Sainton, J. (1934). *Bull. Acad. Med.*, *12*, 56; *Ann. Parasit. Hum. Comp.*, *12*, 371.
Brumpt, E. (1949). *Precis de Parasitologie*, 6th Ed. Masson, Paris.
Bucley, J.J.C. (1947). *Trans. Roy. Soc. Trop. Med. Hyg.*, *41*, 7.
Brygoo, E.R. and Catala, P. (1961). *Arch. Inst. Pasteur, Madagascar*, *29*, 75.
Cameron, T.W.M. (1926). *J. Helminth.*, *4*, 13.
Cameron, T.W.M. (1960). *Parassitologia*, *2*, 381.
Caballero-y-Caballero, E. (1956). *Acta Zool. Mexicana*, *1*, 1.
Clapham, P.A. (1941). *J. Helminth.*, *19*, 84.
Cook, B.R. (1963). *Proc. 1st Intl. Congr. Parasit. Rome*, *2*, 764.
Corkum, K.C. (1966). *J. Parasit.*, *52*, 444.
Correa, F.M.A., Ferrioli, J.F., Forjaz, S. and Martelli, N. (1962). *Riv. Inst. Med. Trop. Sao Paulo*, *4*, 838.
Coudert, J., Euzeby, J. and Garin, J.P. (1970). *Lyon Med.*, *224*, 293.
Cox, R.S. (1965). *East Afr. Med. J.*, *42*, 319.
Cross, J.H. (1963). *J. Parasit.*, *49*, 154.
Cruz, H. (1948). *J. Helminth*, *22*, 73.
Deiana, S. (1962). *Riv. Parassit.*, *23*, 267.
Deiana, S. (1971). *Parassitologia*, *13*, 173.
Deve, F. (1927). *C. R. Soc. Biol.*, *107*, 1130.
Deve, F. (1933). *C. R. Soc. Biol.*, *113*, 1443.
Deve, F. (1934). *C. R. Soc. Biol.*, *115*, 1025.
Deve, F. (1946). *Echinococcose secondaire.* Masson, Paris.
Deve, F. (1949). *Echinococcose primitive.* Masson, Paris.
Diesing, K.M. (1854). *Sitzber Akad. Wiss. Wien. Math. Naturw. Klasse* (Abt. 1), *13*, 555.
Dinnik, J.A. and Dinnik, N. (1969). *Inform. Med. Vet.*, (No. 2) p. 108.
Dixon, J.B. (1973). *Vet. Rec.*, *93*, 255.
Dollfus, R.Ph. (1959). *Parassitologia*, *1*, 143.
Dumon, H., Delmont, J., Ranque, Ph. and Quilici, M. (1971). *Maroc Med.*, *110*, 357.
Epstein, E. (1959). *S. Afric. Med. J.*, *33*, 602.
Euzeby, J. (1960). *Rev. Hyg. Med. Soc.*, *8*, 428.
Euzeby, J. (1967). *Journées Lyonnaises Hydatidologie*, p. 13.
Euzeby, J. (1968). *Maroc Med.*, *48*, 643.
Fain, A. (1952). *Rev. Suisse Zool.*, *59*, 487.
Fain, A., Denisoff, N., Homans, L., Questiaux, G., Van Laere,

L. and Vincent, M. (1956). *Ann. Soc. Belge. Med. Trop., 36*, 679.
Fain, A. (1958). *Nature, 178*, 1352.
Fain, A. and Piraux, A. (1959). *Bull. Soc. Path. Exot., 52*, 804.
Faust, E.C., Campbell, H.E. and Kellog, C.R. (1929). *Amer. J. Hyg., 9*, 560.
Faust, E.C, (1970). *In Craig and Faust's Clinical Parasitology*, 8th Ed., Lea and Febiger, Philadelphia.
Fay, F.H. and Rausch, R.L. (1964). *Proc. 1st Intl. Congr. Paras. Rome, 2*, 765.
Ferro, A. (1953). *Arch. Intern. Hidat., 13*, 223.
Forsek, Z. and Rukavina, J. (1959). *Veter. Sarajevo, 8*, 479.
Gall, Z. and Wikerhauser, T. (1969). *Vet. Arhiv., 39*, 51.
Gall, Z. and Wikerhauser, T. (1970). *Inst. Pat. Terap. Doma Zivotinja.*, p. 1035.
Gailliard, H. (1946). *Ann. Parasit. Hum. Comp., 21*, 146.
Garcia, O.N. (1961). *Rev. Venez. San Assit. Soc., 26*, 69.
Gemmel, M.A. (1962). *Immunology, 5*, 496.
Gemmel, M.A. (1966). *Immunology, 11*, 325.
Gemmel, M.A. and Soulsby, E.J.L. (1968). *Bull. Wld. Hlth. Org., 39*, 45.
Gemmel, M.A. (1968a). *Bull. Wld. Hlth. Org., 39*, 57.
Gemmel, M.A. (1968b). *Bull. Wld. Hlth. Org., 39*, 122.
Gemmel, M.A. (1968c). *Vet. Rec., 82*, 252.
Gemmel, M.A. (1970). *Austr. Vet. J., 46*, 366.
Gleason, N.N. (1960). *J. Parasit., 46*, 230.
Gribel, T.G. (1970). *Amer. J. Trop. Med. Hyg., 19*, 255.
Guilhon, J., Simic, Tsch., Savin, Z. and Bordjoski, A. (1967). *Bull. Acad. Vet., 42*, 327.
Harant, H. and Midrouille, T.R. (1949). *Bull. Soc. Path. Exot., 42*, 173.
Harkema, R. and Miller, G.C. (1964). *J. Parasit., 50*, 60.
Hermos, J.P. (1970). *J. Amer. Med. Ass., 213*, 1461.
Houdemer, E. (1933). *Bull. Soc. Med. Chir. Indochin., 11*, 425.
Ijma, A. (1905). *J. Coll. Sci. Imper. Univ. Tokyo, 20*, 1.
Iwata, S. (1934). *Jap. J. Zool., 6*, 139.
Iwata, S. (1936). *Zool. Mag., 48*, 665.
Iwata, S. (1972). *Progress of Medical Parasitology in Japan*, (Meguro Parasitological Museum, Tokyo), *4*,583.
Johnstone, H.G. (1950). *Amer. J. Trop. Med. Hyg., 30*, 431.
Jones, D.W. (1962). *Brit. J. Ophth., 46*, 123.
Joyeux, Ch. and Houdemer, E. (1927). *Bull. Soc. Path. Exot., 20*, 226.
Kiremerwa, D.N., Byaruhanga, D.B. and Raper, A.B. (1956). *E. Afric. Med. J., 33*, 37.

Kurashvili, B.E. (1964). *Proc. 1st Intl. Congr. Paras. Rome*, *2*, 747.
Leiby, P.D. and Kritsky, D.C. (1972). *J. Parasit.*, *58*, 1213.
Leon, L.A. (1972). *J. Pravas.*, *58*, 184.
Le Van Hoa (1967). *Bull. Soc. Path. Exot.*, *60*, 66.
Lubke, R. (1968). *Helminthologia*, *8/9*, 305.
Lubke, R. (1972). *Tierartzl. Umsch.*, *27*, 28.
Madyarov, S.D. quoted by Abdulaze *et al.* (1971).
Malczewski, A. (1963). *Bull. Acad. Polon, Sci.*, *11*, 296.
McCristell, T. (1967). *N. Z. Nat. Hyd. Counc.* (7th Ann. Rep.) p. 24.
McIntosh, A. (1937). *J. Pravas.*, *23*, 313.
Meillon, B. and Leech, R.L. (1943). *S. Afric. Med. J.*, *17*, 289.
Moore, J.T. (1915). *Amer. J. Trop. Dis.*, *2*, 518.
Movsesijan, M., Sokolic, A. and Mladenovic, Z. (1967). *Vet. Arhiv.*, *37*, 384.
Movsesijan, M., Sokolic, A. and Mladenovic, Z. (1968). *Brit. Vet. J.*, *124*, 425.
Movsesijan, M. and Mladenovic, Z. (1970). *Vet. Glasn*, *24*, 189.
Moya, V. and Blood, B.D. (1964). *Bol. Chil. Parasit.*, *19*, 7.
Mueller, J.F. and Coulston, F. (1941). *Amer. J. Trop. Med. Hyg.*, *21*, 399.
Mueller, J.F. (1963a). *Ann. NY Acad. Sci.*, *113*, 217.
Mueller, J.F. (1963). *J. Parasit.*, *49*, 294.
Mueller, J.F. (1964). *Proc. 1st Intl. Congr. Paras., Rome*, *2*, 815.
Mueller, J.F. (1965). *J. Parasit.*, *51*, 523.
Mueller, J.F. (1966). *J. Parasit.*, *52*, 437.
Mueller, J.F. (1972). *J. Parasit.*, *58*, 438.
Murray, H. (1971). *Med. J. Austral.*, *2*, 779.
Nelson, G.S. and Rausch, R.L. (1963). *Ann. Trop. Med. Paras.*, *57*, 136.
Nelson, G.S., Pester, F.R.N. and Rickman, R. (1965). *Trans. Roy. Soc. Trop. Med. Hyg.*, *59*, 507.
Orihel, T.C., Gonzalez, F. and Beaver, P.C. (1970). *Amer. J. Trop. Med. Hyg.* *19*, 255.
Ortlepp, R.J. (1934). *Onderst. J. Vet. Sci. Anim. Husb.*, *3*, 97.
Ortlepp, R.J. (1938). *Onderst. J. Vet. Sci.*, *10*, 253.
Pampiglione, S. (1965). *Nuov. Ann. Ig. Microb.*, *16*, 345.
Panorazi, J. (1971). Quoted by Dumon, H. *et al.* (1971).
Perez-Fontana, V. (1961). *Bull. Off. Intern. Epiz.*, *55*, 694.
Quilici, M., Dumon, H. and Ranque, Ph. (1972). *Nouv. Presse Med.*, *1*, 2768.
Railliet, A. and Henry, H. (1915). *Bull. Soc. Path. Exot.*, *8*,

173.
Railliet, A. and Henry, H. (1919). *Bull. Soc. Path. Exot.*, *12*, 223.
Ranque, J. and Nicoll, R.N. (1955). *Ann. Parasit. Hum. Comp.*, *30*, 22.
Raper, A.B. and Dockeray, G.C. (1956). *Ann. Trop. Med. Paras.*, *50*, 121.
Rausch, R.L. (1953). *Thapar. Comm. Volume* Ed. J. Dayal), p. 233.
Rausch, R.L. (1960). *Arch. Intern. Hidatid*, *19*, 859.
Rausch, R.L. (1967). *Ann. Parasit. Hum. Comp.*, *42*, 19.
Rausch, R.L. (1968). *Bull. Wld. Hlth. Org.*, *39*, 1.
Rausch, R.L. and Bernstein, J.J. (1972). *Z. Tropenmed. Parasit.*, *23*, 25.
Read, C.P. (1952). *J. Parasit.*, *38*, 29.
Rodriguez-Gallego, C. (1957). *Nota. Prev. Iber. Parasit.*, *17*, 109.
Roger, H. (1942). *Rev. Neurol.*, *74*, 319.
Romano, Cl. (1970). *D.M. Thesis, Paris-Creteil* (1970).
Rudolphi, C.A. (1810). *Entozoorum sive Vermium intestinalium historia naturalis II*, (Part 1), Amsterdam.
Rudolphi, C.A. (1819). *Entozoorum synopsis cui accedunt mantissa Duplex et Indices Locupletissimi*, Berolini.
Rukavina, J. (1957). *Veter. Sarajevo*, *6*, 46.
Ryzenkho, G.F. (1971). *Sbornik Robot Gelm posvyaschen Akad. K. I. Skrjabin*, p. 338.
Sadykov, V.H. (1965). *Trud. Subek Nauk Issled. Inst. Vet.*, *17*, 180.
Sadykov, V.H. (1971). *Moscou Izdatelstvo Kolos K. I. Skrjabin* p. 334.
Sambon, B. (1907). *Proc. Zool. Soc.*, *19*, p. 282.
Sandars, D.F. (1954). *Med. J. Austral.*, (year 41), *2*, 817.
Sandars, D.F. (1959). *Med. J. Austral.*, *41*, 817.
Schantz, F.M., Lord, R.D. and Zavaleta, O. de (1972). *Ann. Trop. Med. Paras.*, *66*, 479.
Schultz, R.S. (1962). *Med. Parazit. Moscow*, *31*, 272.
Schwabe, C.S. and Daoud, K.A. (1961). *Amer. J. Trop. Med. Hyg.*, *10*, 374.
Shortt, R.B. and Lewis, A.L. (1964). *J. Parasit.*, *50*, 800.
Sokolova, A. (1961). *Medit. Parazit. Parazitarn. Bol. Moscow*, *70*, 106.
Stiles, H.H. (1908). *Hyg. Lab. Bull.*, *40*, 7.
Sulimov, A.D. (1965). *Trud. omsk. Vet. Inst.*, *23*, 67.
Sweatman, G.K. and Williams, R.J. (1962). *Trans. Roy. Soc. N.Z. Zool.*, *2*, 221.
Sweatman, G.K. and Williams, R.J. (1963). *Parasitology*, *53*, 339.

Swartzwelder, J.C., Beaver, P.C. and Hood, M.W. (1964). *Amer. J. Trop. Med. Hyg. 13*, 43.
Szidat, L. (1960). *Neotropica Buenos Aires, 6*, 13.
Szidat, L. (1963). *Z. Parasitenk., 23*, 80.
Taramelli, R. and Dubois, A. (1931). *Ann. Soc. Belge Med. Trop., 11*, 151.
Templeton, A.C. (1968). *Trans. Roy. Soc. Trop. Med. Hyg., 62*, 251.
Templeton, A.C. (1971). *Trop. Geogr. Med., 23*, 105.
Thatcher, V. and Sousa, O.E. (1966). *Ann. Trop. Med. Parasit. 60*, 405.
Thatcher, V. (1972). *Ann. Trop. Med. Parasit., 66*, 99.
Turner, E.L., Berberian, D.A. and Dennis, E.W. (1936). *Proc. Soc. Exp.Biol. Med., 30*, 618.
Turner, E.L., Berberian, D.A. and Dennis, E.W. (1936). *J. Parasit., 22*, 14.
Turner, E.L. (1959). *Trans. Roy. Soc. Trop. Med. Hyg., 13*, 23.
Vanderick, F., Fain, A., Langi, S. and van Balen, J. (1964). *Ann. Soc. Belge. Med. Trop., 44*, 1077.
Vogel, H. (1960). *Z. Tropenmed. Parasit., 11*, 36.
von Linstow, C.F.O. (1902). *Zentralb. Bakt., 32*, 882.
Wainright, J. (1957). *J. Path. Bact., 73*, 347.
Watson, K.C. (1955). *Lancet, ii*, 1321.
Williams, R.J. and Sweatman, G. (1963). *Parasitology, 53*, 391.
Williams, J.F. and Trejos, A. (1970). *Res. Vet. Sci, 11*, 392.
Williams, J.F., Colli, C.W. and Leid, R.W, (1973). Papers presented at the 6th International Symposium of the World Association for the Advancement of Veterinary Parasitology, Vienna, 1973.
Wilson, V.C.L., Wayxe, R.D.M. and Addae, P.O. (1972). *Trans. Roy. Soc. Trop. Med. Hyg., 66*, 611.
Wirth, W.A. and Farrow, C.C. (1961). *Amer. J. Trop. Med. Hyg., 9*, 192.

PERSPECTIVES ON THE ERADICATION OF SEVERAL HELMINTHOZOONOTIC DISEASES IN THE USSR

A. S. Bessonov

The All-Union K.I. Skryabin Institute of Helminthology, Moscow, USSR

INTRODUCTION

The eradication of helminthoses and particularly helminthozoonotic diseases is a very difficult task. Despite the fact that the veterinary and public health services have a great variety of means and techniques at their disposal for the control of helminthozoonotic diseases, their use is limited by a number of factors. Among these are the local habits, traditions and practices of people in the cooking of food, in the management and feeding of domestic animals and in religious ceremonies, etc. Other factors include adaptation potential of the helminths themselves especially their ability to adapt to the changing conditions of their habitats, such as to hamper the control against them.

In considering the above factors, it is apparent that the success in the control of helminthozoonotic diseases will be connected: (1) with the changes in the technology of management of animals, (2) with the improvement of veterinary and public health programmes (improved diagnosis, therapy, etc.), (3) with the improvement of sanitary practices among people and the gradual elimination of habits and religious ceremonies which favour the distribution of the helminths (the use of semi-raw meat, etc.).

In the USSR, marked progress has been achieved in these areas, but the most important influence has been the changes in the technology of management of animals and the effect of these and the sanitation of farm animals.

The present trend to industrialize all the methods of management of animals, to establish indoor and semi-indoor types of management makes it possible for example to break links in the life cycles of *Echinococcus*, *Trichinella* and other helminths. Thus it may be possible to achieve successful control of some helminthozoonotic diseases in the near future.

CYSTICERCOSIS

Statistical data indicates a steady decline in the global incidence of cysticercosis cellulosae in pigs. In Hungary, for example, the incidence of pig cysticercosis decreased during 1927-1967 from 0.48% to 0.0002% (i.e. 2400 times) (Bodrossy, 1972). A similar trend was observed in the USSR where the incidence decreased from 0.16% to 0.02% (i.e. 8 times) during 1961-1971 (Fig. 1).

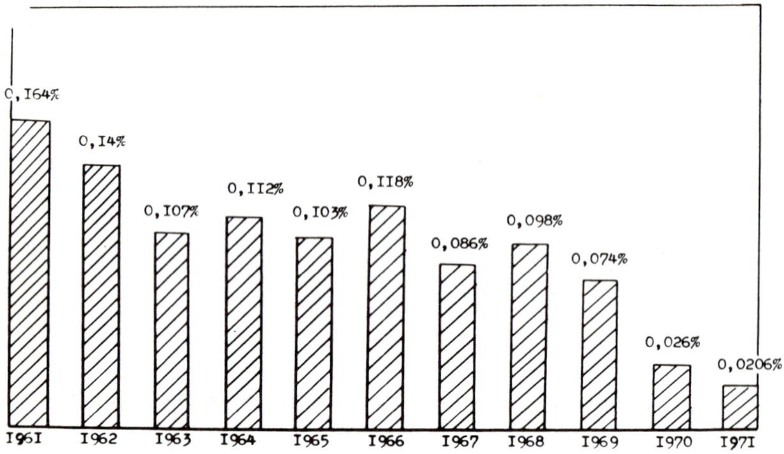

Fig. 1. The prevalence of cysticercosis cellulosae in swine in the USSR during 1961 to 1971.

The main cause of the steady decline of the incidence of *C. cellulosae* in pigs lies in the enlargement of pig farms and in the keeping of pigs indoors which leads to the restriction of contact between pigs and human faeces. Successful control of this disease is favoured also by the fact that *C. cellulosae* cysts are readily detected in swine (in contrast to *Cysticercus bovis* in cattle) since swine are usually heavily infected, possibly due to their coprophagous habits.

Serious problems are observed in the world with bovine cysticercosis (*Cysticercus bovis*). Table 1 indicates the present prevalence of *C. bovis* in different countries of the world. Prevalence is maintained at a steady level or is increasing both in areas where sanitation is deficient (developing countries, mountain and eternal frost regions, etc.) and also in areas with high sanitary standards occur. Thus an increase in cattle cysticercosis is observed in the German Democratic Republic (Hiepe *et al.*, 1967), in the Federal Republic of Germany (Pawlowski and Schultz, 1972), in Romania, (Cironeanu *et al.*, 1970), in Hungary (Bodrossy, 1972) and in other countries. In France during the period from 1968 to 1971 the number of infected carcasses increased from 5683 to 25441 (i.e. about 4.5 times) (Soule *et al.*, 1972).

Table 1

Prevalence of Cysticercus bovis *in cattle in various countries (Data from Pawlowski and Schultz, 1972)*

Country	Cattle infected (%)
Australia	0,21
Argentina	0,62
Bulgaria	0,62
Brazil	about 1
Cuba	0,16
Chad	more than 10
Czechoslovakia	1,385
Equador	0.7
Ethiopia	more than 10
France	0,19
German Democratic Republic	2,63
Federal Republic of Germany	2,06
Guatemala	1,72
Holland	about 1
Hungary	0,224
India	1,4
Ireland	from 0,1 to 10
Kenya	more than 10
Libya	more than 10
Poland	0,56-0,58
Sudan	more than 10
Sweden	about 1
USA	0,04-0,08 (in California - 20 times more)

Consult Pawlowski and Schultz (1972) for references to data for individual countries. These authors also state that bovine cysticercosis is increasing in most of the countries listed.

In the USSR, a marked decrease in bovine cysticercosis has occurred during the last few years. From 1964 to 1972 the number of infected carcasses decreased from 1.09% to 0.38% (Fig. 2), i.e. 2.8 times. This has resulted from a campaign, conducted by health and veterinary authorities, to explain the etiology of the disease, to improve the diagnostic procedures and to provide mass treatment of the population. The eradication of bovine cysticercosis is less affected by the recent developments in the technology of industrialized cattle raising. Cattle due to their physiological peculiarities still frequently use pastures or are fed grass mown on these pastures. Thus little may be changed which affects the life cycle of the tapeworm responsible for the infection.

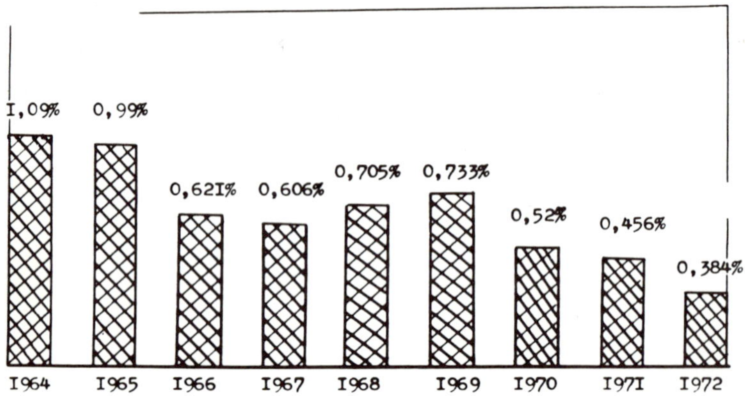

Fig. 2. The prevalence of bovine cysticercosis in the USSR during 1964 to 1972.

Indeed industrialization of animal husbandry and scientific progress even favour the distribution of *C. bovis*. The wide spread use of pastures irrigated by town sewage and increased tourism may increase pollution of pastures with human fecal material. The dispersion of *Taenia saginata* eggs on pastures (through sewage waters) or during fodder preparation may lead to light infection in 90% or more of animals exposed to such infection (Sitov *et al.*, 1969; Prat, 1971; Gladkov, 1972). Such light infections are difficult to detect by routine meat inspection methods. It has been estimated that meat inspectors may miss every fourth infected carcass, even when they are aware of the infection in a group of animals (Dewhirst *et al.*, 1967). The effectiveness of meat inspection can be increased by additional cuts in the meat in a larger number of muscle groups, but this makes the inspection more costly and renders the meat less valuable.

In the development of programmes for the eradication of bovine cysticercosis and human *Taenia* infection, the development of reliable and cheap methods for antemortem and postmortem diagnosis of *C. bovis*, the improvement of treatment of patients and wide educational programs to improve sanitary practices are of paramount importance.

ECHINOCOCCOSIS

Echinococcosis is still widely distributed in the world. The prevalence of larval echinococcosis in sheep, cattle and pigs in some countries reaches 40-70% and higher (Schantz and Schwabe, 1969) (Table 2). In the USSR the prevalence is also quite high with a tendency to a slow decline (Fig. 3). In spite of big efforts conducted in many countries only Iceland and Holland are at present near the goal of eradication (Schantz and Schwabe, 1969).

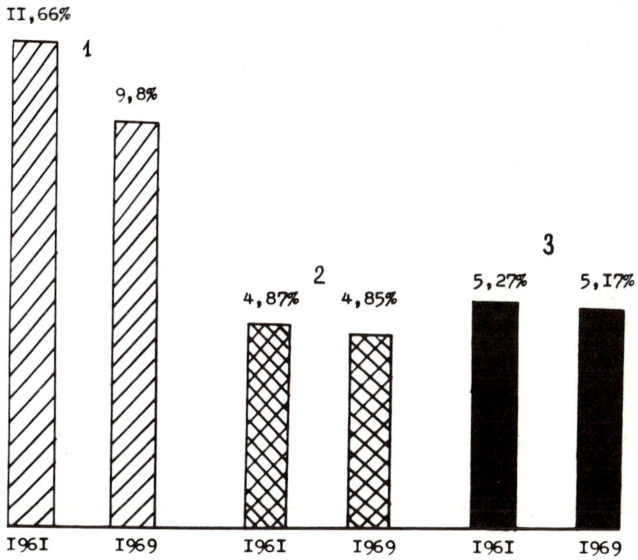

Fig. 3. The prevalence of larvae E. granulosus *in sheep (1), cattle (2) and pigs (3) in the USSR during 1961 to 1969.*

Epidemiological data on the distribution of echinococcosis shows that its prevalence remained at nearly the same level during the last several decades. Probably the prevalence will remain the same until marked changes take place in the host-parasite interrelationships and, particularly, in the technology of animal husbandry (Arundel, 1972). Industrialization of animal husbandry leads to marked changes in traditional habits and methods of management of animals. For example, mechanized sheep raising farms with indoor management, in the USSR and other countries has produced marked changes in host-parasite interrelationships by the elimination of the use of dogs for herding purposes. Eradication of echinococcosis in

Table 2

The prevalence of Echinococcus granulosus *in various countties (Data from Schantz and Schwabe, 1969).*

Countries	Animals infected (%)		
	Sheep	Cattle	Pigs
Algeria	21,8	30,5	-
Argentina	about 90,0	-	-
Australia[x]	-	31,01	-
Bulgaria	67,3	41,1	-
Chile	40,3	58,7	50,9
France[xx]	25,0-30-0	25,0-30,0	3,0
India	21,75	60,9	7,7
Iraq	29,5	13,9	-
Italy[xxx]	76,11	60,7	26,9
Yugoslavia	20,1	19,9	20,5
Lebanon	23,1	37,8	33,0-66,0
Morocco	2,3-80,0	43,0	-
Peru	40,0	-	-
Poland	-	-	20,1-35,5
Spain	10,8	39,8	8,8
Tunisia	20,0-60,0	about 100,0	-
Turkey	52,0	47,4	-
Uruguay	38,1-100,0	60,0	69,8

x Queensland xx Pyrenees xxx Sardinia

(Consult Schantz and Schwabe (1969) for references to data from individual countries).

these circumstances is possible. The same results can be achieved on sheep farms using a system of plot grazing, on industrial pig farms, or on fattening, breeding or dairy cattle farms where direct contact between animals and dogs is eliminated or reduced to a minimum.

The introduction of new technology in animal management will not lead to a rapid eradication of echinococcosis since it may take many years to put new methods of management into practice all over the world. Nevertheless a decline in echinococcosis incidence is to be expected in the near future as the technological methods are introduced into animal husbandry. However, with animal husbandry in remote and inaccessible areas, the prevalence of echinococcis is likely to remain high for many years.

TRICHINELLOSIS

Trichinellosis is widely distributed in the world and particularly in the northern hemisphere, but where also it has shown a tendency to decline gradually. In USA, after the introduction of the regulations for obligatory boiling of meat scraps used as food for pigs, the incidence of trichinellosis declined sharply (Zimmermann, 1971). A marked decrease has also been observed in the USSR. Thus the prevalence in pigs during 1962-1971 decreased 3.7 times. (Fig. 4).

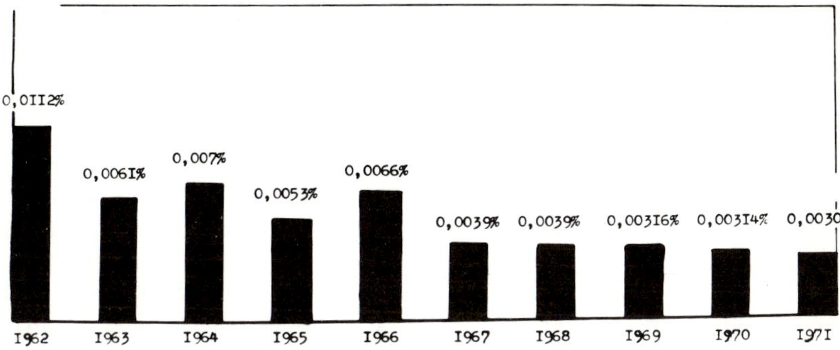

Fig. 4. The prevalence of Trichinella spiralis *in swine in the USSR during 1962 to 1971.*

The technology of industrial pig breeding in indoor farms where cereal food is used only for fodder has practically excluded all possibilities of infection of pigs. Trichinellosis still occurs where food (meat) scraps are used on pig farms and fur-bearing animal farms. On such farms, meat scraps and animal carcasses should be boiled before use.

With trichinellosis in wild animals, the possibility of infection of man and domestic animals from meat of game animals, remains at the same level. Indeed in some areas, with mass tourism and sport hunting its prevalence may become higher. Consequently, at present, total eradication of tricinellosis is possible only on pig farms.

SUMMARY

The present trends in animal husbandry, in our opinion, favour the eradication of pig cysticercosis *(C. cellulosae)*, echinococcosis, to a lesser extent cattle cysticercosis *(C. bovine)* and trichinellosis. For the last two zoonotic infections it is necessary to devise more adequate measures of control and prophylaxis and to increase educational programs to improve sanitary practices in areas where these infections occur.

REFERENCES

Arundel, J.H. (1972). *Austr. Vet. J. 48,* 140.
Bodrossy, L. (1972). *Magyar allatorv. lapja, 27*, 401.
Cironeanu, I., Popa, N. and Iliut, I. (1970). *Rev. Zootehn. Med. Vet., 20,* 81.
Dewhirst, L.W., Cramer, J.D. and Sheldon, J.J. (1967). *J. Amer. Vet. Med. Ass., 150,* 412.
Gladkov, G.N. (1972). *Proc. 8th Conf. Parasit. Ukrainian sssr,* part 1: 201.
Hiepe, T., Farchmin, G. and Buchwalder, R. (1967). *Dtsch. Gesundh. Wes. 22,* 371.
Pawlowski, Z. and Schultz, M.G. (1972). *Adv. Parasit. 10,* 269.
Prat, J. (1971). *Bull. Soc. Vet. France 55,* 161.
Schantz, P.M. and Schwabe, C. (1969). *J. Amer. Vet. Med. Ass. 155,* 2104.
Sitov, K.E., Avdeenko, P.I., Timofeev, E.P., Mulimarov, P.S. and Hairov, N.N. (1969). *Conf. USSR Helminth Soc.* (part 1) 268.
Soule, C., Chevrier, L. and Pantaleon, J. (1973). *Bull. Acad. Vet. France, 45,* 509.
Zimmermann, W.J. *Iowa St. Univ. Vet. 33,* 93.

IMMUNOLOGICAL STUDIES ON EXPERIMENTAL INFECTIONS WITH THE LARVAL STAGE OF *TAENIA SAGINATA*

M. M. H. Sewell and G. J. Gallie

Department of Tropical Animal Health, Royal (Dick) School of Veterinary Studies, Easter Bush, Roslin, Midlothian, Scotland.

Despite the development of efficient and acceptable taeniacidal drugs for use against the adult *Taenia saginata* tape worm in the human host, cysticercosis caused by the larval stage in cattle continues to be of considerable zoonotic and economic importance. The incidence is believed to be increasing in several European countries and its economic importance is particularly serious in those developing countries which possess, or are seeking to establish, a cattle rearing industry for which exports form an important part of the market.

Unfortunately the well-known techniques for controlling this parasite by treatment or hygienic measures designed to prevent the establishment of continuation of infection in man appear to be of limited efficacy, especially in poorly developed rural areas. There are several reasons for this, including the low pathogenicity of the parasite, the almost invariable need to modify long-standing dietary and social practices if hygienic control measures are to be successful and the tendency for existing hygiene facilities to become overloaded and inefficient with increasing populations.

Accordingly effective methods for controlling the infection in the bovine are greatly needed but there is to date no drug which will kill the cysts in cattle and, as there is no reliable means of ante-mortem diagnosis, present techniques to prevent transmission from cattle to man are based almost exclusively on routine post-mortem meat inspection procedures. In view of the very small proportion of the musculature examined such inspection must fail to detect the cysts in many of the epidemiologically significant but lightly infected carcases (Mann and Mann, 1947). Immuno-diagnostic methods have shown promise of affording a means of ante-mortem diagnosis in areas where the infection is not prevalent (Dewhirst *et al.*, 1967) but have been disappointing (Froyd, 1963) in areas where the incidence of the parasite is high and management conditions are such that many calves become infected at a very young age (Urquhart, 1961).

Nevertheless the immunological approach still seems to afford the most likely means of developing a useful technique for ante mortem diagnosis and it might also be possible to stimulate the host to react against and destroy the cysts in its musculature.

At one time, it seemed that this latter procedure would be quite simple. Penfold, Penfold and Phillips (1936) had shown in Australia that the cysticercus larvae of *T. saginata* do not survive in mature infected cattle for more than 9 months and that such cattle were thereafter solidly resistant to reinfection. It seemed therefore that adequate control would be attained by ensuring that cattle were exposed to infection more than 1 year before they were slaughtered for human consumption.

However, Dewhirst, Cramer and Pistor (1963) later found that cysts may survive for up to 639 days in calves first infected at 4-6 months of age. Furthermore, although Soulsby (1963) failed to find any viable cysts in calves slaughtered 9 months after initial infection at 4-6 months of age, such cysts were present in calves slaughtered 9 months after they had been infected during their first few days of life. Moreover, these calves not only failed to destroy their initial burden of cysts, but also failed to resist a challenge infection given at 9 months of age. Also, in contrast to the animals initially infected at 4-6 months of age, these younger calves developed only a weak complement fixing antibody response, with a median maximum titre of 1:10 as opposed to 1:160 in the older animals (Soulsby, 1963).

Yet all these observations conflicted with the experience in the field in areas where this infection is prevalent. In these circumstances many adult animals carry viable cysts, usually in small but epidemiologically significant numbers (Mann and Mann, 1947), and in Kenya, such cysts are known to survive in cattle for at least 2 years (Froyd, 1964a). Nevertheless, also in Kenya, Urquhart (1961) and Froyd (1964b), have both shown that calves become almost completely resistant to reinfection by about 4 months of age. An investigation of this apparently anomalous situation in which the cattle do not destroy their existing burden but are strongly resistant to reinfection is being undertaken with the ultimate two-fold aim of developing a procedure which will cause such calves to destroy the cysts in their musculature and also a method of ante mortem detection of calves which are long-term carriers of this parasite. Most of the techniques used in these studies, and the results, have been described in detail by Gallie and Sewell (1972, 1974a & b).

The first experiment was designed to study the development of resistance to *T. saginata* in calves first infected at 3 months of age. There were 3 calves in the infected group and

2 in the challenge control group. The initial infection comprised 100,000 *T. saginata* eggs and the challenge infection of 150,000 eggs were given to the animals at 1 year of age. A previously uninfected 10 day old calf was given a dose of 10,000 eggs from the same pool as that used for the challenge infection. All six animals were slaughtered 3-5 weeks after challenge. The proportion of the challenge infection that became established in the young calf was 13.7%, which is very similar to the mean figure of 13.8% for the challenge controls. This suggests that age per se has little effect on resistance to an initial infection with *T. saginata* and is thus in agreement with the observations described by Penfold, Penfold and Phillips (1936) and by Urquhart (1961). However the mean proportion of the challenge dose which became established in the previously infected calves was only 3.4 ± 2.1% and most of the cysts in these animals were clearly degenerating. This degeneration was occurring in both the challenge and the pre-challenge cysts, only three of the latter cysts appearing superficially normal.

It therefore appears that these calves, which were first infected at 3 months of age, were in the process of developing their ability both to acquire resistance to reinfection with *T. saginata* and to destroy cysts present in their muscles, but that they were not as competent in either of these functions as the adult cattle infected by Penfold, Penfold and Phillips (1936) or calves first infected when they were 4-6 months old by Soulsby (1963). Schoop and Lamina (1970) have also shown that small numbers of cysts survive for at least 11 months in calves first infected at 8-10 weeks of age.

It seemed possible that the difference between the field observations and those in experimental animals arises because of the continual but probably low-level challenge under the former circumstances. An experiment was therefore designed to replicate the field situation in this respect (Gallie and Sewell, 1972). A total of 16 calves was used and 11 of these received a dose of 10,000 *T. saginata* eggs at 2-3 days of age. One of these calves was killed 5 weeks later and was found to contain 497 cysts, thus demonstrating the infectivity of the eggs used for this initial dose. Five of the remaining calves formed the serial infection group and received 500 *T. saginata* eggs each week for 1 year. The other 5 calves formed the single neonatal infection group. Finally, when they were 1 year old, all 10 calves plus 5 previously uninfected calves - the challenge control group - received a challenge infection with 50,000 *T. saginata* eggs and were killed 18-32 days later.

In the group of calves that had received the single neonatal infection, 12.1 ± 5.9% of the challenge dose of eggs developed to form cysts and this proportion was not significantly different from that of 16.3 ± 6.0% recovered from the calves in the challenge group. Thus, as had been previously shown by Soulsby (1963), the single neonatal infection had not rendered the calves significantly more resistant to later reinfection. In contrast the calves which had received the serial infections were strongly resistant to reinfection, the only reinfection cysts observed in such calves being 8 dead cysts in one animal. On the other hand, both the single neonatal infection and the serial infections led to the presence of small numbers of pre-challenge cysts in the calves, although there was no significant difference between the two groups as regards either the total numbers of pre-challenge cysts or the proportion that were alive. One calf in the single neonatal infection group contained no pre-challenge cysts and two further calves in each group contained only dead pre-challenge cysts.

The results of indirect haemagglutination assays (Boyden, 1951) on the sera from animals in these two experiments are shown in Fig. 1. The antigen used in these assays was a saline extract of *T. saginata* strobila.

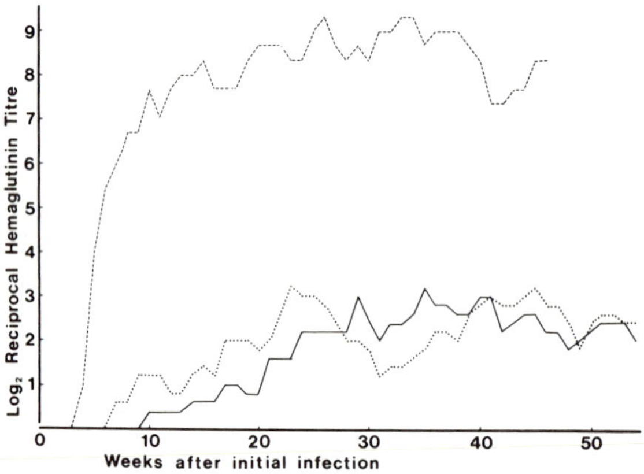

Fig. 1. Mean haemagglutination titres of sera from calves infected with the larval cysts of Taenia saginata.

----- *3 calves infected with 100,000 eggs at 3 months of age.*
····· *5 calves neonatally infected with 10,000 eggs.*
——— *5 calves neonatally infected with 10,000 eggs and also with 500 eggs each week for 1 year.*

The titres rose more slowly and tended to be lower in the calves receiving the neonatal infection than in the calves first infected at 3 months of age. Thus the peak titres in the latter calves ranged from 1:128 to 1:4000, whereas only one calf in the group which had received the single neonatal infection developed a titre of 1:256, the second highest peak titre in this group was 1:64 and the maximum titre in any of the calves receiving the serial infection was 1:32. One calf in each of the neonatally infected groups failed to develop any haemagglutinins although both of these calves contained pre-challenge cysts when they were killed. By the end of the experiment the titres were tending to fall in the other calves in both these groups and by that time haemagglutinins could not be detected in two calves from each group.

There was no correlation between the haemagglutinin titres and resistance to reinfection in either experiment or between these titres and the numbers or viability of the pre-challenge cysts in the neonatally infected calves.

The infected calves also developed precipitating antibodies against the same antigenic preparation but immunochemical studies have shown that these involve different antigenic components to those in the haemagglutination reaction. These precipitins tended to be weaker and less complex in the neonatally infected calves. One of the control animals in the first experiment also developed precipitating antibodies, which gave a reaction of identity in a micro-gel diffusion test (Crowle, 1958) with one of the lines formed by the sera from the calves first infected at 3 months of age. Again there was no consistent difference between the precipitin responses in the calves receiving the single neonatal infection or the serial infections. Only one calf failed to develop any detectable precipitins, this animal being in the serially dose group.

Thus it appears that the serial dosing had replicated the field situation sufficiently well to cause the calves to become strongly resistant to infection with *T. saginata*, without necessarily destroying the cysts already in their muscles and without developing a strong serological response. In particular, the neonatal infection had not resulted in the calves developing a tolerance to reinfection.

As a first step towards attempting to use immunological means to stimulate calves to destroy neonatally acquired *T. saginata* cysts, studies have been undertaken on methods of vaccinating 6 month old and 1 month old calves. These were in large measure replicating and extending the studies described by Wikerhauser, Zukovic and Dzakula (1971).

In the first of these experiments there were 4 groups of 3 six month old calves in each group. These groups included a challenge control group, an infected control group which had received an oral dose of 25,000 *T. saginata* eggs, one experimental group which had received an intra-muscular injection of 22,000 living hatched *T. saginata* oncospheres and a second experimental group given a non-living vaccine consisting of a saline homogenerate of *T. saginata* strobila incorporated in Freund's adjuvant. All the groups were challenged orally 3 months after vaccination with 30,000 *T. saginata* eggs and killed and examined after a further 3 months.

The calves in the challenge control group contained 1849 ± 1351 cysts, but both the oral infection and the living vaccine caused the calves to become totally resistant to reinfection and the non-living vaccine had virtually the same effect, as only one dead cyst was found in any of the calves in this group. This last was a surprising result as such vaccines are not commonly effective in inducing resistance to helminths. Accordingly, the observation requires confirmation. The pre-challenge cysts in the group, which had received the living vaccine, were all located at the injection site. As compared with the orally infected calves, there was a strong serological response in the calves which had received the non-living vaccine, but only a weak response in the calves which had received the living vaccine.

The second of these experiments was a pilot study concerned with the possibility of vaccinating 1 month old calves and there were only 2 calves in each of the 3 groups. The calves in the vaccinated group and the vaccine control group each received 25,000 living hatched *T. saginata* oncospheres by intra-muscular injection. Six weeks later the calves in the vaccinated group and those in the third group - the challenge control group - were each given 25,000 *T. saginata* eggs orally. All the calves were killed and examined 12 weeks later.

Moderate numbers (31 - 849) of small cysts were found closely packed together at the injection sites in all the vaccinated calves. A small number of the injected oncospheres (1 and 15) had migrated from the inoculation site in the vaccine controls and were dispersed throughout the musculature. Such migration has been seen in other young calves. Similar numbers (1 and 35) of dispersed cysts were found in the calves in the vaccinated group and their origin cannot be determined with certainty, although the numbers are not inconsistent with these also being derived from the vaccine. On the other hand both the animals in the challenge control group contained over 3,000 cysts dispersed throughout their musculature. Thus, despite the small numbers of animals, it would seem that the vaccinated calves had at least acquired a strong resistence to reinfection.

It is intended that future studies will include investigations on the effect of such vaccines on the viability of pre-existing cysts in neonatally infected calves and on the effect of various infection schedules on the numbers of cysts surviving for a prolonged period in the musculature of calves.

ACKNOWLEDGEMENTS

We would wish to acknowledge the financial support of the Overseas Development Administration of the Foreign and Commonwealth Office and the facilities provided at the Centre for Tropical Veterinary Medicine by Professor Sir Alexander Robertson. We are also most grateful for the regular supplies of gravid segments and strobila of *T. saginata* from Dr. I. Mann of A.H.I.T.I., Kenya and his colleagues Mr. and Mrs. Leegwater, and for further supplies of such material from Professor Z. Pawlowski of Poznan, Poland, and Mr. A.V.H. Allen of the Hospital for Tropical Diseases, London.

REFERENCES

Boyden, S.V. (1951). *J. exp. Med.*, *93*, 107.
Crowle, A.J. (1958). *J. Lab. clin. Med.*, *52*, 784.
Dewhirst, L.W., Cramer, J.D. and Pistor, W.J. (1963). *J. Parasit.* *49*, 297.
Dewhirst, L.W., Cramer, J.D. and Sheldon, J.J. (1967). *J. Amer. Vet. Med. Ass.* *150*, 412.
Froyd, G. (1963). *Bull. epiz. Dis. Afr.* *11*, 303.
Froyd, G. (1964a). *Brit. Vet. J.* *120*, 205.
Froyd, G. (1964b). *Res. Vet. Sci.* *5*, 434.
Gallie, G.J. and Sewell, M.M.H. (1972). *Vet. Rec.* *91*, 481.
Gallie, G.J. and Sewell, M.M.H. (1974a). *Trop. Anim. Hlth. Prod.* (In press)
Gallie, G.J. and Sewell, M.M.H. (1974b). *Trop. Anim. Hlth. Prod.* (In press)
Mann, I. and Mann, E. (1947). *Vet. J.* *103*, 239.
Penfold, W.J., Penfold, H.B. and Phillips, M. (1936). *Med. J. Aust.* *i*, 417.
Schoop, G. and Lamina, J. (1970). *Dtsch. tierärztl. Wschr.* *77*, 153.
Soulsby, E.J.L. (1963). *Proc. 17th Wld. vet. Cong., Hannover*, 761.
Urquhart, G.M. (1961). *J. Parasit.* *47*, 857.
Wikerhauser, T., Zukovic, M. and Dzakula, N. (1970). *Expt. Parasit.* *30*, 36.

IMMUNIZATION OF CALVES AGAINST THE INFECTION WITH *TAENIA SAGINATA*. INTRAMUSCULAR AND SUBCUTANEOUS VACCINATION WITH THE HOMOLOGOUS ONCOSPHERES AND EGGS

T. Wikerhauser, M. Žuković, N. Džakula and B. Maran

Veterinary Faculty, University of Zagreb, Zagreb, Yugoslavia

In previous small-scale experiments, we have demonstrated that calves can be immunized against cysticercosis (*Cysticercus bovis*) by intramuscular injection of artificially hatched, homologous, oncospheres. A post-vaccinal colony of cysticerci that developed at the site of injection apparently protected the animal against subsequent oral challenge. However, it also caused some damage to the affected muscles. Since a subcutaneous localization of post-vaccinal cysticerci might cause less damage, the present study compared the value of subcutaneous vaccination with that of intramuscular. Additionally the immunizing effect of eggs was compared with that of hatched oncospheres.

Twenty calves, of a few weeks of age, were divided into 5 groups of 4 animals. Four groups were vaccinated intramuscularly or subcutaneously in the neck region with 25,000 hatched oncospheres or eggs of *Taenia saginata* respectively and one group served as controls. Hatched oncospheres was produced *in vitro* by artificial digestion fluids. Two weeks later all animals were challenged orally with 150,000 viable eggs of *T. saginata*. The calves were slaughtered 17-18 weeks after the challenge. At the post-mortem examination muscles and organs were sliced and all living and dead cysts counted.

The results are presented in Table 1. Complete protection was induced in 2 calves which were vaccinated intramuscularly with hatched oncospheres and which developed cysticerci at the site of injection (Fig. 1). In the subcutaneously vaccinated group however, in spite of the establishment of a post-vaccinal colony of cysticerci, complete protection did not occur. In calves vaccinated with the eggs, neither a post-vaccinal colony of cysticerci nor immunity was observed. In the non-vaccinated control calves, a marked variation in cyst numbers was evident.

In the two completely resistant calves (no. 3 and 4) and in 2 calves with a low degree of infection (no. 2 and 20) the liver had gross lesions which on the histologic examination showed traumatic eosinophilic hepatitis. Similar lesions were found also in 2 calves with severe cysticercosis (no. 5 and 19) indicating that these lesions were not related to the

Table 1

Number of Cysts Found 17-18 Weeks After Feeding 150,000 Eggs of Taenia saginata *to Calves Vaccinated 2 Weeks Previously With 25,000 Hatched Homologous Oncospheres of Eggs, and to Controls.*

Group	Calf	Vaccination	Number of cysts: At inoculation site	Number of cysts: In other muscles and organs
I	1	Hatched	16* (15)	280 (244)
	2	oncospheres	52 (52)	146 (112)
	3	i/m.	300 (300)	0
	4		218 (193)	0
II	5	Hatched	145 (145)	1584 (1417)
	6	oncospheres	32 (32)	661 (477)
	7	s/c.	250 (25)	67 (60)
	8		41 (41)	2423 (2207)
III	9	Eggs	0	729 (624)
	10	i/m.	0	887 (90)
	11		0	1250 (941)
	12		0	739 (739)
IV	13	Eggs	0	412 (353)
	14	s/c.	0	1315 (1087)
	15		0	1963 (1716)
	16		0	2023 (1421)
V	17			283 (244)
	18			1041 (978)
	19			1714 (342)
	20			13 (1)

*Figures in parenthesis indicate the number of viable cysts.

state of immunity of the infected animal. The mean percentage of dead cysts was markedly higher in the heart than in the skeletal muscles. In the heart this percentage was 58.41 whereas in the skeletal muscles it was 20.16.

SUMMARY

Intra muscular immunization with living oncospheres in-

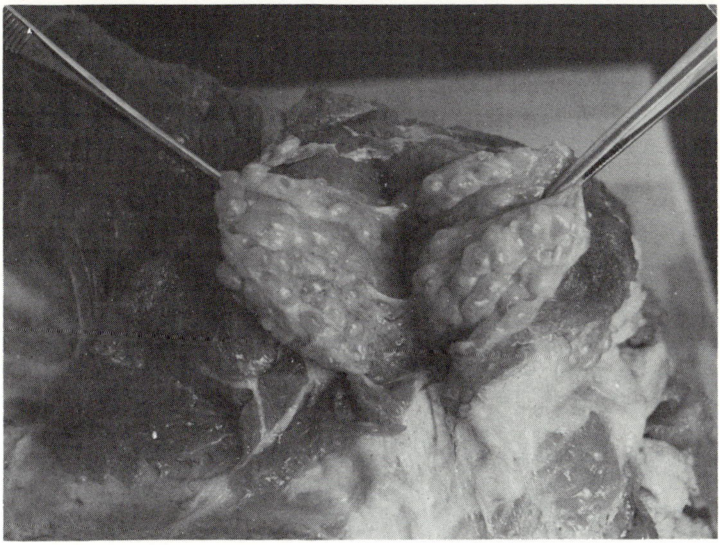

Fig. 1. Post-vaccinal colony of cysticerci at the site of infection of hatched oncospheres x 2/3.

duced complete protection against oral challenge with *T. saginata* eggs in 2 of 4 calves. Calves immunized by subcutaneous injection of oncospheres did not resist a challenge infection. In all calves injected with oncospheres, a focus of cysticerci developed at the site of injection.

Calves vaccinated with unhatched eggs did not develop a focus of cysticerci at the site of injection, neither did they show evidence of immunity to the challenge infection.

ACKNOWLEDGEMENT

This research was supported by the U. S. Department of Agriculture PL 480 Grant FG-YU-216.

REFERENCES

Wikerhauser, T., Žuković, M. and Džakula, N. (1971). *Expt. Parasit. 30,* 36.

Wikerhauser, T., Zuković, M., Dzakula, N. and Maran, B. (1971) *Proc. 1st Collg. Europ. Parasit.* Rennes p. 39

CYSTICEROCOSIS IN PIGS DUE TO INFECTION WITH *TAENIA SOLIUM* LINNAEUS, 1758.

I. V. HERBERT AND CARLOS OBERG

Department of Applied Zoology, University College of North Wales, Bangor, United Kingdom and Instituto de Patologia Animal, Facultad de Medicina Veterinaria, Universidad Austral de Chile, Valdivia, Chile.

An increasing interest is currently focused on zoonoses caused by the taeniid cestodes, not only on account of the disease problems they cause in humans, but also because of the serious economic losses they incur in animal production. The FAO/WHO Animal Health Yearbook (1973) records the prevalence of various zoonotic taeniid cestode infections in farm livestock, from those countries that produce statistics. However, it is clear that this represents estimates of infections rather than those which actually exist. The persistence of these infections, frequently on a grand scale, in humans, domesticated animals or wild animals is a continual reminder of the ineffectiveness of existing methods for the detection of these infections as well as of a failure to produce workable legislation to prevent infection.

This paper presents a review of present information and the results of preliminary studies into the pathogenesis of *Taenia solium* cysticercosis (*Cysticercus cellulosae*) in pigs, with particular reference to the post-mortem detection of infection and the correlation of these findings with serological studies performed in the living animal during the course of infection. This study represents the only attempt, the authors are aware of, to study these parameters in experimentally infected animals.

The serological diagnosis of metacestode infections in domesticated animals has long proven difficult. This is due to the marked cross-reactivity found between infections with one taeniid metacestode and another (Kagan, 1968). In Chile the other cestode infections commonly found in pigs are *Taenia hydatigena* and *Echinococcus granulosus*. Studies on the serological specificity of different diagnostic tests are clearly necessary, as is an understanding of the scope of the problem of *T. solium* cysticercosis.

Stoll (1947) estimated that 2.5 million people in the world were infected with *T. solium*. Though it seems likely that the number of infected persons has decreased since that time in certain countries, it is clear that the infection is still widespread in India, Indo China, China, U.S.S.R., South Africa, Mexico, and much of Central and South America. With the advent of satisfactory drugs to eliminate the taeniid parasites in humans it is probable that many infections are treated by medical practitioners without the prevalence or the identification of the parasite being noted. The work of Proctor (1972) has shown that the differential diagnosis of human infections with adult *T. solium* or *T. saginata* based on the numbers of lateral uterine branches of a gravid proglottid passed in faeces is no longer tenable. Proctor (1972) has described other features of use in the true identification of gravid proglottids in human faeces.

The importance of human cysticercosis has recently been reviewed by Marquez-Monter (1971).

Life history and epidemiology

Taenia solium infection is described as an obligatory cyclozoonosis (Schwabe, 1969), an anthropozoonotic helminthiasis (Sprent, 1969) or euzoonosis (Garnham, 1958). Each classification holds in common the fact that man is one of the essential, or usual, hosts involved in the life cycle. Man is the usual definitive host, though experimental infection of the lar gibbon (*Hylobates lar lar*) in Thailand has been described (Cadigan *et al.*, 1967). Nelson *et al.*, (1965) states that the adult worm will develop to some extent in the dog. Sandground (1936) considered that the taenias can persist as adults for 20 - 34 years.

Ripe onchospheres will hatch only following passage through the stomach of a suitable host. They hatch in the duodenum and penetrate the blood vessels of the tunica propria. The young cysticerci are visible in the muscles and organs between 6 and 12 days after infection where they grow and become cystic (Yoshino, 1933). The young cysts may migrate through the liver, causing linear haemorrhages in the parenchyma (Herbert, Oberg and Gonzales, unpublished). The 'bladder worm' is considered to be fully developed and infective within the musculature after 60 days (Yoshino, 1933) or 110 days (von Ostertag, 1897). Slais (1970) considers that the cysticercus is essentially a parasite of the lymphatic system and eventually locates in those regions where it lodges as an embolus. In heavy infections cysticerci may locate in the liver, lungs, subcutaneous fat and in the lymph nodes.

Mature proglottids are frequently shed in non-motile ribbons and not as single motile proglottids as is the case for *T. saginata*. This fact alone can explain the common finding of massive cysticercosis in pigs compared with the relatively low density of *T. saginata* infections in bovines (Viljoen, 1937).

Man, primates, wild carnivores and domestic dogs, wild hogs, some deer, even sheep and cats have been reported to harbour the cysticercus, though the development and infectivity of the cysticercus in animals other than man, pigs, domestic dogs and the spider monkey (*Ateles geoffroyi*) has not been described. Dogs may play an important role in the infection of S.E. Asia and the Malagasy Republic where dogmeat is eaten by humans. Reports of infections in dogs in South America are those of Hernandez *et al.*, (1966) in Peru, and Gallo and Vogelsang (1951) in Venezuela.

Man can be infected with the cysticercus in two ways. He may ingest onchospheres which contaminate his food and drink, or ripe proglottids of an established adult worm may pass to the stomach by a process of retro-peristalsis where eggs are stimulated to hatch following contact with the gastric juices. When onchospheres reach the small intestine, they hatch and subsequently invade the musculature or brain tissue. For this reason, infection with an adult *T. solium* is a potentially serious condition deserving special attention.

Man usually harbours only one taenia though Bull (1962) found 4 specimens in one patient in Concepcion, Chile and Donckaster and Donoso (1960), also in Chile, recorded a mixed infection of *Taenia solium* and *T. saginata*.

Figure 1., taken from an official agency of the Chilean government (SOCOAGRO), shows the prevalence of *T. solium* cysticercosis as detected in the abattoirs in Chile controlled by this agency. These are the only reliable statistics available. They also describe, for comparison, the infections due to other metacestodes of pigs, *Echinococcus granulosus* and *Taenia hydatigena (Cysticercus tenuicollis)*. A continuing low level of infection with *T. solium* cysticercosis has been maintained over the period of available records. Infection with this parasite results in total condemnation of the carcass, whereas this rarely happens with the other two infections. Consequently, the loss of meat for human consumption is much greater, even though the incidence is less than the other two forms of cysticercosis.

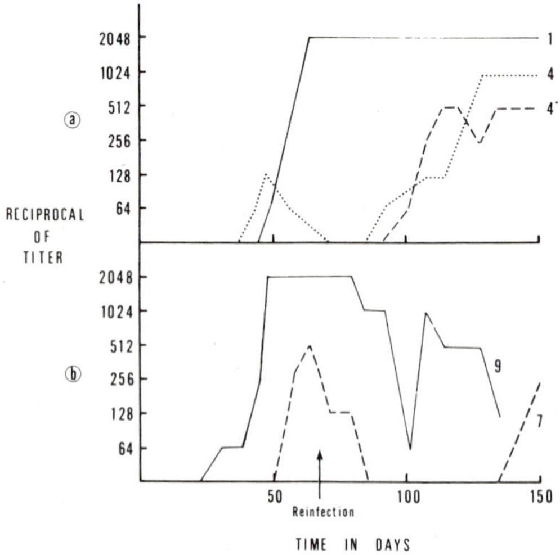

Fig. 1. The prevalence of hydatidosis, cysticercosis (Taenia solium) *and cysticercosis* (Taenia hydatigena) *in pigs in Chile 1965 - 1972. Data from SOCOAGRO and S.A.G. Ordinate: Percentage of infected animals slaughtered in the abattoirs of SOCOAGRO.*

Table 1 shows the findings of cysticercosis from human autopsies and of clinical cases of taeniasis observed in the hospital of the University of Chile in Santiago. Adult *T. solium* is found much less frequently than *T. saginata*, despite the fact that bovine cysticercosis *(T. saginata)* is an extremely rare finding in Chilean abattoirs.

This situation is due probably to several factors including incorrect differentiation of ripe proglottids (see Proctor, 1972), the failure to diagnose some cases of bovine cysticercosis in the abattoir, the eating of non-inspected meat, and the importation of infected meat from abroad. Proctor points out that, in South Africa, *T. solium* cysticerosis is common but the finding of the adult tapeworm is relatively rare. Nelson *et al.*, (1965) consider that many cysticerci identified as *C. cellulosae* are incorrectly identified.

The persistence of the adult *T. solium* in man and cysticercosis in man and pigs is due to several social and economic factors. Pigs would not become infected if man did not leave his faeces around for them (and dogs) to scavange. In many parts of the world, in the absence of water closets, people defaecate out in the open. Even if they have privies they have periodically to empty them, which they do frequently by distributing the faecal material over the land as fertilizer. In South America, and undoubtedly elsewhere, many

Table 1

INCIDENCE OF TAENIASIS AND CYSTICERCOSIS IN MAN IN THE HOSPITAL OF LA UNIVERSIDAD DE CHILE

A. Adult Tapeworm Infections

	T. saginata	*T. solium*	RATIO *T. saginata* : *T. solium*
1952*	not recorded	not recorded	25 : 1
1961**	176	15	14 : 1
1961-68***	573	70	8 : 1
1967	24	7	34 : 1
1968	72	11	6.5 : 1
1969	63	26	2.4 : 1
1970	66	22	3 : 1

Data from Doncaster and Donoso (1960*), Faiguenbaum (1961**) and Reyes (Personal Communication***)

B. Larval Cestode Infections

1939-1966**** (of 5,132 autopsies)	0	39
1947-1966***** (of 41,799 autopsies)	0	16

Data from Barrientos *et al.*, (1967****) and Schenone & Reyes (1968*****).

families of farmworkers have their own small group of free-ranging pigs which are fed household scraps but are left, in the main, to scavange anything else available. Such animals are slaughtered at home for home consumption or sold to aid the family budget. This situation is found also on state-owned farms (Asentamientos) in Chile. Such animals never enter official statistics concerned with either livestock production or with prevalence of infection. How much of this non-inspected food finds its way into restaurants and the like is open to conjecture.

A major source of infection is inadequately treated human excretment used as fertilizer or when, in aqueous suspension, used in the irrigation of vegetable or other crops. Men work amongst and handle such crops, as do the vendors and purchasers. The crops may be eaten raw after 'washing'.

The eggs of *Taenia solium* readily stick to hands and other surfaces and infection may be passed by persons infected with the adult worm by contamination of foodstuffs. Cysticerci readily stick to the hands and in the case of persons handling fresh meat, oral infection with cysticerci may readily occur.

IMMUNOLOGY OF LARVAL T. SOLIUM *INFECTIONS*

In vivo Manifestations

The immunological responses to metacestode infections have been reviewed by Gemmell and Macnamara (1972). It is clear that little is known of the response either of the pig or man to *T. solium* cysticercosis. The 'pre-encystment' and 'post-encystment' (Gemmell and Soulsby, 1968) immune responses described for the other metacestode infections have not been described.

The writers experimentally infected 7 of a litter of 9 pigs with *T. solium* eggs as described in Table 2.

Table 2

Number of eggs of Taenia solium *administered to pigs*

No. of pigs	*Taenia solium* 1st dose	*Taenia solium* 2nd dose	Time of slaughter or death after infection	Cysts found at necropsy as percentage of eggs fed
1	6,300	0	5 months	2.2
2	0	0	5 months	-
3	4,500	0	5 months	1.71
4	2,250	0	5 months	6.31
5	0	0	5 months	-
6	2,250	10,000	5 months	0.106
7	4,500	10,000	10 months	0.00
8	2,250	10,000	10 months	0.37
9*	6,750	10,000	9½ months	0.00

* died at 9½ months of age

No clinical signs were seen in any of these animals. Four of the 7 infected animals were reinfected 2 months after the initial infection. Five months after the initial infection, or 10 months later in the case of the reinfected animals, the animals were slaughtered and examined for cysticerci by means of serial cuts made in the heart, tongue, maseter, intercostal, anconial and ham muscles. The brain was also examined. Though it is probable that not all cysts were observed the percentage of eggs fed which were recovered as cysts after 5 months varied from 1.71 - 6.31%, the highest figure being from the animal receiving the lowest dose. Only 2 of the reinfected animals showed cysticerci at slaughter, 0.106% and 0.37% of eggs fed were recovered as cysticerci. It is emphasised that there are preliminary results based on small numbers of experimental animals and needing further corroboration, but the recovery was highest where the number of onchospheres fed was least, and the results from the reinfected animals suggest either a gradual elimination of cysticerci with time or that the reinfection accelerated cysticercus degeneration and absorption. The latter explanation would be supported by the findings from infections with other metacestodes. Leikina *et al.*, (1964) and Gemmell (1970) found that superinfection with *T. saginata* in bovines and of *T. hydatigena* in sheep, respectively, may cause the death of the initial infection. It is noteworthy that here the *T. solium* cysticerci were found in those reinfected animals which had received the lowest initial infections. Doubtless differences from this situation, but the longevity of cysticerci in single or multiple infections needs to be further investigated.

In all of the necropsy findings quoted by the writers, the number of cysticerci found varied from 13 to 142. Viljoen (1937) considered that the finding of 10 cysticerci or more in an animal constituted a heavy infection, though numbers greatly in excess of this are frequently found in nature.

Various authors (Neumann, 1892; von Ostertag, 1934; Viljoen, 1937; Slais, 1970; Herbert and Oberg, 1972) have seen degenerating cysticerci in pigs. It is now known if an immunological reaction is involved though the results presented above indicate that it may be. Slais considered that the cysticerci of *T. solium* die of senility, though he thought that the high antibody levels found in bovines infected with the cysticercus of *T. saginata* destroy ingested larvae immediately following reinfection.

Host response to the cysticercus of *T. solium* during life is slight (Meyenburg, 1923) and pathological manifestations are said to be associated with the death of the parasite (Smyth and Heath, 1970). A different situation may pertain depending upon whether the cysticerci are located in the musculature or in a vital part of the brain (Slais, 1970; Hernandez - Jauregui *et al.*, 1973). Death of the cysticercus is said to lead to resorption, caseation and calcification. Neumann (1892) refers to 'dry measles' which are hard, compact, grain-like, calcified cysticerci which remain in the flesh. The writers occasionally observed such grainlike structures from the infected pigs and these frequently stuck to the hands during dissection.

It seems reasonable to suppose from the results of the single infections detailed here that the cysticerci of *T. solium* degenerate gradually. Viljoen (1937) quotes von Ostertag as stating that cysticercus degeneration occurs simultaneously throughout the body though Viljoen found degenerated and viable cysticerci in the same animal.

Such is the low level of host reaction against *C. cellulosae* that at low infection levels the host response may be one of tolerance. Such cysticerci may die of senility. Higher levels of infection may provoke a host response which reduces the longevity of the cysticerci.

Gemmell and Macnamara (1972) have drawn attention to the similarity of host derived and metacestode derived antigens and the possibility that some of these may be involved in permitting the long term survival of the parasite. It is possible that such a situation is widespread in infections with metacestodes.

In Vitro Manifestations

The *in vitro* manifestations of immunity in the pig have been studied by various workers, including Soltys, (1936); Trawinsky (1936); Biagi and Tay, (1958); Biagi *et al.*, (1961); Proctor and Elsden-Dew (1966) and Herbert and Oberg (1972). All, with the exception of Herbert and Oberg (1972), have studied serological responses in natural infections, comparing their findings with post-mortem data. The precipitin tests have not given satisfactory results, since they are not sufficiently sensitive. The complement fixation test was thought by Biagi *et al.*, (1961) to give too many false positive reactions. Indeed, the complement fixation reaction involving porcine serum and helminth antigen has frequently been unreliable due to the unusual stability of the C_3 fraction of porcine complement and the pro or anti complementary action of helminth antigens. Biagi *et al.*, (1961) considered the indirect haemaglutination reaction (IHR) to be of greatest use and this test has been used by subsequent investigators, even though positive reactions have been found in animals in which cysticerci were not found at slaughter. This finding may be explained, however, by the elimination of an established infection in some pigs.

In our study of experimental infections with *T. solium* (see Table 2) and *T. hydatigena* (unpublished) infections in pigs we have followed the course of infection by means of various serological tests. Immediate 'wheal and flare' skin tests were used 119 days after initial infection of pigs with *T. solium* eggs to see if it was possible to diagnose infection by this test. The test gave anomolous results and passive cutaneous anaphylaxis tests (PCA) were done using the sera from these animals. The IHR, modified from W. J. Herbert (1973) but using porcine red blood cells and porcine serum as diluent, was also used to follow the course of infection. The antigens used were saline extracts and the specificity of the serological reactions were examined by using antigens prepared from the cysticerci of *T. solium* and *T. hydatigena* and by cross reacting these with sera taken from animals infected with either parasite.

The results of the immediate 'wheal and flare' skin test bore little relationship with the results of the other serological tests. The reactions were non-specific, and false positive and false negative results occurred. The PCA reaction, which can be used to identify the same antibody (i.e. reaginic or homocytotropic antibody) bore out these findings (see Table 3).

Table 3

The PCA Reaction in 7 pigs Infected with eggs of T. solium *and 3 Infected with Eggs of* T. hydatigena, *Using the Cyst Antigen of* T. solium. *The Antigen was Intravenously Injected 4 Hours after the Intradermal Injection of the Test Sera into Recipient Pigs.*

Pig No.	Days post infection	Treatment of serum	Reaction	Diameter of reaction (mm)
2	157	-	-	-
3	157	-	+	5
4	30	-	-	-
4	92	-	+	4
4	157	-	-	-
6	92	-	+	3
6	157	-	+	3
6	157	56°C for 2 hours	+	2
7	251	-	-	-
8	251	-	-	-
8	251	56°C for 2 hours	-	-
9	137	-	+	4
9	137	56°C for 2 hours	+	5
63*	64	-	-	-
89*		-	-	-
92*	57	-	-	-
Rabbit 2			+	7
Rabbit 4			+	5

* Infected with *T. hydatigena*

The PCA reaction, where antigen challenge was performed 72 hours after intradermal injection of test sera into recipient pigs, were all negative. The PCA tests done 4 hours after intradermal injection showed a positive response of a low order. Table 3 summarizes these results. Though these results are a preliminary indication of the need for a wider study, it is of interest that the earliest PCA reaction occurred 92 days after infection, and had disappeared by day 251 in two animals (7 and 8) which had been reinfected (see Table 2). No false positive reactions were seen where sera from *T. hydatigena* infected animals was included in the test. Serum from rabbits sensitised to the antigen, when included in the PCA test reactions, showed a heterocytotropic antibody response.

These findings require further examination. Brunner (1928) reported a positive (though low grade) P.K. reaction in *T. solium* infected humans, though he did not state what the time interval was between injection of serum and challenge with antigen. Further Herbert, Rumpus and Smith (unpublished) have shown that some pigs may not produce homocytotropic antibody which is demonstrable in PCA tests during infections with *Hyostrongylus rubidus* even though the majority of pigs do so.

The IHR results are detailed in Fig. 2.

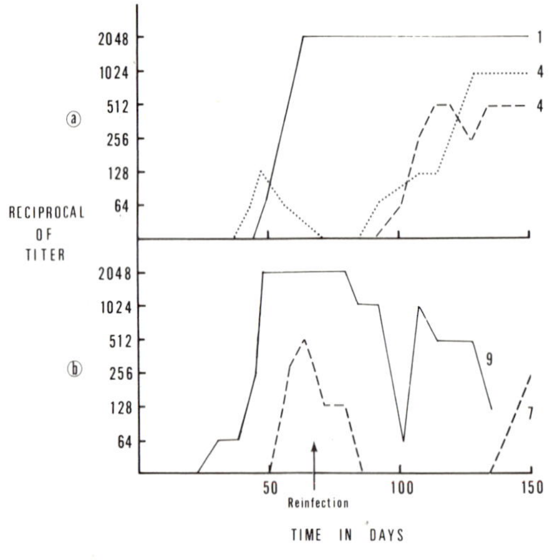

Fig. 2. The IHA titres of pigs infected with eggs of T. solium, *taken during the first 150 days of infection. (Details of the infection: see Table 2). A titre of 1:64 is arbitrarily accepted as a positive titre.*
Titres above 1:2048 are not recorded.
(a) Once infected animals. 4 = Serum from animal No. 4. reacted against* C. cellulosae *antigen. 4 Serum from animal No. 4 reacted against* C. tenuicollis *antigen.*
(b) Reinfected animals.

Comparison of these results with the finding of cysticerci at necropsy (see Table 1), showed that the titres rose to a maximum during a period of 50-100 days after infection, the height of the titre and its duration being related to the level of initial infection. The titres gradually fell and there was no evidence of an anamnestic response in those animals which were reinfected except in one instance (pig no. 7). One of the non-infected control animals gave a positive response more than 100 days after the time the other animals had been infected and one of the infected animals never developed a titre of more than 1:64. Such titre would be regarded as negative by Proctor and Elsdon-Dew (1966). Such anomalous responses have been described for other metacestode infections (see Kagan 1968).

The IHR, using *T. hydatigena* cyst antigen gave positive reactions, though the titres recorded during the infection varied from those obtained with the homologous antigen.

The anomalous results seen in the above tests were probably due to the crude nature of the antigen used and the differing reactivity to infection of different pigs. Cross reactivity between different metacestode antigens in serological tests is well documented (Kagan, 1968). The IHR is a useful test but it must be refined for use in this and related systems. It is a highly sensitive reaction, but it is not sufficiently specific. The cysticercus antigen may not be the best antigen to use and other antigens may demonstrate a different serological response. It will be necessary to extend these preliminary studies to determine the duration of the IHR in *T. solium* cysticercosis. In addition to refinement, the technique, using standarised red cells, diluent and specifically reacting antigen, will be advantageous.

The results do show that (a) positive results may be found in animals in which no cysts are found at slaughter, this being an indication that the cysts are resorbed (b) positive results are present at the time when the developing cysticercus is infective to humans (i.e. 60 days, Yoshino, 1933; 100 or more days according to von Ostertag, 1896), (c) some pigs may give false negative results.

Conclusions

There is ample evidence of the need to re-examine the epidemiology, and pathogenesis of *T. solium* infection in pigs. There is a need to understand more about the immunological responses, both in *vivo* and *in vitro* and their importance in the epidemiology and pathogenesis of natural infections. In particular, it is desirable that the factors concerned with the establishment and longevity of the cysticercus be examined in light, heavy, single and multiple infections. The

The development of a specific diagnostic test for cysticercosis is desirable since it is clear that light infections are frequently missed at the time of meat inspection. It is considered that the use of crude antigens in serodiagnostic tests is one of the main reasons for the unpredictable serological responses. Finally, the immunological (including serological) response may be associated with the location of the cysticercus as well as the numbers present. This factor may also explain the variable responses seen in individual animals.

Acknowledgements

This work was supported in part by the Overseas Development Administration of the United Kindgom Government. We wish to thank them as well as our collegues at the Universidad Austral for their help.

REFERENCES

Barrientos, J., Schirmer, E., Schenone, H., Aranda, R., Concha, L. and Rojas, A., (1967). *Bol. Chil. Parasit.*, *22*, 150.

Biagi, F.F. and Tay, J. (1958). *Am. J. Trop. Med. Hyg.*, *7*, 63.

Biagi, F.F., Navarrette, F., Pina, A., Santiago, Ana Maria, and Tapia, L. (1961). *Rev. Med. Hosp. Gen.*, *25*, 501.

Brunner, M. (1928). *J. Immunol.*, *15*, 83.

Bull, F. (1962). *Bol. Chil. Parasit.*, *17*, 80.

Cadigan, F.C. Jr., Stanton, J.S., Tanticharoenyos, P. and Chaicumpa, V. (1967). *J. Parasit.*, *53*, 844.

Donckaster, R. and Donoso, F. (1960). *Bol. Chil. Parasit.*, *15*, 83.

Faiguenbaum, J. (1961). *Bol. Chil. Parasit.*, *16*, 71.

FAO/WHO (1973). *Animal Health Yearbook.*, 1972. F.A.O. Rome, Italy.

Gallo, P. and Vogelsang, E.G. (1951). *Rev. Med. Vet. Parasit. Caracas.*, *10*, 3.

Garnham, P.C.C. (1958). *J. Trop. Med. Hyg.*, *61*, 92.

Gemmell, M.A. (1970). *Austral. Vet. J.*, *46*, 366.

Gemmell, M.A. and Macnamara, F. N. (1972). *In Immunity to animal parasites*. (Soulsby, E.J.L. Ed.) Academic Press. New York, London.

Gemmell, M.A. and Soulsby, E.J.L. (1968). *Bull. Wld. Hlth. Org.*, *39*, 45.

Herbert, I.V. and Oberg, C. 1972. (unpublished)

Herbert, W. J. (1973). Passive haemagglutination with special reference to the Tanned cell technique. *In Handbook of experimental immunology*. (Weir, D.M. Ed) Blackwell Oxford.

Hernandez, J., Guerrero, J., Tabacchi, L., Guerrero, C. (1966). *Rev. Med. Vet. Lima., 18, 19, 20,* 263-8.
Hernandez-Jauregui, P.A., Marquez-Monter, H., and Sastre-Ortiz, S. (1973). *Am. J. Vet. Res., 34,* 451.
Kagan, I. G. (1968). *Bull. Wld. Hlth. Org., 39,* 25.
Leikina, E.S., Moskuin, S.N., Sokolovskaya, O.M., and Poletaeva, O.G. (1964). *Med. Parazitol. Parazit. Bol., 33,* 694.
Marques-Monter, H. (1971). *In Pathology of Protozoal and Helminths diseases.* (Marcial-Rojas, R.A. Ed.) Williams Wilkins, Baltimore.
Meyenburg, H. von (1923). Die quergestreifte Mustulatur. *In Handbuch der speziellen pathologischen Anatomie und Histologie., 9.* Band 1. Teil, 11. Springer. Berlin.
Nelson, G.S., Pester, F.R.N. and Rickman, R. (1965). *Trans. Roy. Soc. Trop. Med. Hyg., 59,* 507.
Neumann, L.G. (1892). *Treatise on the parasites and parasitic diseases of domestic animals.* Transl. By Fleming. Bailliere, Tindall and Cox.
von Ostertag, R. (1897). *Z. Fleisch. Milch. Hyg., 8,* 1.
von Ostertag, R. (1934). *Textbook of meat inspection.* Bailliere, Tindall and Cox. London.
Proctor, E.M. (1972) *S. African. Med. J., 46,* 234-8.
Proctor, E.M. and Elsdon-Dew, R. (1966). *S. African J. Sci., 62,* 264.
Sandground, J.H. (1936). *J. Parasit., 22,* 52-3.
Schenone, H. and Reyes, H. (1968). *Bol. Chil. Parasit., 23,* 62.
Schwabe, C.W. (1969). *Veterinary medicine and human health.* Williams and Wilkins Co. Baltimore.
Slais, J. (1970). *The morphology and pathogenicity of the bladder-worms Cysticercus cellulosae* and *Cysticercus bovis.* W. Junk The Hague.
Smyth, J.D. and Heath, D.D. (1970). *Helminth. Abstr.* Series A *39,* 1.
Soltys, M.A. (1936). *Prz. Weteryn., 41,* 393.
Sprent, J.F.A. (1969). *Helminth. Abstr., 38,* 333.
Stoll, N.R. (1947). *J. Parasit., 33,* 1.
Trawinsky, A. (1936). *Zblt. Bakt. Parasitk. Infkr.* 1 Abt. Orig. *136,* 116.
Viljoen, N.F. (1937). *Onderst. J. Vet. Sci. An. Ind., 9,* 337.
Yoshino, K. (1933). *J. Med. Ass. Formosa., 32,* 1717.

STUDIES ON ANTIGENS COMMON TO *CYSTICERCUS BOVIS* AND *TAENIA SAGINATA*

Barbara Machnicka

Polish Academy of Sciences, Department of Parasitology, Warsaw, Poland

INTRODUCTION

A reciprocal antigenic relationship between the larval and adult forms of tapeworms has been known for many years. Thus Campbell (1936) reported the presence of common antigens in *Taenia taeniaeformis* and *Cysticercus fasciolaris* and he showed that a protein fraction of *T. taeniaeformis* produced immunity in rats to a subsequent infection with *C. fasciolaris*. Campbell (1938a,b) found that immunity could be transferred by serum taken during the second week after infection or immunization. The protective capacity of serum could be removed by absorbtion with larval or adult worm tissues. Heyneman (1962) in experiments with *Hymenolepis nana* in mice induced protection with cysticercoids against egg infection and Németh (1971) demonstrated an antigenic identity between *Taenia pisiformis* and *Cysticercus pisiformis*.

Oncospheres from adult cestodes have been used to induce immunity to metacestodes. Thus Gemmell (1964, 1965) injected sheep intramuscularly with hatched oncospheres of *Taenia hydatigena* or *Taenia ovis* and induced immunity to homologous and heterologous infection. Wikerhauser *et al.*, (1971) immunized calves against bovine cysticercosis by intramuscular injection of artificially hatched oncospheres of *Taenia saginata* and *T. hydatigena*. Incomplete larval development, attained by X-irradiation of eggs is sufficient to protect against infection. Thus Dow *et al.*, (1962) immunized mice against *C. fasciolaris* by oral infection with X-irradiated *T. taeniaeformis* eggs and Urquhart *et al.*, (1963) obtained a high degree of protection in calves against *C. bovis* infection following oral infection with X-irradiated eggs of *T. saginata*.

The present study examined the antigenic relationship between *C. bovis* and *T. saginata*. Sera of calves infected with *C. bovis* of humans infected with *T. saginata* and anti-sera prepared in rabbits were used for the studies.

MATERIALS AND METHODS

Antigens.

Cysticerci were obtained from calves infected at the age of two weeks and slaughtered 2.5 and 3.5 months later. Two antigenic preparations of *C. bovis* were used. One was a buffered saline (pH 7.2) extract of homogenized scolices and membranes and contained 7.2 mg/ml of protein. The other was cyst fluid and it contained 12 mg/ml of protein. A crude somatic antigen of *T. saginata* consisted of the supernatant from a buffered saline (pH 7.2) extract of fresh proglottids. Further antigenic fractions of *T. saginata* were obtained and chemically determined as described by Machnicka-Roguska (1965). In the present study polysaccharide, protein and nucleoprotein fractions were used.

Immune sera.

Sera was obtained at weekly intervals from calves experimentally infected with *C. bovis*. Human sera were obtained from patients, with proven *T. saginata* infection, at the District Consulting Center in Gdynia. Antisera to *T. saginata* was produced in rabbits by 6 subcutaneous injections at weekly intervals. Each injection consisted of 20 mg of lyophilized crude *T. saginata* antigen in Freund's complete adjuvant. Antisera to *C. bovis* were prepared in rabbits by three injections at weekly intervals of 0.5 ml of antigen.

Gel precipitation tests were performed according to Ouchterlony (1949), immunoelectrophoresis was done according to Grabar and Williams (1953) passive hemagglutination tests with untreated erythrocytes exposed to antigen were performed by the method described by Netor *et al.* (1956) and passive hemagglutination tests with antigen treated, tannic acid exposed, erythrocytes were done following the procedure of Stavitzky (1954) using formalinized erythrocytes as recommended by Weinbach (1959). The indirect immunofluorescence test with *T. saginata* oncospheres was done as described by Machnicka (1973). Oncospheres hatched and activated according to Silverman (1954) were incubated for 30 min with test serum, washed, incubated with conjugate, washed, and then treated with counterstain. Rabbit anti-bovine gamma globulin serum conjuncted with fluorescein isothiocyanate was used in studies with bovine sera and rabbit anti-human gamma globulin serum similarly conjugated was used to examine human sera.

RESULTS

The sera of calves experimentally infected with *C. bovis*

reacted with homologous antigens. Passive hemagglutination responses were obtained 3 weeks after infection in calves infected with 80,000, 125,000 and 150,000 eggs and 2 weeks after infection in a calf infected with 180,000 eggs (Fig. 1). Higher titres were obtained with the fluid of cysticerci than with the extract prepared from scolices and membranes.

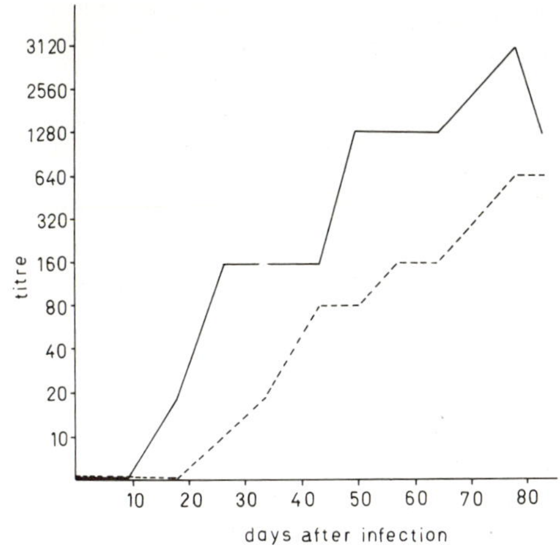

Fig. 1. Passive haemagglutination tests with Cysticercus bovis *fluid antigen (continuous line) and an antigenic fraction of* Taenia saginata *(dotted line) with the serum of a calf infected with 180,000 eggs of* T. saginata.

Indirect immunofluorescence tests with activated oncospheres of *T. saginata* were usually positive at higher dilutions of sera than those which reacted with the passive hemagglutination tests. Specific immunoflourescence of oncospheres was detectable as a distinct fluorescence of the cells of the hexacanth embryo (Fig. 2 and 3).

The majority of human sera from persons infected with *T. saginata* showed positive passive haemagglutination tests with untreated erythrocytes exposed to the crude extract of *T. saginata*. This confirms the previous findings of Machnicka-Roguska and Zwierz (1966). Serum titers increased after treatment with anthelmintics. The highest titres were obtained in passive hemagglutination tests with the fractions C_F, $N_{0.1}$, B_1 and C respectively of Macknicka-Roguska (1965). The same fractions but in a different order (B_1, $N_{0.1}$, C_F, C) were the most active in the complement fixation test. In intradermal tests on individuals infected with *T. saginata* Machnicka-Roguska and Zwierz (1970) noted that fraction C_{alk} was the best allergen.

Rabbit antisera to *C. bovis* antigen reacted in agar precipitation test with all the antigenic fractions of *T. sagi-*

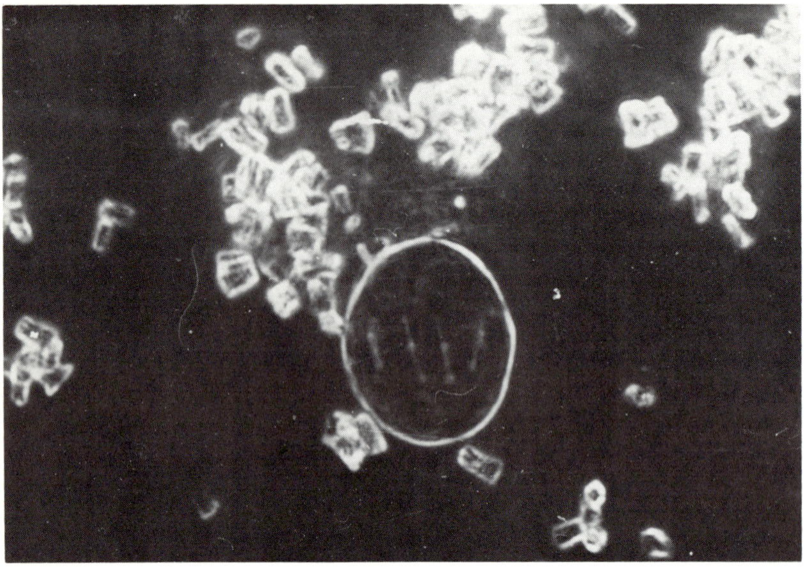

Fig. 2. Oncosphere of Taenia saginata *showing a negative indirect immunofluorescence reaction.*

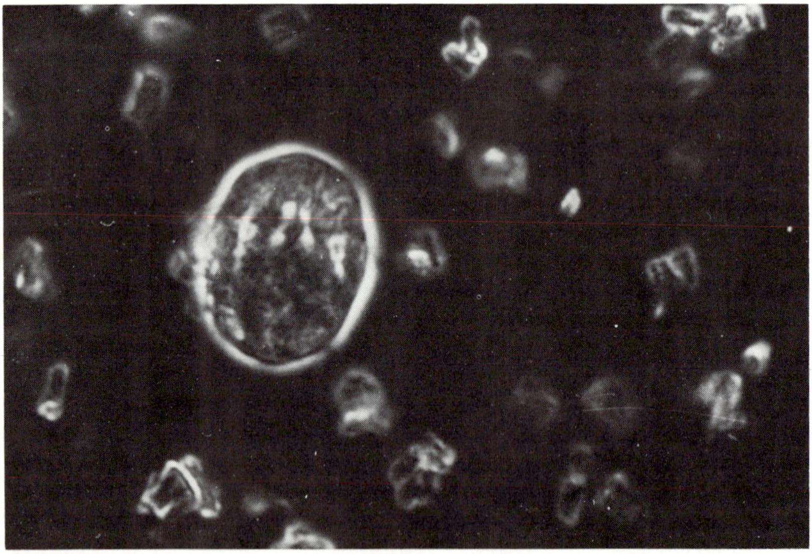

Fig. 3. Oncosphere of Taenia saginata *showing positive indirect immunofluorescence reaction.*

nata. Common precipitin bands occurred with fractions C and $N_{0.1}$ as well as with fractions B_1 and B_2. Rabbit antisera to *T. saginata* showed 6 precipitin bands with the extract of *C. bovis* scolices and membranes and 4 bands with *C. bovis* fluid. When diffused together, antisera to *C. bovis* and *T. saginata* produced reactions of identify with some of the antigens of the extract of *C. bovis* scolices and membranes and of the *C. bovis* fluid (example Fig. 4).

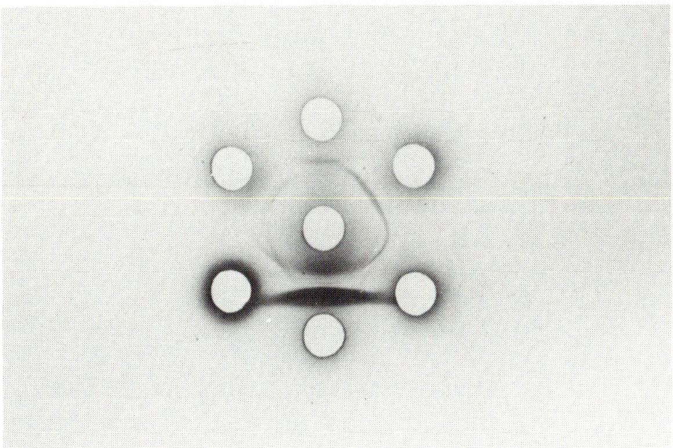

Fig. 4. Gel precipitation test with Cysticercus bovis *fluid antigen (Central well) with rabbit antisera to* Cysticercus bovis *(wells 1, 3, 5) and rabbit antisera to* Taenia saginata *(wells 2, 4, 6). Well numbering starts at 2 o'clock, hence 12 o'clock = well no. 6.*

The sera of calves infected with *C. bovis* and the serum of humans infected with *T. saginata* were examined by haemagglutination and gel precipitation using antigens from *T. saginata* and *T. bovis* respectively.

The sera of calves infected with *C. bovis* gave precipitin reactions with crude *T. saginata* antigen and with the antigenic fractions of *T. saginata*. Single precipitin bands were obtained with fractions C, C_F, $N_{0.1}$, B_1, B_2. With fraction C_{alk} three faint precipitin lines were formed. With passive hemagglutination tests using *T. saginata* antigen absorbed onto untreated erythrocytes the highest serum titres were obtained with fractions C_{alk} and C; fractions C_F, $N_{0.1}$. B_1 gave lower serum titres (Fig. 2). In passive hemagglutination test with tannic acid treated erythrocytes, the sera of calves infected with *C. bovis* reacted only with fraction $N_{0.1}$ of *T. saginata* and to a lower titre than with homologic antigens (Fig. 1).

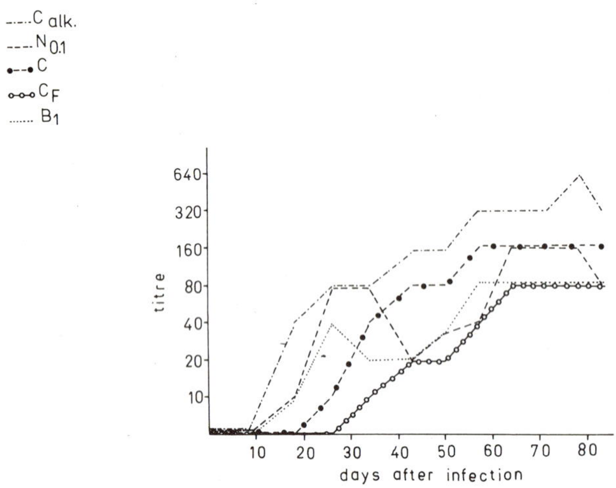

Fig. 5. Passive hemagglutination tests with Taenia saginata *antigenic fractions absorbed on untreated erythrocytes with the sera of a calf infected with* C. bovis.

Human sera from *T. saginata* infected patients did not give precipitin reactions in agar gel with antigens of *C. bovis*, even used concentrated sera. In passive hemagglutination tests with tannic acid treated erythrocytes coated with *C. bovis* antigens, human sera reacted in low dilutions (1:10 to 1:40). Of 40 sera examined 37 were positive. Higher serum titres were obtained with the *C. bovis* fluid antigen than with the supernatant of *C. bovis* scolices. Comparatively higher titres were obtained when the antigenic fraction $N_{0.1}$ of *T. saginata* was used as antigen, the lowest titre being 1:80. With immunofluorescence tests using *T. saginata* oncospheres, weak reactions only were obtained with low serum dilution.

DISCUSSION

A distinct antibody response occurred in calves infected with *C. bovis*. This confirms the work of others. Antibodies were detectable by passive haemagglutination, by gel precipitation and by immunoelectrophoresis (Fig. 6).

The time after infection when antibodies can be detected depends on the infective dose. In a calf infected with 180,000 eggs, antibodies were demonstrable in the third week

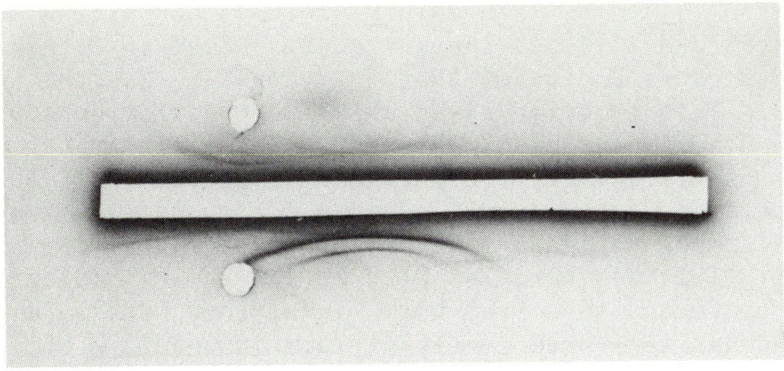

Fig. 6. Immunoelectrophoresis of Cysticercus bovis *antigens with the serum of calf infected with* C. bovis. *Upper well: antigen of* C. bovis *scolices and membranes; lower well:* C. bovis *fluid.*

of infection while calves given smaller doses of eggs showed a response one week later. A higher reactivity with *C. bovis* fluid was noted in gel precipitation tests with sera of infected calves then with the homogenate from *C. bovis* scolices and membranes. This may be related to the apparent greater antigenic complexity of the cyst fluid, since it gave more lines of precipitation with the sera of infected calves than the extract of scolices and membranes.

It is interesting to note that the antigens of *C. bovis* can be used only in passive haemagglutination tests with tannic acid treated erythrocytes. They cannot be absorbed onto untreated erythrocytes, which would indicate that they are protein in nature.

The positive results with the indirect fluorescence test using *T. saginata* oncospheres concur with the results of Silverman (1955) who reported that precipitins were formed when hexacanth embryos were incubated with immune sera. However, in the present experiments specific immunofluorescence occurred in the cells of the hexacanth embryo and not on the membrane. Indeed fluorescence under the oncospheral membrane, often observed after incubation with normal sera was considered as unspecific.

Sera of patients infected with *T. saginata* showed an elevation of passive hemagglutination titres after the treatment with anthelmintics. This might be ascribed to the removal of antigens which would bind antibodies to the parasite. *Taenia saginata* antigenic fractions C_F, $N_{0.1}$, B_1 and C were the most active in passive hemagglutination test with human sera. The fraction C_F and C were polysaccharides containing a small amount of protein (0.14% and 0.25% of N respectively). The fractions $N_{0.1}$ and B_1 were mainly proteins containing some sugar (4.5% and 21.5%). The intradermal test in *T. saginata* infected persons indicated that fraction C_{alk} was the best allergen. This fraction is an aklaline preparation and contains 76.0% of sugar and 1.95% of N. The other fractions did not react satisfactorily in intradermal tests.

Antisera to *C. bovis* and *T. saginata* produced in rabbits revealed common antigens in the larval and adult form of the tapeworm. This was verified with sera of calves infected with *C. bovis* and sera from human infections with *T. saginata*.

Of the antigens used in the various immunodiagnostic tests, high titres were obtained with fractions C_{alk} and $N_{0.1}$ of *T. saginata* with sera from calves infected with cysticerci, and in man, fraction C_{alk} was the most satisfactory allergen. However, in spite of the common antigenic components in *C. bovis* and *T. saginata* the sera of humans infected with *T. saginata* response poorly to *C. bovis* antigens. This may suggest that the antigens which induce the antibody response in *T. saginata* infection in man are different from those which constitute the cross reacting antigens between *C. bovis* and *T. saginata*.

REFERENCES

Campbell, D.H. (1936). *Amer. J. Hyg.*, *23*, 104.

Campbell, D.H. (1938a). *J. Immunol.*, *35*, 195.

Campbell, D.H. (1938b). *J. Immunol.*, *35*, 205.

Dow, C., Jarret, W.F.H., Jennings, W.F., McIntyre, W.I.M., Mulligan, W. (1962). *Amer. J. Vet. Res.*, *23*, 146.

Gemmell, M.A. (1964). *Immunology*, *7*, 489.

Gemmell, M.A. (1965). *Immunology*, *8*, 281.

Grabar, P. and Williams, C.A. (1953). *Biochim. Biophys. Acta*, *10*, 193.

Heyneman, D. (1962). *Amer. J. Trop. med., Hyg.*, *11*, 46.

Machnicka-Roguska, B. (1965). *Acta Parasit. Pol.*, *13*, 337.

Machnicka-Roguska, B. and Zwierz, Cz. (1970). *Acta Parasit. Pol.*, *17*, 293.

Machnicka, B. (1973). *Bull. Acad. Pol. Sci.*, *21*, 743.

Németh, I. (1971). *Acta Vet. Hung.*, *21*, 319.

Neter, E., Westphal, O., Lüderitz, O. and Gorzyński, E.A. (1956). *Ann. NY Acad. Sci.*, *66*, 141.

Silverman, P.H. (1954). *Ann. Trop. Med. Parasit.*, *48*, 207.

Silverman, P.H. (1955). *Nature*, *176*, 598.

Stravitzky, A.B. (1954). *J. Immunol.*, *72*, 360.

Urquhart, G.M., McIntyre, W.I.M., Mulligan, W., Jarret, W.F.H. and Sharp, N.C.C. (1963). *Proc. 17th World Vet. Congr.*, *1*, 769.

Weinbach, R. (1959). *Schweitz. Ztschr. Allg. Path.*, *22*, 1.
Wikerhauser, T., Zuković, M., Dzakula, N. (1971). *Expt. Parasit.*, *30*, 36.

INTRADERMAL TESTS WITH ACID SOLUBLE PROTEIN FRACTIONS OF CESTODE ANTIGENS IN THE DIAGNOSIS OF CEREBRAL CYSTICERCOSIS IN MAN

Wanda Zapart, Wiesław Ślusarski and Jerzy Ptasiński

Intestinal Diseases Consulting Unit, Department of Parasitology, Polish Academy of Sciences; and Clinic of Neurosurgery, Medical Academy, Warsaw, Poland

INTRODUCTION

In the world literature there are over 200 papers dealing with at least 2,500 cases of cerebral cysticercosis in man (Bojarski and Waleszkowski, 1963). Cerebral cysticercosis has been reported from a large number of countries, but its incidence varies greatly. The disease is by no means rare in Poland. Stepień (1962) reported 132 cases of cerebral cysticercosis in all the Polish neurosurgical clinics from 1936 to 1961. The number of cases has not shown a decrease in recent years.

The differential, pre-operative, diagnosis of cerebral cysticercosis, though based on several recognized pathognomonic signs and clinical criteria, is by no means easy. It is one of the more serious problems in neurosurgery, neurology, psychiatry and related medical sciences and as a rule only a presumptive diagnosis can be made. Supporting evidence for a positive diagnosis includes ventriculographic findings, the presence of cysticerci in muscles or retina, a history of intestinal infection with a cestode, the presence of the blood eosinophilia, typical changes in the cerebrospinal fluid, or calcification recorded by radiography of the skull.

An early and accurate diagnosis may be decisive for the fate of a patient. Because of this there have been extensive studies aimed at developing ancillary diagnostic methods, and immunodiagnostic techniques have been widely studied for the diagnosis of such cestode infections. Serological examination of blood and cerebrospinal fluid in human cerebral cysticercosis is a common adjunct in diagnosis. The complement fixation and the ring precipitation tests are most frequently used, however, there is a difference of opinion as to the usefulness of these tests for the diagnosis of cysticercosis of the brain. Some writers have stressed a close correlation between positive complement fixation tests and the proven brain cysticercosis (e.g., Pinto Pupo *et al.*, 1947; Spina-Franca, 1956; Lombardo and Mateos, 1961). Such tests are made by examining either the blood or the cerebrospinal fluid (Nieto, 1956; Tolosa, 1954; Jeziorańska and Zapart, 1959). Unfortunately, only in a few cases have the results been verified surgically or by post-mortem examination (Nieto, 1956; Voznaia, 1953).

Knowledge concerning the hypersensensitivity responses in cerebral cysticercosis is rather poor, though allergic host reactions induced by complex cestode antigens do occur with the tissue cestode infections such as echinococcosis and cysticercosis.

The detection of these hypersensitive responses by intradermal tests with crude antigens prepared from a parasite are of little practical value in the diagnosis of cestode infections, since the allergic reactions obtained are variable and often non-specific. However, recent reports (Zapart *et al.*, 1969; Machnicka-Roguska and Zwierz, 1970; Slusarski and Zapart, 1971) have suggested that intradermal tests using antigenic fractions (e.g., polysaccharide and acid soluble protein fractions) instead of the crude antigens may offer advantages in the diagnosis of infections with adult cestodes in man. This superiority of antigen fractions for the detection of adult parasites prompted further search for parasite antigenic fractions which would be sensitive and specific in skin tests for tissue cestode infections. This paper presents an evaluation of the diagnostic usefulness of an acid soluble protein fraction with known nitrogen content, in a defined group of individuals showing clinical manifestations of cerebral infections with cestode larvae.

MATERIALS AND METHODS

Antigens

Three different antigens, consisting of the acid soluble protein fraction, were prepared respectively from freshly eliminated mature proglottides of *Taenia saginata*, viable cysts of *Taenia solium (Cysticercus cellulosae)* and *Echinococcus granulosus* protoscolices. The modified Melcher (1943) technique of fractionation was used and the nitrogen content was determined by the micro-Kjeldahl analysis, using the apparatus recommended by Markham (1942). The details of preparation of antigens, technique of performing, reading and evaluating results are given elsewhere (Slusarski and Zapart, 1971). Antigens for intradermal tests were prepared in physiological salt solution to a nitrogen content of 20 ug/ml.

Patients

The tests were performed on three groups of patients.

Group A comprised 17 patients hospitalized at the Neurosurgical Clinic, Medical Academy, Warsaw, at different periods between 1969 and 1972. Clinically they were suspected of cysticercosis or echinococcosis of the brain, eye or muscles. The patients were aged from 11 to 55 years, 10 were male and 7 were female and 5 were under 30. All the patients had had at least two routine stool examinations for intestinal parasites and except for two were free of intestinal parasite infections. The two exceptions were infected with *Trichuris trichiura* and *Ascaris*, respectively, and both were infected with *Enterobius*. Three patients had a history of infections with cestodes, *Enterobius, Trichuris* or *Ascaris*.

Two different control groups were also used. *Group B* comprised 27 persons in which cysticercosis or echinococcosis had been excluded in clinical examination. Of this group two were with epilepsy, one with polyneuritis, twelve with "disc syndrome" and twelve were hospitalized for cranial injuries. *Group C* contained 50 healthy persons, who were free from helminth infections, as determined by serodiagnostic and fecal examination. Persons in this group were not hospitalized.

Test Technique and Reading

Exactly 0.05 ml of each antigen solution and the control fluid (physiological salt solution) was injected intradermally on the median region of the forearm. Control persons were treated similarly. The area of the wheal was measured 15 min after injection. The criterion of a positive reaction was an increase of wheal area at least twice that of the wheal produced by the control solution.

RESULTS

The results of intradermal tests performed on patients in Group A are summarized in Table I.

Group A

Case 1. Male,aged 46; hospitalized for internal hydrocephalus. A complement fixation titre of 1:4 with cysticercus antigen was present. Intradermal tests with all the three antigens were negative. The patient received non-operative medication.

Case 2. Female, aged 34; surgery in 1969 revealed positive echinococcosis of the left-side frontal lobe. A marked positive intradermal reaction with *C. cellulosae* antigen was evident prior to operation.

Case 3. Female, aged 32; with clinical signs of internal

Table 1

Distribution of positive intradermal tests with three antigens in patients of Group A suspected of brain cysticercosis

Antigens	Positive of 17 patients	Total	No. of operated or necropsied verified infestation of the brain	
			Echinococcus	Cysticercus
At least one antigen	14	7	2	5
Ts only	-			
Eg only	-			
Cc only	2		1	
Ts + Eg	-			
Ts + Cc	4		1	2
Eg + Cc	2			1
Three antigens simultaneously	6			2

Ts = *Taenia saginata*, Eg = *Echinococcus granulosus*, Cc = *Cysticercus cellulosae*

hydrocephalus and epilepsy. A marked positive intradermal reaction with *C. cellulosae* antigen was present. The patient received non-operative treatment.

Case 4. Female, aged 54, clinically diagnosed as cysticercosis of the brain and muscles. The ring precipitation test was positive at 1:2 dilution. Marked positive intradermal reactions were obtained with *C. cellulosae* and *Taenia saginata* antigens. The patient died due to lung abscess, pheumothorax and epilepsy. Post-mortem examination revealed extensive cysticercosis of the brain and muscles.

Case 5. Female, aged 45; hydrocephalus, with suspected cerebral cysticercosis. The intradermal test was positive with *I. saginata* antigen and strongly positive with *C. cellulosae* antigen. At surgery an echinococcus cyst located at the posterior cranial region of the brain was found.

Case 6. Male, aged 15; admitted in 1970 for epilepsy, with previous surgical history of cerebral cysticercosis in 1964. The complement fixation test with the *C. cellulosae* antigen was doubtful. Intradermal tests were negative with all antigens. The patient received non-operative medication.

Case 7. Female, aged 32; symptomatic epilepsy with suspected cerebral cysticercosis. A history of infection with intestinal parasites 6 years previously. Three stool examinations proved negative. Intradermal tests with all three antigens were positive. Symptomatic treatment given.

Case 8. Male, aged 55; Jacksonian epilepsy with right sided motor paralysis; encephalopathy and cerebral cysticercosis were diagnosed. A history of cured taeniasis was present. Marked positive intradermal reactions with all antigens were noted. Symptomatic medication was applied.

Case 9. Male, aged 11; hospitalized in 1970 with meningitis and Jacksonian epilepsy; a previous history of cysticercosis of the brain, treated surgically in 1960. Intradermal tests with all antigens were negative. Symptomatic medication applied.

Case 10. Male, aged 55; suspected of cerebral cysticercosis with menigitis, internal hydrocephalus, Jacksonian epilepsy, unilateral hemiparesis and a history of taeniasis. Marked positive intradermal reactions with all three antigens were obtained. Symptomatic medication applied.

Case 11. Female, aged 16; suspected cerebral cysticercosis with a history of taeniasis. The ring precipitation test with *C. cellulosae* antigen showed a titre of 1:4. Positive intradermal reactions were obtained with *E. granulosus*, *T. saginata* and *C. cellulosae* antigens. Symptomatic medication was applied.

Case 12. Female, aged 14; diagnosed as left-sided frontal epilepsy. *Trichuris trichiura* eggs present in the stool. Intradermal tests with *C. cellulosae* and *T. saginata* antigens were positive. Frontal, left-sided, lobectomy was performed but no helminths were detected.

Case 13. Male, aged 43; suspected of cerebral cysticercosis. A history of infection with *Ascaris* and *Enterobius* was present. Marked positive intradermal reactions with *C. cellulosae* and *T. saginata* antigens were present. At surgery cysticercosis of the cerebellum was detected.

Case 14. Male, aged 23; hospitalized in 1972 with the diagnosis of frontal right-sided epilepsy. A history of ascariasis, trichuriasis and taeniasis, cured in 1964 was present. Positive intradermal tests were obtained with *C. cellulosae* and *E. granulosus* antigens. At surgery a "cystic tumour" of the left hemisphere of the cerebellum proved to be a cysticercus.

Case 15. Male, aged 31; hospitalized for a vision defect in the left eye and suspected of cysticercosis of the eye. Intradermal tests with *E. granulosus* and *C. cellulosae* antigens were markedly positive. The patient received non-surgical medication.

Case 16. Male, aged 45; hospitalized with suspected cerebral cysticercosis and showed left-sided convulsions of the Jackson type. Ventriculography suggested a tumour of the left ventricle. Positive intradermal reactions were obtained with all the antigens used. The patient died after surgery.

At autopsy, cysticercosis of the brain was observed.

Case 17. Male, aged 59; diagnosed as cerebral cysticercosis, internal hydrocephalus and meningitis. The patient died with the symptoms of decerebration. At autopsy a structural obliteration of the brain base associated with unequal thickening of meninges covering the optic nerves was noted, as well as hydrocephalus of the fourth ventricle. A cyst, 2 cm in diameter, containing a cysticercus was found in the fourth ventricle.

Groups B and C

Patients of these groups showed negative intradermal tests with all three antigens, except for two cases with epilepsy (Group B), one of which was also infected with *Lamblia*. However, it must be emphasized that the positive reactions in both the cases were insignificant, compared with the reactions obtained with individuals in Group A.

Control intradermal tests with saline, in all patients in all groups were negative.

DISCUSSION

Table I gives the distribution of positive intradermal reactions with the three antigen preparations. As a rule, intradermal reactions were more marked with homologous than heterologous antigens in proven cases of cerebral cysticercosis. However, the results indicated that a combination of antigens in the intradermal test was advantageous. The antigens used in this study were from closely related forms and their combination probably served to broaden the range of antigens available for reactivity in the intradermal test.

The results support earlier findings by Zapart *et al.* (1969) and Slusarski and Zapart (1971) on the usefulness of acid soluble protein fraction antigens for intradermal tests for the immunodiagnosis of parasitic infections. Generally, this type of antigen is the most sensitive and it is particularly useful for intradermal tests since it can be standardized and hence results obtained with it can be compared objectively. A saline extract suffers from diverse and varying component ratios and standardization of the source parasitic material used, the method of preparation and preservation procedures may vary greatly (Kagan, 1963).

In the present study, intradermal tests proved to be a valuable adjunct in the clinical diagnosis of cerebral cysticercosis or hydatidosis. However, it is recognized that the antigens employed were still complex mixtures of polysaccharides and proteins each of which may show different antigenic activities (Kent, 1963). Therefore, further studies are needed to isolate fractions which would be more sensitive and specific for the diagnosis as cysticercosis. For the time being however the Melcher type antigen can be employed in the intradermal test as an ancillary method in the diagnosis of cysticercosis or echinococcosis of the brain in man.

REFERENCES

Bojarski, Z. and Waleszkowski, J. (1963). *Wiad. Parazyt.*, *9*, 571.

Jeziorańska, A. and Zapart, W. (1959). *Polski Tyg. Lek.*, 133.

Kagan, I.G. (1963). *Am. J. Hyg.*, (Mon. Ser.), *22*, 133.

Kent, J. F. (1963). *Am. J. Hyg.*, (Mon. Ser.), *22*, 35.

Lombardo, L. and Mateos, J.H. (1961). *Neurology*, *9*, 2311.

Machnicka-Roguska, B and Zwierz, C. (1970). *Acta Parasit. Pol.*, *17*, 293.

Markham, M. (1942). *Biochem. J.*, *36*, 790.

Melcher, L.B. (1943). *J. Infect. Dis.*, *73*, 31.

Nieto, D. (1956). *Neurology*, *6*, 725.

Pinto Pupo, P., Cordoso, W., dos Reis, J.B. and da Silva, C.P. (1947). *Arq. Assist. Psicopat.*, Sao Paulo, *3*, 10.

Spina-França, A. (1956). *Rev. Paul. Med.*, *47*, 59.

Ślusarski, W. and Zapart, W. (1971). *Acta Parasit. Pol.*, *19*, 445.

Stepien, Z. (1962). *J. Neurosurg.*, *6*, 505.

Tolosa, E. (1954). *Rev. Neurol. Paris.*, *90*, 187.

Voznaia, A. (1953). *Vop. Neurokhir.*, *1*, 36.

Zapart, W., Adonajło, A. and Gancarz, Z. (1969). *Wiad. Parazyt.*, *15*, 77.

THE PASSIVE TRANSFER OF IMMUNITY TO THE METACESTODE OF *TAENIA TAENIAEFORMIS**

Sheelagh Lloyd and E. J. L. Soulsby

Department of Pathobiology, School of Veterinary Medicine, University of Pennsylvania, Philadelphia, U.S.A.

Acquired immunity is stimulated by infections with larval cestodes (metacestodes) (Gemmell and Soulsby, 1968). The immune response to metacestode infections may be divided into two phases: "Pre-encystment" immunity and "post-encystment" immunity. "Pre-encystment" immunity operates early in infection and probably is functional in the intestinal lumen or in the intestinal mucosa. Examples of this are the studies by Heath (1970) who reported that the oncospheres of *Echinococcus granulosus* failed to penetrate the intestine of sheep immunized against this parasite and those of Leonard and Smith (1939), Froyd and Round (1960) and Heath (1970) who reported that animals resistant to oral infection could be infected by parenteral injection of artificially activated oncospheres. "Post-encystment" immunity is active against the developing metacestode in the tissues.

Immunity to metacestodes appears largely due to humoral antibody since passive transfer of immunity with serum or colostrum has been reported. Thus the passive transfer of humoral immunity has been demonstrated with rats infected with *Taenia taeniaeformis* (Miller, 1932a; 1934; Miller and Gardiner, 1932a, 1932b; Campbell, 1938a, 1938b; Leid and Williams, 1973), rabbits infected with *Taenia pisiformis* (Miller and Gardiner, 1934; Kerr, 1935; Campbell, 1938c) and mice infected with *Hymenolepis nana* (Hearin, 1941). The maternal transfer of this immunity to the offspring, both *in utero* and via colostrum, has been demonstrated with *T. taeniaeformis* infections in rats (Miller, 1932b, 1935) and *H. nana* infections in mice (Larsh, 1942, 1944).

Passive transfer of immunity in metacestode infections in ruminants has shown variable results. For example, neither Urquhart (1961) nor Froyd (1964) were able to demonstrate passive transfer of immunity to *Taenia saginata* infections in calves. However, preliminary studies (Lloyd and Soulsby,

---

* Studies supported by USPHS Grant AI-06262 and the Pennsylvania Plan to Develop Scientists in Medical Research (S.L.).

unpublished) suggest a reduction in the number of cysts in calves receiving large amounts of immune serum and Gemmell *et al.* (1969) reported the transfer of a low degree of resistance to the metacestode of *Taenia hydatigena* with colostrum from hyperimmunized ewes. Recently, the passive protection of lambs against *Taenia ovis* infection via the colostro-intestinal route has been demonstrated (Rickard and Arundel, 1974).

The present study examines the protective immunological response to *T. taeniaeformis* metacestodes in mice, the sources of antibodies to this parasite (e.g. colostral, intestinal or systemic) and the role played by the individual immunoglobulin classes in protection. The system provides a satisfactory laboratory model for infection of the bovine with metacestodes of *T. saginata.*

MATERIALS AND METHODS

Taenia taeniaeformis eggs were obtained from Dr. J. A. Dvorak (National Institutes of Health, Washington, D.C.). CF1-S mice (Carworth Farms) were infected with the eggs and the livers of these mice were used to infect three parasite-free cats. After patency of the tapeworm, eggs were collected daily, washed in 0.15M saline containing penicillin and streptomycin and they were stored in this solution at 4°C until required. For the infection of mice, eggs, collected over a period of three days, were pooled and their viability was assessed morphologically.

Neonatal mice were obtained from CF1-S females bred at 10 weeks of age. "Neonates born of infected females" were derived from mice which had received a series of four oral infections or intramuscular injections of 100 viable *T. taeniaeformis* eggs each at weekly intervals, beginning at 6 weeks of age. Males were then introduced and the females were immunized twice more during pregnancy.

Serum and intestinal immunoglobulins were obtained following oral infection of 6 week old female mice with 100 viable *T. taeniaeformis* eggs at weekly intervals for 6 weeks. One week after the last infection the animals were exsanguinated and serum collected. Intestinal immunoglobulins were collected by homogenization of the small intestine, inactivation of the intestinal enzymes at 56°C for 30 minutes and centrifugation at 2,000 g for 30 minutes. Colostral whey was obtained by centrifugation (2,000 g, 30 minutes) of the colostrum clot obtained from the stomachs of 1-10 day old neonates which had suckled on female mice that had been orally infected with 100 viable *T. taeniaeformis* eggs weekly for 6 weeks. Immunoglobulins were separated from the serum, colostral whey and intestinal extract by ammonium sulphate precipitation.

In the first two experiments mice were infected with 100 viable *T. taeniaeformis* eggs via stomach tube at 12, 21 and/ or 42 days of age. In the third experiment seven groups of 11 day old neonates, born of normal mothers, were fed via stomach tube with 5 mgms of serum, intestinal or colostral immunoglobulins, or saline, at 18, 12 and 3 hours prior to and 3 hours after a dose of 100 viable *T. taeniaeformis* eggs (time 0). All animals were killed 3 or 4 weeks after infection and their livers examined for the presence of cysticerci.

Taenia taeniaeformis antigen was prepared from protoscolices extracted from the cysticerci from the livers of Fisher rats. The protoscolices were lyophilized and them extracted by homogenization in Tris-HCl buffer. The suspension was allowed to extract for 12 hours at 4°C and then the supernatant antigen collected after centrifugation at 140,000xg for 60 minutes at 4°C.

Specific rabbit anti-mouse heavy chain antisera to μ, α, γ_1 and γ_2 heavy chains were prepared from mouse serum and colostrum (Lloyd and Soulsby, to be published).

Immunofluorescence was performed by a sandwich technique following that of Holborow and Johnson (1967). Sections of the jejunum of 12 day old mice that had been suckled on normal or orally infected mothers were cut on a cryostat at-20°C. The sections were fixed in methanol and stained with *T. taeniaeformis* antigen, rabbit anti-*T. taeniaeformis* antibody and fluorescent goat anti-rabbit immunoglobulins (Cappel Labs.). All preparations were inactivated at 56°C for 30 minutes and adsorbed with acetone dried mouse liver powder prior to use. Controls included inhibition of the reaction with mouse anti-*T. taeniaeformis* serum and by omission of antigen in the staining procedure.

Indirect haemagglutination was performed as described by Khoury (1973). After the results had been read the cells in each tube in the dilution series were washed three times in phosphate buffered saline and enhancement of haemagglutination was performed in microtitre haemagglutination trays. The immunoglobulin-antigen coated, three times washed, sheep red blood cells from each dilution were added to the wells in the trays and a 1:20 dilution of the specific rabbit anti-mouse heavy chain antiserum (complement inactivated and adsorbed with gluteraldehyde-treated and gluteraldehyde-treated-antigen-coated sheep red blood cells) was added to each well.

RESULTS

Maternal Transfer of Antibody

120 mice born of normal or orally infected females were challenged orally with 100 viable *T. taeniaeformis* eggs at 12, 21 and 42 days of age.

The results are presented in Table I. The offspring of infected females were protected against infection when they were challenged at 12 and 21 days of age ($p < 0.005$). By 42 days of age this maternally transferred immunity had waned.

TABLE I

The Mean Number of T. taeniaeformis *Metacestodes Found in the Offspring of Normal Mice, or Mice Infected Orally with* T. taeniaeformis, *Following Challenge with 100 Eggs of* T. taeniaeformis.

	Age of Litters in Days		
	12	21	42
Litters Born of Normal Females	17.4 ± 0.61*	30.1 ± 0.57	50.8 ± 1.07
Litters Born of Infected Females	0.8 ± 0.24†	1.0 ± 0.24†	46.8 ± 0.93

* Mean Number of Metacestodes ± S.E.
† $p < 0.005$

Placental and Transmammary Transfer of Immunity

120 neonatal mice were obtained from normal females (40), orally infected females (40) or intramuscularly injected females (40). At birth half of the neonates were left with their mothers. The other half, born of normal females, were given to infected females to suckle and half of those born of infected females were given to normal females to be suckled. All the neonates were challenged at 12 days of age with 100 viable *T. taeniaeformis* eggs.

The results are presented in Table II. Immunity was passively transferred from orally infected females both through the placenta and the colostrum. Thus a significant reduction in the number of metacestodes was found in the neonates born of normal females but suckled on infected females compared to similar neonates suckled on normal females. Neonates born of infected females but suckled on normal females showed a similar significant reduction of metacestodes. The offspring of intramuscularly injected females and suckled on these females or orally infected females also demonstrate a significant level of protection ($p < 0.005$).

TABLE II

The Mean Number of T. taeniaeformis *Metacestodes Found in Neonatal Mice Following Prenatal and Postnatal Transfer of Immunity.*

	Litters Suckled on Normal Females	Litters Suckled on Orally Infected Females	Litters Suckled on Intramuscularly Injected Females
Litters Born of Normal Females	15.9 ± 0.85*	1.0 ± 0.38†	ND
Litters Born of Orally Infected Females	1.3 ± 0.45†	0.2 ± 0.13†	ND
Litters Born of Intramuscularly Injected Females	ND	0.7 ± 0.26†	3.2 ± 0.61†

* Mean Number of Metacestodes ± S.E.
† $p < 0.005$
ND = Not Done

Passive Transfer of Immunity by Serum, Intestinal and Colostral Immunoglobulins

140, 11 day old neonatal mice, born of normal mothers, were divided into seven groups of 20 mice each. They were fed normal or immune serum, intestinal or colostral immunoglobulins, or saline, from 18 hours prior to and 3 hours after an oral infection of 100 viable *T. taeniaeformis* eggs (See Materials and Methods). They were killed 4 weeks later.

The results are presented in Table III. No significant difference was found in the number of metacesotdes found in the livers of those animals given saline, normal serum, normal intestinal or normal colostral immunoglobulins. The neonates fed serum, intestinal or colostral immunoglobulins extracted from infected mice all had a significant reduction in the number of metacestodes found in their livers ($p < 0.005$). A striking feature was the degeneration of 74% of the metacestodes found in the livers of the animals fed serum immunoglobulins compared to 7% and 17% degeneration of the metacestodes in those animals that were fed intestinal or colostral immunoglobulins respectively.

TABLE III

The Numbers of T. taeniaeformis *Metacestodes Found in Neonatal Mice Receiving Serum, Intestinal or Colostral Immunoglobulins from* T. taeniaeformis *Infected Mice.*

	Immunoglobulin Extracted From			
	Serum	Intestinal	Colostral	Saline
Extracted from Normal Mice	20.8±0.92*	20.3±0.63	22.0±0.68	19.2 ± 0.85
Extracted From Infected Mice	6.8±0.61† (74%)[a]	8.4 ± 0.5† (7%)	7.5±0.47† (17%)	

* Mean Number of Metacestodes ± S.E.
† $p < 0.005$
a Percent Dead Metacestodes

Indirect Haemagglutination and Enhanced Hemagglutination

As seen in Table IV all the classes of immunoglobulins (IgM, IgA, IgG_1 and IgG_2) were involved in the haemagglutination of *T. taeniaeformis* coated sheep red blood cells by serum immunoglobulins. IgA and IgG_2 were predominant in intestinal extracts while in colostrum IgA predominated. The indirect haemagglutination test was inhibitable by soluble antigen, and the enhanced haemagglutination reactions were inhibited by immunoglobulins of the same class as the antiserum used but not by those of other classes.

TABLE IV

Indirect Haemagglutination and Enhanced Haemagglutination Titres of the Serum, Intestinal and Colostral Immunoglobulins Extracted from T. taeniaeformis *Infected Mice.*

	Indirect Haemagglutination	Enhanced Haemagglutination with Antisera to			
		IgM	IgG_1	IgG_2	IgA
Serum Immunoglobulins	4*	16	64	64	128
Intestinal Immunoglobulins	2	2	4	8	16
Colostral Immunoglobulins	8	4	8	16	1048

* Reciprocal of Titer

Antibody to T. taeniaeformis *on the Intestinal Wall of Neonatal Mice.*

Mouse anti-*T. taeniaeformis* antibody could be detected by the indirect fluorescent antibody technique on the intestinal mucosa of 12 day old neonates which had suckled on orally infected mice. This was evident as areas of especially bright fluorescence against a diffusely fluorescent background (Fig. I). Such areas of bright fluorescence were not detectable in the intestine of neonates suckled on normal females. The reaction could be inhibited by the addition of mouse anti-*T. taeniaeformis* antibody or by the omission of antigen from the staining procedure. A diffusely fluorescent background was found in all controls and this was probably due to naturally adsorbed immunoglobulins on the surface of the neonatal intestine.

DISCUSSION

The passive transfer of immunity to *T. taeniaeformis* infections in neonatal mice has been examined as a model system for the study of the passive transfer of immunity to *T. saginata* infections in calves.

These experiments demonstrate the natural passive transfer of immunity to the offspring of *T. taeniaeformis* infected mice.

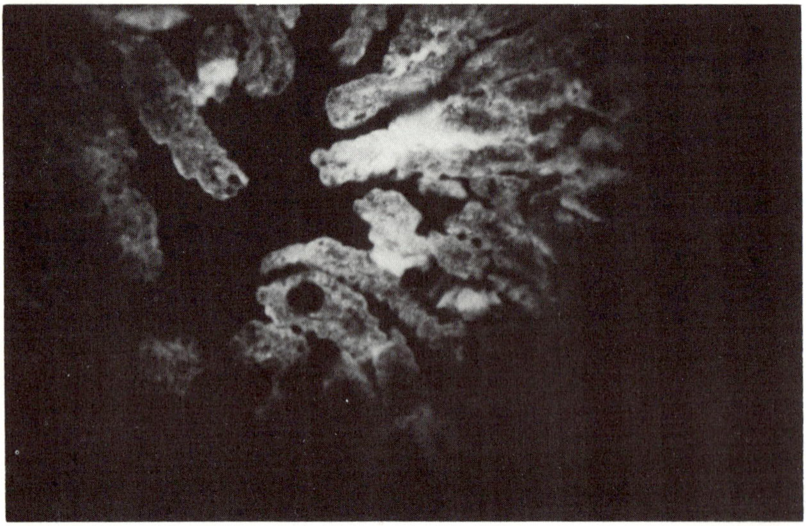

*Fig. 1. Fluorescent micrograph of the intestine of a 12 day old neonatal mouse showing areas of fluorescence indicating the presence of anti-*Taenia taeniaeformis *antibody.*

This transfer of immunity takes place both prenatally and postnatally. The prenatal transfer of immunity could be associated with antibodies in the IgG class of immunoglobulins as these are known to cross the mouse placenta (Fahey and Barth, 1965; Grey *et al.*, 1971). Since IgG immunoglobulins have a half-life of 2.7 - 5 days (Fahey and Sell, 1965) antibodies of this class would be expected to be still in the circulation of 12 day old neonates. IgG_{2a} immunoglobulins, with a half-life of 5 days (Fahey and Sell. 1965), have been demonstrated to confer protection against *T. taeniaeformis* infections in rats (Leid and Williams, 1973).

IgA is the predominant immunoglobulin im mouse colostrum as compared to IgM and IgG (Fahey and Barth, 1965; Lloyd and Soulsby, to be published). Since this immunoglobulin was largely responsible for the haemagglutination of antigen coated red blood cells it is possible that the postnatal transfer of immunity to neonatal mice is due to antibodies in this class of immunoglobulins. However, further studies are needed to assess the ability of purified IgA antibodies to confer protection.

Gemmell and Macnamara (1972) have suggested that the inability of *E. granulosus* to penetrate the intestine of immunized sheep may be due to an humoral effect at the level of the intestine, since immunity to sheep metacestodes can be transferred by serum or colostrum to non-immune recipients (Blundell *et al.*, 1968; Gemmell *et al.*, 1969). The present study indicates that protective immunoglobulins can be extracted from the intestinal tissue of *T. taeniaeformis* infected mice, but whether these antibodies have their activity within the intestinal lumen, in the intestinal mucosa or systemically has not yet been elucidated. However, antibody to *T. taeniaeformis* can be detected on the intestinal wall of neonatal mice suckled on infected mothers and this might suggest that the intestine acts as a first line of defence against a metacestode infection.

The antibodies on the intestinal epithelium might be expected to be of the IgA class of immunoglobulins but it is possible that IgA antibodies alone are not the sole means of protection within the intestine. The experiments of Heath (1970) were performed on animals immunized intramuscularly and this route of immunization would not be expected to raise high levels of antibodies of the IgA class.

The demonstration that mouse colostral antibodies do confer protection against neonatal infection with *T. taeniaeformis* and that the major *in vitro* antibody activity in colostrum is due to the IgA class of immunoglobulins has led to the examination of the role of this class of immunoglobulins in the passive transfer of immunity to *T. saginata* infections in the bovine. Lascelles and McDowell (1970) have demonstrated that IgA antibody can be produced by local immunization of the mammary glands of ewes, and this technique is being examined as a means of producing protective antibodies for *T. saginata* infections in neonatal calves.

REFERENCES

Blundell, S.K., Gemmell, M.A. and Macnamara, F.N. (1968). *Exp. Parasit.*, *23*, 79.

Campbell, D.H. (1938a). *J. Immunol.*, *35*, 195.

Campbell, D.H. (1938b). *J. Immunol.*, *35*, 205.

Campbell, D.H. (1938c). *J. Immunol.*, *35*, 465.

Fahey, J.L. and Barth, W.F. (1965). *Proc. Soc. Exp. Biol. Med.*, *118*, 596.

Fahey, J.L. and Sell,S. (1965). *J. Exp. Med.*, *122*, 41.

Froyd, G. (1964). *Res. Vet. Sci.*, *5*, 434.

Froyd, G. and Round, M.C. (1960). *Res. Vet. Sci.*, *1*, 275.

Gemmell, M.A. and Macnamara, F.N. (1972) in "Immunity to Animal Parasites," ed. Soulsby, E.J.L., Academic Press, p. 235.

Gemmell, M.A. and Soulsby, E.J.L. (1968). *Bull. Wld. Hlth. Org.*, *39*, 45.

Gemmell, M.A., Blundell-Hassell, S.K. and Macnamara, F.N. (1969). *Expt. Parasit.*, *26*, 52.
Grey, H.M., Hirst, J.W. and Cohn, M. (1971). *J. Exp. Med.*, *133*, 289.
Hearin, J.T. (1941). *Amer. J. Hyg.*, *33*, Sec. D, 71.
Heath, D.D. (1970). Cited by Gemmell, M.A. and Macnamara, F.N. (1972) in "Immunity to Animal Parasites" ed. Soulsby, E.J.L., Academic Press, p. 235.
Holborow, E.J. and Johnson, G.D. (1967) in "Handbook of Experimental Immunology," ed. Weir, D.M., F. A. Davis, p. 571.
Kerr, K.B. (1935). *Amer. J. Hyg.*, *22*, 169.
Khoury, P.B. (1973). Ph.D. Thesis, University of Pennsylvania, Philadelphia, U.S.A.
Larsh, J.E. (1942). *Amer. J. Hyg.*, *36*, 187.
Larsh, J.E. (1944). *Amer. J. Hug.*, *39*, 129.
Lascelles, A. K. and McDowell, G.H. (1970). *Immunology*, *19*, 613.
Leid, R.W. and Williams, J.F. (1973). Abstr. "Amer. Soc. Parasit." p. 50.
Leonard, A.B. and Smith, A.E. (1939). *J. Parasit.*, *25*, 30.
Miller, H.M. (1932a). *Proc. Soc. Exp. Biol. Med.*, *30*, 82.
Miller, H.M. (1932b). *Proc. Soc. Exp. Biol. Med.*, *29*, 1124.
Miller, H.M. (1934). *Amer. J. Hyg.*, *19*, 270.
Miller, H.M. (1935). *Amer. J. Hyg.*, *21*, 456.
Miller, H.M. and Gardiner, M.L. (1932a). *Science*, *75*, 270.
Miller, H.M. and Gardiner, M.L. (1932b). *Proc. Soc. Exp. Biol. Med.*, *29*, 779.
Miller, H.M. and Gardiner, M.L. (1934). *Amer. J. Hyg.*, *20*, 424.
Rickard, M.D. and Arundel, J.H. (1974). *Aust. Vet. J.*, *50*, 22.
Urquhart, G.M. (1961). *J. Parasit.*, *47*, 857.

IMMUNOGLOBULIN LEVELS IN PATIENTS INFECTED WITH *TAENIA SAGINATA**

Kathryn H. Nepote,** Z.S. Pawlowski*** and E.J.L. Soulsby**

**Department of Pathobiology, School of Veterinary Medicine, University of Pennsylvania and ***Clinic of Parasitic Diseases Medical Academy of Poznan, Poland.

INTRODUCTION

The human tapeworms *Taenia saginata* and *Taenia solium* may survive for several years in the lumen of the bowel. This suggests that immunological rejection mechanisms for these infections are poorly developed. With the exception of the hymenolepid tapeworms, the immune response to infection with the adult tapeworms has received little study. Experimental studies indicate that purely lumen dwelling cestodes induce little immune response. Thus, while *Hymenolepis nana* (which can undergo autoinfection via a cysticercoid stage in the villus) induces good immunity and a good antibody response, the related parasite, *Hymenolepis diminuta*, which does not migrate into the villi, fails to do so (Chadler, 1940). However, adult cestodes which become closely associated with the crypts of the intestinal mucosa (e.g. *Echinococcus granulosus*) will induce immunity to reinfection (See Gemmell and Soulsby, 1968).

Several workers have reported the detection of antibodies in patients infected *Diphyllobothrium latum* or *T. solium* (Isaac and Velden, 1904; Ghedini, 1913, Jerlov, 1919), but, others obtained positive serological reactions only in isolated instances in such patients (Basson, 1911; Voille and Saint Rat, 1919). Immediate hypersensitivity reactions to intradermal tests reported in patients infected with *T. saginata* and *D. latum* (Ramsdell, 1927, Brunner, 1928) may be interpreted as indicating the presence of immunoglobulin E class antibodies in these infections since elevated levels of IgE have been reported in humans infected with other parasitic helminths (Johannson, *et al.*, 1970). The ability of parasitic helminths to stimulate reaginic antibodies with characteristics similar to those of human IgE in experimental animals is well known (Sadun, 1972). However, there has been little

---

*Studies supported by U.S. Public Health Service Grants 05-3342 (Center for Disease Control), AI06262, and NIH GM02051-05.

study of immunoglobulin E levels in humans following treatment and removal of the parasite associated with increased levels of the immunoglobulin. In the present studies an opportunity was available to determine immunoglobulin levels before and after treatment in patients infected with *T. saginata*.

MATERIALS AND METHODS

Serum samples were taken from *T. saginata* infected patients before treatment, and one week and four months after treatment with "Niclosamide" or tin compounds and from uninfected blood donors in the vicinity of Poznan, Poland. Serum was either lyophilized or frozen and sent to Philadelphia for examination.

Levels of serum immunoglobulins G,M, and A were determined by the Mancini technique using heavy chain specific goat anti-human immunoglobulin sera (Mancini, Carbonara and Hereman, 1965). The amount of immunoglobulin per ml. of serum was calculated using known standards for each immunoglobulin. Immunoglobulin E levels were determined by radioimmunoassay (Gleich, Averbeck and Svedland, 1971) in which anti-IgE covalently bound to Sephadex particles is used to determine the capacity of a sample of serum to inhibit the binding of a standard ^{125}I IgE.

Differences in the immunoglobulin levels between the 3 groups of sera from infected persons and sera from uninfected persons were analyzed using the Kruskal-Wallis test for differences in ranked data. This nonparametric method of analysis was used since the variance of the data was so great as to prevent the use of standard parametric analysis. Significance was determined using the calculated H value and the Chi-square table at 3 degrees of freedom (number of groups minus 1) (Sokal and Rohlf, 1969). Linear regression analysis was used for those infected individuals for whom IgE levels had been determined in 3 serum samples taken prior to, one week and four months after treatment, respectively.

RESULTS

Immunoglobulin levels for 113 serum samples were determined. Sixty-three serum samples were obtained from 28 patients infected with *T. saginata*. Comparison of the mean immunoglobulin levels between infected and uninfected groups indicated little change in IgM or IgG levels (Table 1). Prior to treatment the mean IgA level in infected patients was lower than the mean level of uninfected individuals and increased to the uninfected mean level following treatment. In comparison, the mean IgE level was greater in infected individuals and declined with time after treatment so that it approached that of the uninfected group at 4 months after treatment (Table 1).

Table 1

Mean Serum Immunoglobulin Levels During the Course of Taenia saginata *Infection*

Group	IgA (mgm%)	IgG (mgm%)	IgM (mgm%)	IgE (ngm/ml)
Before Treatment n=28	273.5±29.0*	1216.9±70.0	144.7±13.9	1107.6±323.5
1 week After Treatment n=23	283.4±26.5	1328.0±85.5	128.9±12.1	1233.0±385.7
4 months After Treatment n=12	313.3±29.8	1227.5±94.9	116.3±97.3	508.8±164.2
Uninfected n=50	381.8±29.0	1233.0±86.2	166.7±17.7	356.6± 84.8 **

* Mean ± Standard Error ** N = 28

Analysis of the results by the Kruskal-Wallis test is presented in Table 2. The general trends noted upon examination of the means are reflected in the levels of significance of differences between groups. Thus, the differences between groups were significant with IgA ($p<0.05$) and highly significant with IgE ($p<0.005$).

Table 2

Comparison of T. saginata *Infected and Uninfected Individuals according to the Kruskal-Wallis Test for Ranked Data (See Table 1).*

Immunoglobulin Class	H value	Significance (d.f.=3)
IgA	8.6	p<0.05
IgG	2.1	nonsig.
IgM	4.8	nonsig.
IgE	17.8	p<0.005

Mean Ranks Between Groups (IgA and IgE)

Group	IgA	IgE
Before treatment	47	54
1 week after treatment	48	56
4 months after treatment	60	41
Uninfected	66	31

With 11 of the infected patients it was possible to obtain

serum samples taken before treatment, 1 week and 4 months after treatment (33 samples). The immunoglobulin levels of these samples were examined to see if they reflected the same trends noted in the total 63 samples from infected persons (Table 3).

Table 3

Mean Serum Immunoglobulin Levels of 33 Serum Samples from 11 Infected Individuals

Time with respect to Treatment	IgA (mgm%)	IgG (mgm%)	IgM (mgm%)	IgE (ngm/ml)
Before	309.1±22.7	1315.0±140.8	132.3±30.3	1424.5±656.8
1 week After	316.5±45.1	1272.7± 79.2	145.8±23.2	1411.4±656.4
4 months After	318.0±32.3	1205.9±101.3	120.3±18.4	440.5±163.5

Only the IgE levels appeared to differ significantly. The IgE levels were greatest before treatment and lowest 4 months after treatment. A scatter graph of the IgE levels in these individual sera illustrates the trend noted (Fig. 1).

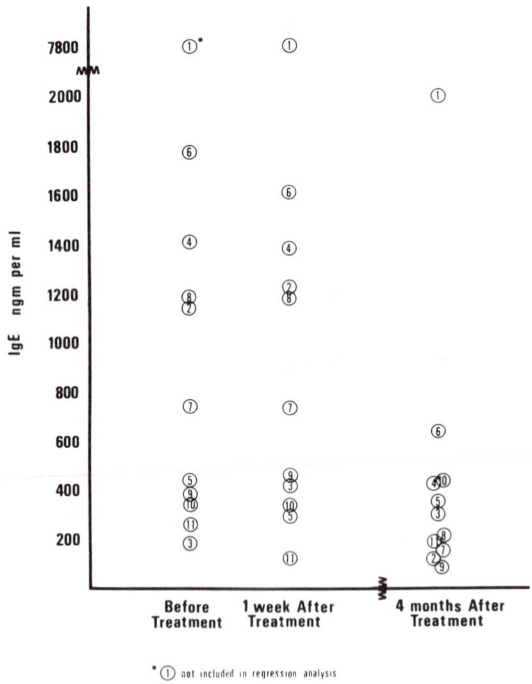

Fig. 1. Serum IgE levels of 33 progressive serum samples from 11 Taenia saginata *infected individuals.*

Analysis of regression was calculated for the IgE levels of 10 of these 11 individuals. One infected individual, though reflecting the general trend in IgE levels (7800 ngm/ml before and 1 week after treatment, 2000 ngm/ml 4 months after treatment) was not included in the regression analysis because the serum IgE levels were so much greater than the others. Linear regression fitted to the data indicated a slope of -31.8973 with a significance of the slope at $p<0.01$.

DISCUSSION

Significant differences in IgA and IgE levels between *T. saginata* infected and uninfected individuals and in the infected individuals following treatment were found. This was especially evident with IgE ($p<0.005$). Since *T. saginata* is a bowel parasite and both IgA and IgE are associated with mucosal surfaces, these results suggest that infection with *T. saginata* may affect the production of these immunoglobulins at such mucosal surfaces.

The IgE trend was consistant with a possible antibody response to infection, with high levels occurring during infection and with a return to low levels once the antigenic stimulus was removed. The significance of the IgE levels in infected individuals and the change in the level of this immunoglobulin following treatment was verified by linear regression analysis of the immunoglobulin levels of 10 individuals from whom serial serum samples were obtained. The wide variance present in these 10 individuals eliminated the use of parametric analysis to test for the significance of the change in IgE. The nature of the sample enabled the use of linear regression analysis of IgE levels over time with respect to treatment. The change in IgE levels was significant as illustrated by the marked slope of the regression line and the high significance of the slope ($p<0.01$).

The fact that 2 different statistical analyses both indicate highly significant differences in the IgE levels in uninfected and infected individuals, and in time after treatment suggests that serum IgE levels are affected by infection with *T. saginata*. Increased IgE levels may explain the immediate hypersensitivity reactions to intradermal tests reported by Ramsdell (1927) and Brunner (1928). Similarly, increased IgE levels may be related to symptoms such as urticaria, pruritis, diarrhea and eosinophilia which have been reported, though infrequently, in *T. saginata* infection (Pawlowski and Schultz, 1972). In the present study there was no correlation noted between IgE levels and eosinophil counts, neither could the symptoms of infected patients be related to

IgE levels.

The IgA profile in this study was the reverse of the IgE levels and is difficult to explain. The significance of the differences in IgA between groups was not as marked as in IgE and might have been a result of the abnormal sample. The variance present in the sample was so great that non-parametric analysis was necessary. Several variables inherent in the sample population such as, age of infected individuals (9-67 years), duration of infection (3-39 months), and number of unsuccessful treatments (0-3) may have contributed to the variance. Therefore, the differences noted in IgA levels though statistically significant may reflect a sampling error not that of the total population. Since the analysis of the immunoglobulin levels of the 11 individuals for whom progressive serum samples were available indicated a distinct difference only in IgE and not IgA, this suggests that the trend noted for IgA with the total sera was not real but a result of the abnormal sample used for analysis.

Though elevated IgE in these individuals does not necessarily indicate the production of an anti-*T. saginata* antibody of the IgE class, the reduction of IgE levels following removal of the tapeworm would suggest a specific stimulation by the parasite. Evidence from other studies (Sadun, 1972) is consistent with the idea that specific IgE antibodies are produced. Nevertheless, further work is necessary to determine if the increased IgE is due to the production of a specific antibody and the functional role of such antibody in the immune response to the parasite.

SUMMARY

IgE was the only immunoglobulin that showed a consistantly significant difference between *T. saginata* infected and uninfected individuals and in infected individuals with respect to treatment. The data suggest that IgE levels are affected by *T. saganita* infection. These results must be interpreted with caution because of the great variation of the sample population used for analysis. Further studies are needed to demonstrate that elevated IgE levels in *T. saginata* infected patients are due to IgE class specific antibody.

ACKNOWLEDGEMENT

It is a pleasure to acknowledge Dr. Donald A. Abt for his advice concerning the statistical treatment of the data.

REFERENCES

Basson, D. (1911). *Zbt. Bakt. (Orig.) (I Abt.) 60,* 426.
Brunner, M. (1928). *J. Immunol. 15,* 83.
Chandler, A.C. (1940). *Amer. J. Hyg. 31.* 17.
Gemmell, M.A. and Soulsby, E.J.L. (1968). *Bull. Wld. Hlth. Org. 39,* 45.
Ghedini, G. (1913). *Gass. Osp. Milano. 34,* 321.
Gleich, G.J. Averbeck, A.K. and Svedlund, H.A. (1971). *J. Lab. Clin. Med. 77,* 690.
Isaac, S. and van der Velden, R. (1904). *Dtsch. Med. Wschr. 30,* (27), 982.
Jerlov, M. (1919). *Immun. Forsch. 28,* 489.
Johannson, S.G.O., Bennich, H., Berg, T. and Hogman, E. (1970) *Clin. Exp. Immunol. 6,* 43.
Mancini, G., Carbonara, C.O. and Hereman, J.F. (1965). *Immunochem. 2,* 235.
Pawlowski, Z.S. and Schultz, M.G. (1972). *Adv. Parasit. 10,* 269.
Sadun, E.H. (1972). *In: Immunity to Animal Parasites* (Ed. Soulsby, E.J.L.) Academic Press, New York.
Sokal, R.R. and Rohlf, F.J. (1969). *Biometry,* W.H. Freeman and Co., San Francisco.
Violle, H. and de Saint-Rat, L. (1919). *C.R. Soc. Biol. 82,* 1033.

IMMUNE MECHANISMS AND HEPATIC FIBROSIS IN FASCIOLIASIS

J. D. Dargie, J. Armour, B. Rushton and Max Murray. Glasgow University Veterinary School. Bearsden, Glasgow, Scotland

INTRODUCTION

Effective vaccines are available against several economically and socially important parasitic diseases of domestic animals including parasitic bronchitis in cattle and sheep (Jarrett *et al.*, 1959; and Jovanovic *et al.*, 1965), canine ancylostomiasis (Miller, 1965), syngamiasis in chickens (Varga, 1968) and coccidiosis in chickens (Hein, 1963). In Great Britain, the three major parasitic problems in domestic livestock are parasitic bronchitis, ostertagiasis and fascioliasis, while in man fascioliasis is an increasingly recognised problem throughout the world. An effective vaccine is now available for parasitic bronchitis and research is in progress towards immunisation against the remaining two.

It is well recognised, both from field and experimental observations that animal hosts have a variable susceptibility to infection with the liver fluke *Fasciola hepatica* (Ross, 1967; Boray, 1967; Nansen *et al.*, 1972). Some, e.g., pigs and cattle, have a high or at least moderate degree of natural resistance, whereas others, e.g., sheep and laboratory animals are highly susceptible. The underlying reason for such differences in host susceptibility is not clear. It has been suggested that natural immunity is expressed both during the migratory-parenchymal and adult-bile duct stages of the infection. The former is considered to be related to the distribution and amount of connective tissue in the host's liver parenchyma; sheep are thought to be highly susceptible because their liver parenchyma contains only small amounts of connective tissue, whereas pigs and to a lesser extent cattle are more resistant because of the relatively large amounts of connective tissue in their livers. Possibly the connective tissue stroma helps to trap young migrating flukes. Similarly the range of susceptibility to reinfection in various hosts may be related to the degree of hepatic fibrosis present. In cattle, the presence of adult flukes in the biliary system is characterised by elimination of a large proportion of the population between 16 and 30 weeks after infection (Doyle, 1971) and this expulsion is preceded by a period of 4 to 6 weeks of reduced biological activity of the flukes manifested by diminished faecal egg output. It has been suggested that these effects are caused by bile duct calcification and that under such conditions the adult flukes are eliminated as a result of starvation.

On the other hand, there is now substantial evidence of experimentally acquired resistance to *F. hepatica* in rats (Thorpe & Broome, 1962; Corba *et al.*, 1971; Hayes *et al.*, 1973, mice (Lang, 1967), cattle (Ross, 1966; Boray, 1967; Doyle, 1971), and to a limited extent sheep (retardation of migration Sinclair, 1971). In such situations it would appear likely that immune mechanisms are operative.

In our studies we have attempted to clarify whether resistance is non-specific, i.e., related to physical factors such as fibrosis and calcification acquired in primary infections or is a reflection of a specific immunological response by the host. To evaluate the relative importance and nature of host defence mechanisms in fascioliasis, we have carried out a series of experiments employing active immunisation procedures in rats, cattle and sheep together with investigations into the role of humoral and cellular components of the immune response. This was combined with a study of the pathogenetic mechanisms underlying the development of hepatic fibrosis in fascioliasis.

IMMUNE MECHANISMS IN FASCIOLIASIS

Acquired resistance

Rats

Recent studies (Armour & Dargie, 1974) have shown that rats previously exposed to normal or irradiated metacercariae of *F. hepatica* can develop a significant degree of resistance to subsequent reinfection by this parasite. For example, in rats infected with 20 metacercariae and treated with anthelmintic 8 weeks later, an average of only 2.6 flukes became established from a challenge infection of 20 metacercariae, compared with a mean recovery of 5.5 parasites from previously uninfected animals. This difference represented a degree of protection in the order of 53% in reinfected animals. Likewise, an equally high level of protection against challenge infection was obtained by prior exposure of rats to 3 doses of 20 irradiated metacercariae given at weekly intervals, 2.4 as against 5.4 flukes representing 56% protection.

Cattle

Although it is well recognised that cattle exhibit high resistance to infection and reinfection with *F. hepatica*, it is only comparatively recently that the nature and extent of this resistance has been studied under controlled experimental conditions. It is now apparent that resistance to fascioliasis in the bovine is expressed at both the parenchymal and bile duct stages of the infection. Thus, Doyle (1971) demonstrated that calves infected with 750 metacercariae of *F. hepatica* and killed 16 weeks later contained significantly higher fluke burdens (mean 126.8 ± 22.2) than animals similarly infected and necropsied 30 weeks later (19.8 ± 6.1 flukes). In a further experiment where calves were infected with 500 metacercariae, it was found that most of the fluke burden was eliminated between weeks 20 and 24, and that this was preceded, beginning at 15 weeks, by a marked drop in faecal egg output (Doyle, 1972). With regard to immunity at the parenchymal level, Doyle (1971) showed that in calves which had been infected with 750 *F. hepatica* metacercariae 17 weeks previously, an average of only 25.3 flukes developed to maturity from a challenge infection of 1650 metacercariae given 13 weeks previously; this compared with 135.8 parasites recovered from challenged controls, representing a reduction in fluke burden of about 80% in reinfected animals.

Despite the high degree of natural and acquired resistance of cattle to liver fluke infection, attempts to vaccinate animals against the parasite have produced rather conflicting results. Bitakeramire (1973) reported that of 7 calves given two doses of 1,000 metacercariae of *F. gigantica* exposed to 3 kr. of gamma rays, only 2 animals had parasites in their bile ducts from a challenge infection of 1,000 normal metacercariae given 14 weeks after the second vaccine dose (10 and 18 flukes respectively, representing a mean "recovery" of 4 flukes for the group); the livers of the remaining animals were found to be normal when examined grossly and microscopically. Challenge controls receiving only normal metacercariae were found to have extensive liver lesions at necropsy and harboured an average of 273 adult *F. gigantica* within their bile ducts. A similar vaccination schedule, i.e., 2 doses of 1,000 metacercariae exposed to 3.5 kr. of gamma rays did not appear to induce a comparable immunity to *F. hepatica* (unpublished results in co-operation with J.J. Doyle). Vaccinated animals, when challenged with 800 metacercariae of *F. hepatica* contained an average of 28 flukes at necropsy compared with an average recovery of 93 flukes in non-vaccinated animals, representing a degree of protection in the order of only 70% compared with over 98% recorded for *F. gigantica*.

Sheep

Although there is little evidence of acquired resistance in the field, and attempts to vaccinate sheep against fascioliasis have proved uniformly unsuccessful, we have recently shown in a small pilot experiment that sheep given 6 doses of 100 irradiated *F. hepatica* metacercariae (3 kr) developed some degree of resistance against a challenge infection of normal metacercariae. Vaccinated animals, when challenged with 750 metacercariae, contained an average of 36 adult flukes compared with an average recovery of 105 parasites from non-vaccinated animals; although marked, (vaccination offered a degree of protection in the order of 66%) the difference between the groups was not statistically significant.

Taken as a whole, the results described above demonstrate that rats, cattle and sheep can develop a significant degree of acquired resistance to *F. hepatica*, but reveal little of the mechanisms involved. There are basically two possibilities, neither of which are mutually exclusive. One explanation is that as a result of the damage caused by the primary infection, the liver environment is rendered unsuitable for further infections; the second possibility is that this resistance is at least partly immune in nature.

Transfer of immunity by cells and serum

It is customary to separate immune responses into cellular and humoral components, and while it is now accepted that this is an artificial dichotomy in that in the disease situation the various components of the immunological system work in cooperation to produce an optimal reaction, it is nonetheless a convenient classification. Since direct evidence for the involvement of sensitised lymphoid cells or serum can be obtained only by transfer of cells or humoral antibody, an attempt was made to evaluate the relative roles of these components in resistance to *F. hepatica* by transfer experiments involving syngeneic or highly inbred animals.

Adoptive transfer of lymphoid cells

The results in Table 1 show that cells taken from the mesenteric and hepatic lymph nodes and spleens of rats harbouring adult flukes were able when transferred to syngeneic recipients to confer a high degree of protection against a primary challenge infection. The extent of the reduction in fluke burden in recipient animals (30 to 81%) was apparently related to the number of flukes in the donor rats and dependent upon the transfer of viable cells.

Likewise, cells from the hepatic lymph nodes of infected donor calves and sheep, when transferred to their monozygous twins (or highly inbred animals in the case of sheep) also conferred a high degree of protection (77 to 97%) as against a primary infection (Table 1).

Table 1

Passive Transfer of Immunity to Fasciola Hepatica by Adoptive Transfer of Lymphoid Cells

Species	Fluke burden in Donor	Age of Donor Infection (weeks)	Number of Lymphoid Cells transferred	Challenge Infection (Metacercariae)	Number of *F. Hepatica* at Necropsy (± S.E.)	Reduction in fluke burden compared with controls (%)
Rat	7	10	3×10^8	20	1.2 ± 0.6	81
			-	20	6.3 ± 0.6	(P<0.001)
	6	10	2.5×10^8	20	1.5 ± 0.7	68
	6	10	2.5×10^8 Freeze/Thawed	20	4.5 ± 0.5	(P<0.001)
			-	20	4.7 ± 0.4	0
	3	10	3×10^8	20	3.1 ± 0.4	30
			-	20	4.4 ± 0.6	(N.S.)
Cattle	110	14	3×10^{10}	1,000	9	93
			-	1,000	155	
	104	14	3×10^{10}	1,000	23	
			-	1,000	113	77
Sheep	0 (6 x 100 irradiated metacercariae (3 kr))	8	3×10^9	500	3 ± 2	97 (P<0.01)
			-	500	105 ± 26	

NOTE: Rat Recipients Necropsied 10 weeks after cell transfer and challenge
Cattle " " 14 " " " " " "
Sheep " " 12 " " " " " "

The role of humoral antibody

Although previous attempts to transfer resistance passively to *F. hepatica* using serum from infected donors have been consistently unsuccessful (see review by Sokolić, 1968), the results of some recent experiments (Armour & Dargie, 1974) have shown that rats can be protected against liver fluke by intraperitoneal injection of antiserum (Table 2). For example, injection of 10 ml. of serum at the time of challenge and again 2 days later resulted in an overall reduction of 67% (mean 1.7 flukes) in the number of parasites which became established compared with the number recovered from challenged rats receiving no serum or similar quantities of serum taken from non-infected donors (mean 5.1 flukes). This effect was achieved both with homologous serum and with serum obtained from infected sheep and cattle.

Table 2

Passive Transfer of Immunity to Fasciola Hepatica in Rats by Serum from Infected Donors

Donor Species	Volume and Type of serum transferred (ML.)	Challenge infection (Metacercariae)	Number of *F. Hepatica* at Necropsy ±S.E. (week 10)	Reduction in fluke burden compared with controls (%)
Rat	2 x 10 ml. Immune Serum Day 0 and Day 2	20	1.6 ± 0.2	71
	-	20	5.6 ± 0.4	(P<0.001)
	2 x 10 ml. Immune Serum Day 0 and Day 2	20	2.6 ± 0.3	57
	-	20	6.1 ± 0.4	(P<0.001)
Cattle	2 x 2.5 ml. Immune Serum Day 0 and Day 2	20	2.0 ± 0.3	29 (N.S.)
	2 x 5 ml. Immune Serum Day 0 and Day 2	20	1.4 ± 0.4	50 (P<0.05)
	2 x 10 ml. Immune Serum Day 0 and Day 2	20	0.6 ± 0.3	79 (P<0.001)
	2 x 10 ml. Normal Serum Day 0 and Day 2	20	3.6 ± 0.5	0
	-	20	2.8 ± 0.5	
Cattle	2 x 10 ml. Immune Serum Day -14 and Day -12	20	4.9 ± 0.6	(N.S.)
	2 x 10 ml. Immune Serum Day 0 and Day 2	20	2.4 ± 0.4	57 (P<0.001)
	2 x 10 ml. Immune Serum Day +12 and Day +14	20	5.2 ± 0.6	(N.S.)
	-	20	5.6 ± 0.5	
Sheep	2 x 2.5 ml. Immune Serum Day 0 and Day 2	20	3.8 ± 0.5	34 (P<0.02)
	2 x 5 ml. Immune Serum Day 0 and Day 2	20	2.4 ± 0.5	59 (P<0.001)
	2 x 10 ml. Immune Serum Day 0 and Day 2	20	2.0 ± 0.2	66 (P<0.001)
	2 x 10 ml. Normal Serum Day 0 and Day 2	20	5.1 ± 0.8	12 (N.S.)
		20	5.1 ± 0.5	

A further feature of these results was the apparent relationship observed between the degree of protection and volume of serum transferred. This was demonstrated by the experiment where immune bovine serum was inoculated into groups of rats in amounts ranging from 0 to 20 ml. The mean number of flukes recovered from a challenge infection of 20 metacercariae was 3.6, 2.0, 1.4 and 0.6 in rats receiving 0, 5, 10 and 20 ml. of serum respectively. Similar results were obtained by transfer of serum from fluke-infected sheep. Although serum given within the first two days of challenge had considerable protective effect, the same serum given either 2 weeks after infection offered no protection (Table 2). Clearly for serum to confer protection it must be present in a high concentration and is only effective against young flukes prior to their entry into the liver.

Attempts to protect cattle and sheep by passive transfer of serum from fluke-infected donors also proved successful, provided large amounts were used (Table 3). Whereas intraperitoneal injection of 3.6 litres of immune serum into a 250 kg. bovine recipient resulted in almost complete protection against challenge of 1000 *F. hepatica* metacercariae (only 1 fluke was recovered at necropsy compared with 155 flukes from the animal receiving no serum), injection of 2.4 litres into an animal weighing 386 kg. offered no significant protection. In sheep, injection of 400 ml. of serum taken from fluke- infected sheep conferred approximately 80% protection against a challenge infection of 750 metacercariae.

Table 3

Passive Transfer of Immunity to Fasciola Hepatica in Cattle and Sheep by Serum from Infected Donors

Species	Volume and Type of serum transferred (ML.)	Challenge Infection (Metacercariae)	Number of *F. Hepatica* (±S.E.) at Necropsy	Reduction in fluke burden compared with controls (%)
Cattle	3,600 ml. Day 0	1,000	1	
	-	1,000	155	99
	2,400 ml. Day 0	1,000	100	
	-	1,000	113	12
Sheep	400 ml. from donor sheep given 6 doses of 100 irradiated metacercariae (3 kr.)	500	20 ± 9	81
	-	500	105 ± 26	(N.S.)

NOTE: Cattle recipients necropsied 14 weeks after serum transfer
Sheep " " 12 " " " "

The pathology of vaccination and passive protection

In all experiments, the degree of hepatic damage was related to the number of fluke recovered. Thus while similar lesions were found in all groups, hepatic fibrosis was considerably less both in vaccinated and cell or serum recipients than in challenge controls, i.e., protection was unrelated to the degree of hepatic fibrosis.

HEPATIC FIBROSIS IN FASCIOLIASIS

In cattle and sheep one of the major consequences of infection with *F. hepatica* is the development of hepatic fibrosis. In some cases the severity of the fibrosis which develops justifies the use of the term cirrhosis. Under certain circumstances the degree of fibrosis is much more severe than apparently can be accounted for by the straightforward destructive effect of the parasite; such a situation arises in animals which have been subjected to certain reinfection procedures (Rushton *et al.*, 1974). Moreover, although fibrosis is an indication of hepatic damage, it has been suggested that it may be beneficial to the host in that it acts as a defence barrier to fluke migration. Thus there is a need to define the types of fibrosis and the possible mechanisms underlying their genesis.

Nature of hepatic fibrosis

Studies on the pathology of fascioliasis indicate that a number of different types of fibrosis exist involving both the parenchyma and the portal canal.

Parenchyma

Post-necrotic scarring

One of the major forms of fibrosis encountered is scarring resulting from organisation and fibrosis of tracts of necrosis caused by fluke migration through the parenchyma. Such areas of fibrosis are extremely irregular and result in considerable distortion of hepatic architecture (Fig. 1). These scars may invest clumps or single hepatocytes and many contain haemosiderin-laden macophages, evidence of previous haemorrhage. In addition, linear septa often radiate from healing and healed fluke tracts to the normal hepatic fibrous framework of adjacent portal canals, hepatic veins and liver capsule.

Fibrosis due to ischaemic necrosis

Bordering the central liquifactive necrotic area of fluke tracts, zones of coagulative necrosis occur; in addition larger areas of coagulative necrosis are occasionally present.

The likely causes of such lesions are thrombi which are often found in the vicinity, and invariably are close to fluke tracts. Organisation and fibrosis follows resulting in further scar formation.

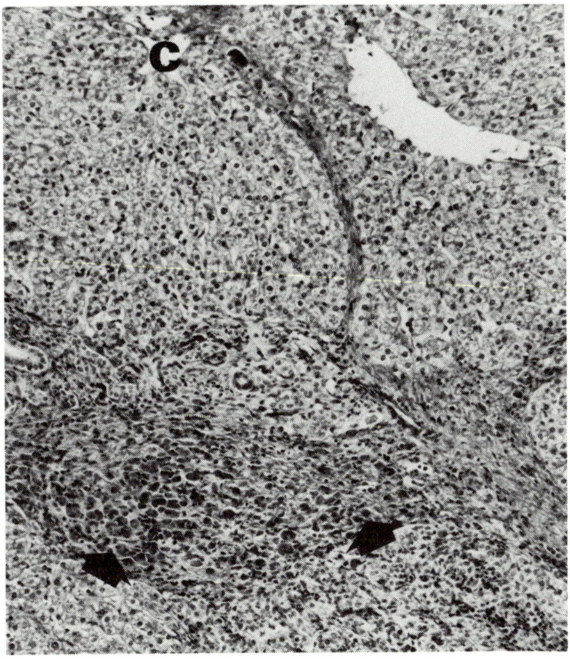

Fig. 1. Post necrotic scar in parenchyma of sheep infected with F. hepatica *16 weeks previously. The irregular scar is distorting hepatic architecture and is enclosing haemosiderin-laden macrophages (arrows). Note the band of fibrous tissue radiating to a central hepatic vein (C). Martius Scarlet Blue. x 150.*

Monolobular fibrosis

Grossly this can be seen as delicate white strands of fibrous tissue demarcating the hepatic lobule (Fig. 2). In fascioliasis, this change is found not only in close proximity to but also in areas apparently fairly distant from healing fluke tracts. Monolobular fibrosis is found mainly in longstanding primary infections, is common in field cases and in animals subjected to certain reinfection schedules (Rushton *et al.*, 1974). Histologically, monolobular fibrosis describes the interconnection of portal canals by fibrous tissue (Fig. 3). Close to healed fluke tracts, the fibrous bands are much thicker and often enclose single or groups of hepatocytes.

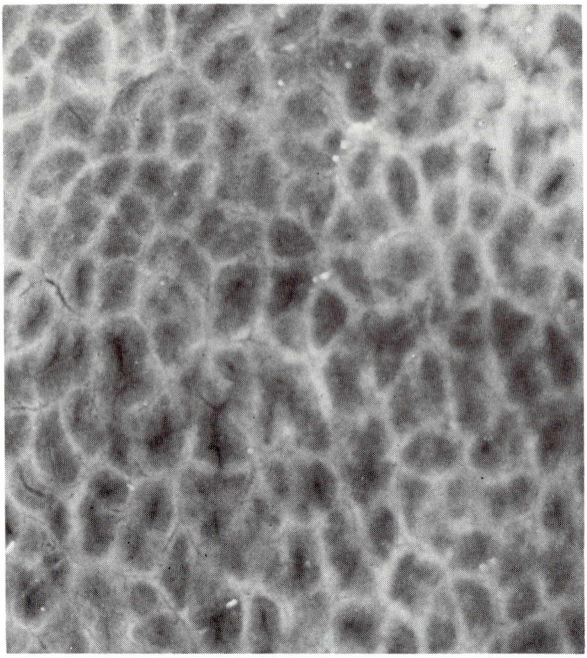

Fig. 2. Monolobular fibrosis in bovine infected with F. hepatica *30 weeks previously. Delicate strands of fibrous tissue are delineating the hepatic lobule.*

Distally the fibrous tissue is more delicate and consists of fine strands of collagen deposited in a perisinusoidal location. Frequently, vascular channels are found in these fibrous bands forming porto-portal vascular anastomoses. A striking feature within such hepatic lobules is stretching and straightening of hepatic plates not only between adjacent portal canals but also between central veins and portal canals. Occasionally hepatic plates are markedly disorganised due to dilatation of adjacent sinusoids.

Portal canal

Peribiliary fibrosis

Following colonisation of the bile ducts about 8 to 12 weeks after inoculation a cholangitis develops. The bile ducts expand to accommodate flukes and a marked inflammatory reaction with congestion, exudation and emigration of cells develops in the adjacent lamina propria. Organisation of such areas results in fibrosis not only in the lamina propria but also in the surrounding adventitia. In addition, in the bovine, pathological calcification develops in the lamina propria. This latter lesion first appears as localised plaques of calcification and ossification in the lamina propria about 5 months after infection and thereafter becomes extensive and erodes the mucosa breaking off into the bile duct lumen. With movement of the adult fluke through the major bile ducts, peribiliary fibrosis comes to affect most of the biliary system.

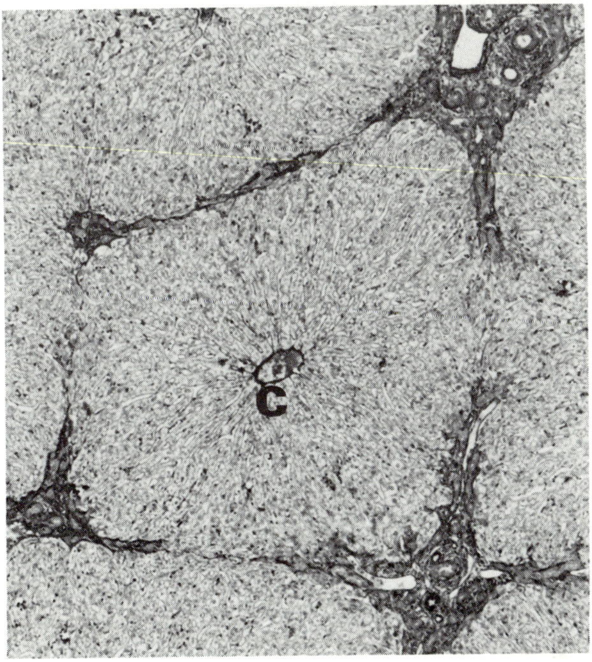

Fig. 3. Monolobular fibrosis in hepatic parenchyma of a sheep infected with F. hepatica *30 weeks previously. The portal canals are interconnected by bands of fibrous tissue. C, central vein. Martius Scarlet Blue. x 50.*

In addition, bile ducts too small to house flukes often develop a striking laminated form of peribiliary fibrosis; the basis of this lesion is unknown. Another factor contributing to biliary fibrosis is found in advanced cases of fascioliasis, at least in sheep, where fluke eggs in the smaller ducts appear to provoke a specific infective granuloma-like reaction resulting in destruction and obliteration of bile ducts and the development of further fibrosis (Fig. 4).

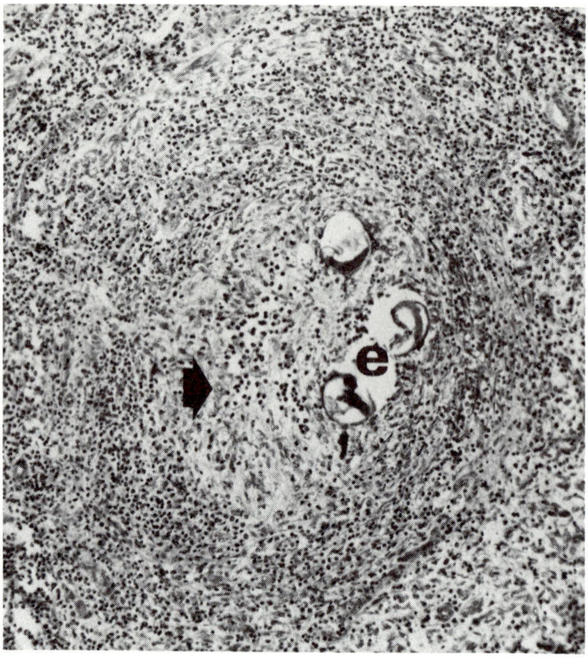

Fig. 4. Portal canal of sheep 30 weeks after infection with F. hepatica. *Fluke eggs (e) are the focus of a granuloma reaction. Occasional bile duct epithelial cells are still present (arrow). Haematoxylin and eosin. x 150.*

Portal canal fibrosis

In addition to the peribiliary changes, fibrous tissue is deposited in and around portal veins and hepatic arteries, and this together with peribiliary fibrosis results in marked expansion of the portal canal (Fig. 5). This lesion is most severe in the vicinity of fluke tracts but even in primary infections tends to involve portal canals in all liver lobes.

Shortly after infection, the portal canals become infiltrated by large pyroninophilic lymphoid cells and later by eosinophils followed by lymphocytes, macrophages and plasma cells. In addition, in advanced primary cases, some field cases and in animals subjected to experimental reinfection, lymphoreticular nodules are encountered. Within the canal, a marked portal vein phlebitis develops. As early as one week after infection, the portal veins become cuffed and infiltrated by large lymphoid cells which are soon replaced by eosinophils. At this time the wall of the vein swollen and oedematous and proliferating endothelial cells are thrown into folds almost occluding the vessel lumen. Later this lesion becomes organised and fibrosed leading terminally to a veno-occlusive effect (Fig. 6). The portal veins most severely affected are the secondary ones particularly those in close proximity to fluke tracts, (for definition of ovine hepatic vascular nomenclature see Rushton, 1974). As a con-

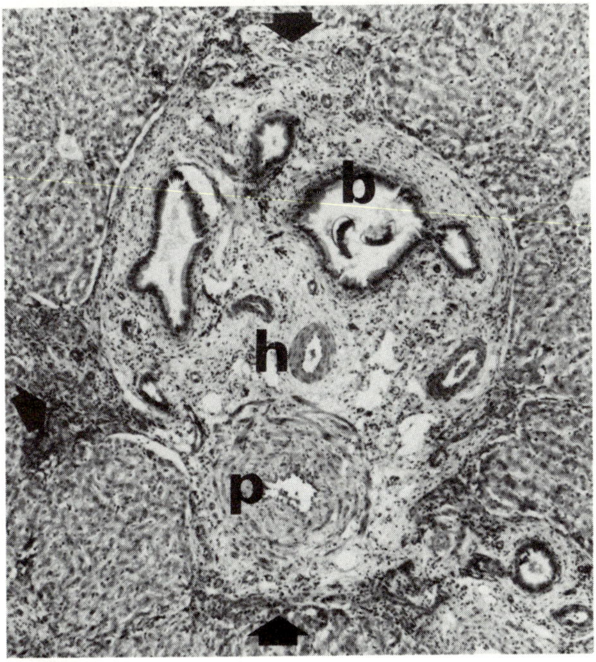

Fig. 5. Portal canal fibrosis in sheep infected with F. hepatica *20 weeks previously. The hepatic limiting plate is partially disrupted and replaced by proliferating bile ductules (arrows). Within the fibrosed portal canal, note the thickened portal vein with narrow lumen (p), the prominent hepatic artery (h) and the hyperplastic dilated bile duct containing fluke eggs (b). Haematoxylin and eosin. x 80.*

sequence the thin-walled tertiary portal veins collapse and become occluded; such a change is also contributed to by the cellular infiltrate and oedema within the portal canal. The tertiary portal vein is the one which traverses the hepatic limiting plate around the portal canal to supply the sinusoids. The result is that the portal blood supply to the hepatic lobule is reduced (Figs. 7 and 8). Accompanying the development of portal vein veno-occlusion, hepatic arteries

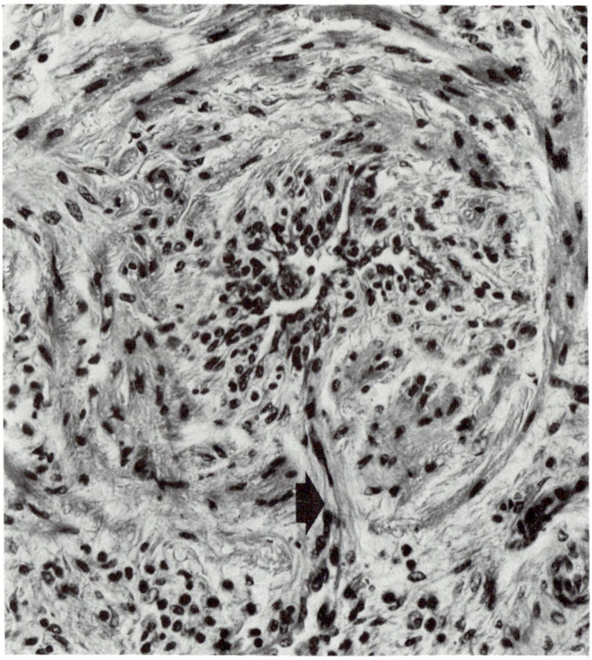

Fig. 6. Terminal veno-occlusive lesion in secondary portal vein of bovine with longstanding F. hepatica *infection. The wall of the portal vein is thickened by fibrous tissue, is infiltrated with eosinophils and the lumen is extremely narrow. Note the associated tertiary portal vein compressed by connective tissue (arrow). Haematoxylin and eosin. x 300.*

of all sizes and in all lobes become progressively thickened and tortuous (Figs. 7 and 8). In addition, fibrosis of central hepatic and sub-lobular veins occurs with occlusion of sinusoidal connections in some areas; this change is diffuse but is most obvious in the vicinity of fluke tracts.

Associated with these cellular and vascular events in the canal, the surrounding limited plate of hepatocytes is disrupted with ensuing degeneration and death of constituent hepatocytes. Fibrous tissue deposition then occurs in conjunction with bile ductule proliferation which apparently arises from the remaining hepatocytes. This connective tissue response surrounds the proliferating bile ductules; it also invests single or clumps of hepatocytes some of which undergo degeneration and necrosis (so-called piecemeal necrosis), while other hepatocytes remain apparently viable. The cellular infiltrate described earlier is also found in the vicinity of these changes.

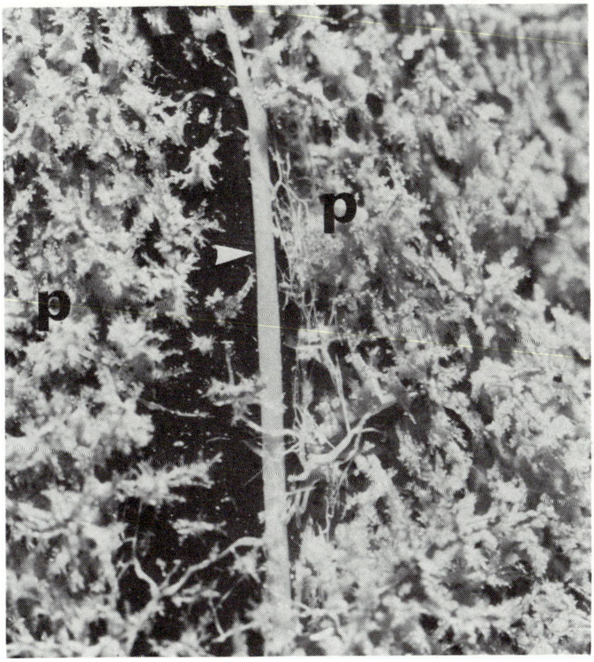

Fig. 7. Acrylic cast showing portal vein and hepatic artery in a normal sheep. Note the extent of the portal sinusoidal blood supply (p) and the straight hepatic artery (arrow).

As a result of the above events, there is progressive deposition of connective tissue in and around the portal canal zone. Associated with severely affected portal canals, bands of fibrous tissue often enclosing vascular channals occasionally radiate to neighbouring fibrous tissue structures, e.g., adjacent canals (monolobular fibrosis), central veins, the capsule of Glisson or post-necrotic scars.

Liver capsule

In fascioliasis, the capsule of Glisson becomes markedly irregular and thickened due to fibrosis. This is due to organisation of the necrotic inflammatory changes induced by fluke migration.

The development of hepatic fibrosis

In sheep, post necrotic fibrous scars appear as early as 4 weeks after infection, are most marked at 12 weeks and

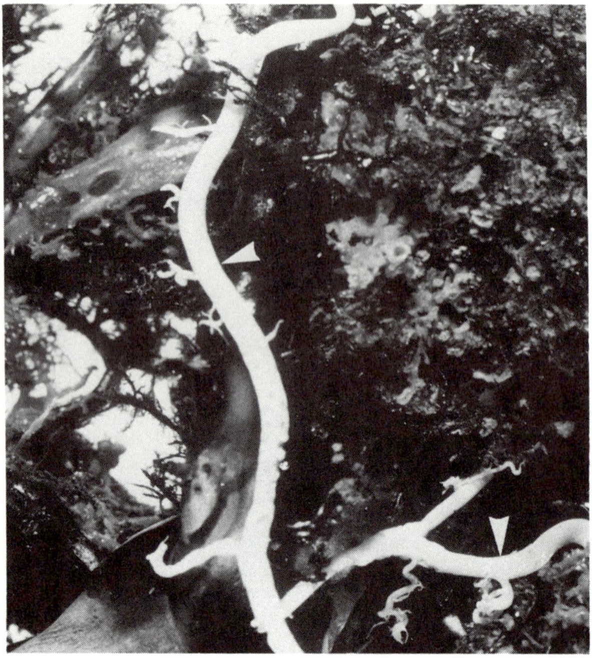

Fig. 8. Acrylic cast showing portal vein and hepatic artery in sheep infected with F. hepatica *for 16 weeks. The portal sinusoidal blood supply has been reduced while the hepatic artery and its branches are dilated and notably tortuous (arrows).*

therefore start to resolve and condense when the fluke burden has moved into the biliary system. Irregular bands of fibrous tissue radiating from the healing and healed tracts appear about the same time. More regular fibrosis (the monolobular type) occurs later in the infection and becomes most prominent in primary infections from 16 to 24 weeks. Deposition of connective tissue in and around portal canals is seen between 6 and 16 weeks. In primary infections all such changes are most severe in the vicinity of fluke tracts and hence are found primarily in the ventral lobe. Peribiliary fibrosis is associated with the presence of adult flukes in the bile ducts and therefore develops from 12 weeks onwards; because of migration of the fluke population, bile ducts in all lobes are eventually affected.

In animals reinfected with *F. hepatica*, the type and distribution of the fibrosis which develops varies according to the regime employed. Sheep which are dosed at 10 weeks to remove the fluke population from the bile ducts and parenchyma and then re-challenged one week later, develop a severe cirrhosis with fibrosis affecting all liver lobes. This fibrosis consists of all the constituent types found in the ventral lobe of primary infections with a noticeable proponderance of monolobular fibrosis. Histological and biochemical data show that this pattern of fibrosis can be attributed to the delayed entry of flukes into the biliary tree and thus a prolonged and diffuse migratory phase (Rushton *et al.*, 1974). In animals not dosed and reinfected at the same time, histological and biochemical data indicate that there is no delay in fluke migration to the bile ducts, healing commencing earlier than in the dosed group and fibrosis being largely confined to the ventral lobe.

In the bovine, the nature, timing and distribution of the various types of hepatic fibrosis is similar to that in sheep. Such differences as exist are only of degree, e.g., fibrous tissue formation is usually more obvious, monolobular fibrosis tends to be more common and peribiliary fibrosis is more marked. In addition, pathological calcification, a major feature of the bile duct reaction in the bovine, does not occur in sheep.

DISCUSSION

The present results demonstrate that immune mechanisms are operative in the acquisition of resistance to *F. hepatica* in rats, cattle and sheep. Both normal and irradiated metacercariae are able to stimulate a considerable degree of host resistance. However, further work in defining the important parameters (see review by Murray, 1973) will be required to determine whether a satisfactory field vaccine can be produced. For example, our studies have shown that "time" is important in the development of acquired resistance in the lymphoid cells transferred from donors 4 weeks after infection have little or no protective effect (Corba *et al.*, 1971; Armour & Dargie, 1974). This might suggest that the adult parasite is the immunogenic stage. However, that this is not necessarily so is shown by the fact that an equal level of protection can be achieved with irradiated metacercariae which do not survive in the host more than 3 or 4 weeks. Another important factor is the quantity of antigenic stimulus provided. The adoptive transfer of lymphoid cells from donors with high fluke burdens confers significantly more protection to recipients than cells taken from rats harbouring few flukes; similarly the quantity of hyperimmune serum transferred has a direct bearing on the level of protection achieved.

In order to engineer an effective protective response, an understanding of the basic immune mechanisms underlying resistance to *F. hepatica* is essential. In this respect our present results indicate that both cellular and humoral components of the immune response can play a part.

Several possibilities exist regarding the function of the transferred immune cells; in our work it must be assumed that the transferred cells were a mixture of T lymphocytes (Thymus-dependent) and B lymphocytes (Bursa-equivalent). Thus it is possible that T lymphocytes, sensitised against parasite antigens initiate a cell mediated immune reaction and in contact with the parasite release cytotoxic and/or lymphokine factors which lead to the destruction of the parasite. This hypothesis is supported by the histological and cell transfer studies of Lang (1967 and 1968) who concluded that acquired resistance in murine fascioliasis was an expression of a delayed-type hypersensitivity reaction.

On the other hand, B lymphocytes are the progenitors of plasma cells and our results using hyperimmune serum indicate that an antibody mediated immunity to *F. hepatica* also exists. It is possible that both mechanisms, i.e., cell-mediated and humoral, operate concurrently. Thus when a high degree of immunity is obtained with immune serum the livers of challenged recipients are almost completely normal, suggesting that the young parasites are destroyed prior to entry to the liver. In this context, by killing rats serially after serum transfer and challenge, we have recently found that the flukes are in fact killed within the peritoneal cavity and not at the gut level (unpublished data). In contrast, a similar level of protection against challenge after lymphoid cell transfer is invariably accompanied by marked liver lesions associated with cellular infiltrates and dead immature parasites. This might suggest that both humoral and cell-mediated mechanisms are implicated in acquired immunity to *F. hepatica*, the latter possibly functioning as a second line of defence. Clearly further work is needed into the humoral and cellular aspects of the immune response involved in protection against *F. hepatica* e.g., the role of the various immunoglobulin classes, the role of T and B lymphocytes if and when suitable cell markers become available in rats, cattle or sheep and lastly to provide some insight into the apparent immunological unresponsiveness to liver fluke exhibited by sheep under field conditions.

While it is not possible to discount the importance of non-specific mechanisms, *viz.*, hepatic fibrosis, in host resistance to fascioliasis, the present results have established that immune mechanisms are involved. As mentioned earlier, in these studies the degree of protection achieved was not related to the extent of hepatic fibrosis. These conclusions are substantiated by work in rats (Hayes *et al.*, 1973) and sheep (Rushton *et al.*, 1974). Rushton *et al.*, (1974) found in sheep reinfected with *F. hepatica* 11 weeks after primary infection that fluke migration to the bile ducts was prolonged in animals treated before reinfection but not in untreated and reinfected sheep. If it is assumed that the degree of hepatic fibrosis was similar in both groups on challenge at 11 weeks, then some factor other than hepatic fibrosis must have been influencing the progress of the fluke through the parenchyma. The results presented in this paper would suggest that this factor is an immunological one. Similarly, the suggestion that in the bovine bile duct calcification is responsible non-specifically for the expulsion of the adult fluke from the bile ducts must be doubted. Doyle (1971) found that 85% of the adult fluke population was expelled between 16 and 30 weeks after infection and that bile duct calcification only started around 20 weeks and took some months to become severe. During this phase of parasite loss the biliary mucosa becomes populated by a range of immunological cell types including plasma cells, lymphocytes, macrophages, eosinophils, mast cells and globule leukocytes making it highly likely that some immunological process at the mucous surface is involved in expulsion. It is known in other systems that similar cellular changes are associated with parasite loss (Murray, 1972).

Hepatic fibrosis has long been recognised as a major consequence of fascioliasis (Urquhart, 1956; Thorpe, 1963; Dow *et al.*, 1967; Dow *et al.*, 1972). While in the field the disease process of anaemia and hypoalbuminaemia is largely attributable to changes in the biliary tree, there is little doubt that cattle and sheep subjected to reinfection can develop severe and extensive hepatic fibrosis or cirrhosis which may lead to chronic liver failure. Only Urquhart (1956) discussed the possible mechanisms operative in the production of hepatic fibrosis. Our results confirm and extend his observations and show that a number of different types of hepatic fibrosis occur in fascioliasis and that several mechanisms are operative in their production.

The fluke itself directly causes marked inflammation and necrosis both of the parenchyma and of the biliary system resulting in post-necrotic scarring, peribiliary fibrosis and diffuse fibrosis of the capsule of Glisson. Fluke migration through the parenchyma also results in vascular damage with resultant thrombosis, ischaemic necrosis and hepatic fibrosis.

The explanation for monolobular fibrosis, irregular parenchymal fibrosis, and portal canal fibrosis is not so obvious.

Such forms of fibrosis are found not only close to but distal from fluke tracts and also are usually more marked in reinfection cases. Thus it would appear that factors other than direct trauma may be operative in their induction. Perhaps the most significant lesions to develop in relation to such changes in the hepatic vasculature with the development of veno-occlusive lesions in the portal and hepatic veins and of thickened tortuous hepatic arteries; such changes in the hepatic artery are indicative of hypertension (Gould, 1968). The aetiology of the portal veno-occlusive lesion remains unknown but the initial presence of large lymphoid cells and later of eosinophils in the vessel wall implicate an immunological reaction. Hypertension in the hepatic artery probably reflects the response to increased intra-hepatic peripheral resistance caused by hepatic fibrosis; it may also be a compensatory response to reduced portal blood supply. Possibly occlusion of the portal vein is responsible for the events associated with connective deposition in the portal canal, namely disruption,degeneration and necrosis of the hepatic limiting plate, piecemeal necrosis of hepatocytes and bile ductule proliferation.

Acrylic resin casts of the portal venous system confirm that the portal vein sinusoidal blood supply is reduced. Moreover the histological findings of stretching and straightening of hepatic plates and sinusoidal dilatation suggest increased intralobular pressure and that the hypertensive hepatic artery has possibly taken over the sinusoidal blood supply. In addition, hepatic vein fibrosis are severing of sinusoidal connections must lead to considerable sinusoidal and hepatic plate changes. Thus it may be that perisinusoidal fibrous tissue is laid between portal canals and between other hepatic structures as a compensatory response to stabilise the hepatic parenchyma and counteract the distorsion produced by these vascular lesions and also by other forms of fibrosis, particularly post-necrotic scarring. In addition, as perisinusoidal fibrous tissue is so often found lining vascular channels, this form of fibrosis may be part of a restructuring programme for vascular shunts to by-pass scar tissue and vascular occlusive lesions.

Another possible explanation is that some cytotoxic immunological reaction may play a part in hepatocyte death in the limiting plate leading to portal and possibly contributing to monolobular fibrosis. Since these forms of fibrosis are predominant in the livers of sheep subjected to certain reinfection prodedures (see earlier), it may be that in these potentially hypersensitive animals fluke migration with hepatic cell necrosis releases liver antigen which stimulates an immune reaction, either of a humoral or cellular nature, directed against the liver. Thus in vicinity of hepatocyte death a variety of immunological cell types may be found including small lymphocytes, large lymphoid cells, macrophages, plasma cells and eosinophils. An investigation into the specificity of the antibody being produced by these plasma cells, *viz.*, is it directed against fluke or the liver itself and also into the nature of the lymphoid cell population might help to clarify this possibility. Preliminary investigations into a putative autoimmune mechanism causing hepatocyte death have proved equivocal.

The lesions conforming to the pattern of specific infective granuloma, which develop in terminal bile ducts in association with fluke eggs, resemble a delayed type hypersensitivity response. These lesions are similar to those described in schistosomiasis where it has been established that such granulomas represent a cell mediated hypersensitivity reaction (Warren *et al.*, 1967). Therefore it would appear that immunological hypersensitivity mechanisms are operative in fascioliasis and are responsible for tissue damage and fibrosis.

CONCLUSIONS

Immunological mechanisms both of a humoral and cellular nature appear to be involved in the development of acquired resistance to infection with the liver fluke *F. hepatica* in cattle, sheep and rats. This resistance can be actively stimulated by exposure to irradiated metacercariae. Thus the production of an effective vaccine must be a possibility.

In infected cattle and sheep a major complication is the development of several types of hepatic fibrosis which involve both the parenchyma and the portal canals. A number of different mechanisms are implicated in the production of hepatic fibrosis including trauma caused by the fluke, vascular lesions and immune hypersensitive reactions.

ACKNOWLEDGEMENTS

This work was supported by grants from the Agricultural Research Council and the Wellcome Trust. Mr. B. Ruston was financed by the Agricultural Research Council.

REFERENCES

Armour, J., and Dargie, J.D. (1974). *Exptl. Parasit.* (In Press).

Bitakaramire, P.K. (1973). *In: Isotopes and Radiation in*

Parasitology III. International Atomic Energy Agency, Vienna. p. 23.
Boray, J.C. (1967). *In: The Reaction of the Host to Parasitism.* (E.J.L. Soulsby, Ed.) Elwert, Marburg, Germany. p. 84.
Corba, J., Armour, J., Roberts, R.T. and Urquhart, G.M. (1971) *Res. Vet. Sci. 12,* 292.
Dow, C., Ross, J.G. and Todd, J.R. (1967). *J. Comp. Path. 77,* 377.
Dow, C., Ross, J.G. and Todd, J.R. (1968). *Parasitology 58,* 129.
Doyle, J.J. (1971). *Res. Vet. Sci. 12,* 527.
Doyle, J.J. (1972). Ph.D. Thesis. University of Glasgow.
Gould, S.E. (1968). *In: Pathology of the Heart and Blood Vessels.* Charles C. Thomas, Springfield, Illinois. p. 925.
Hayes, T.J., Bailer, J. and Mitrovic, M. (1972). *Parasit. 58,* 1103.
Hayes, T.J., Bailer, J. and Mitrovic, M. (1973). *Parasit. 59,* 810.
Hein, E.H. (1963). Ph.D. Thesis. University of Glasgow.
Jarrett, W.F.H., Jennings, F.W., McIntyre, W.I.M., Mulligan, W., Sharp, N.C.C. and Urquhart, G.M. (1959). *Am. J. Vet. Res. 20,* 522.
Jovanovic, M., Sokolic, A., Movsesijan, M., Cuperlovic, K. (1965). *Brit. Vet. J. 121,* 119.
Lang, B.Z. (1967). *J. Parasit. 53,* 21.
Lang, B.Z. (1968). *Am. J. Trop. Med. Hyg. 17,* 561.
Miller, T.A. (1965). *Am. J. Vet. Med. Ass. 146,* 41.
Murray, Max (1972). *In: Immunity to Animal Parasites,* (E.J. L. Soulsby, Ed.) Academic Press, New York and London. p. 155.
Murray, Max (1973). *Vet. Rec. 93,* 500.
Nansen, P., Andersen, S., Harmer, E. and Riising, H.J. (1972). *Exptl. Parasit. 31,* 247.
Ross, J.G. (1966). *Irish Vet. J. 20,* 131.
Ross, J.G. (1967). *In: The Reaction of the Host to Parasitism,* (E.J.L. Soulsby, Ed.), Elwert, Marburg, Germany. p. 96.
Rushton, B., Murray, Max and Armour, J. (1974). (In Preparation)
Rushton, B., (1974). (In Preparation).
Sinclair, K.B. (1971). *Brit. Vet. J. 127,* 125.
Sokolic, A. (1968). *In: Isotopes and Radiation in Parasitology,* International Atomic Energy Agency, Vienna. p. 93.
Thorpe, E. and Broome, A.W.J. (1962). *Vet. Rec. 74,* 755.
Thorpe, E. (1963). *J. Comp. Path. 75,* 45.
Urquhart, G.M. (1956). *J. Path. Bact. 71,* 301.

Varga, I. (1968). *In: Isotopes and Radiation in Parasitology*, International Atomic Energy Agency, Vienna. p. 1.
Warren, K.S., Domingo, E.O. and Cowan, R.B.T. (1967). *Am. J. Path. 51,* 735.

ZOOPROPHYLAXIS WITH SPECIAL REFERENCE TO *SCHISTOSOMIASIS* AND *FILARIASIS*

G. S. Nelson

London School of Hygiene and Tropical Medicine,
Keppel Street, London, U. K.

INTRODUCTION

What is Zooprophylaxis?

Although there are still a few biologists who interpret the term zoonosis in the literal sense to mean diseases of animals, most public health orientated scientists have now accepted the much more restricted WHO/FAO (1967) definition of the zoonoses as "those diseases and infections naturally transmitted between vertebrate animals and man". The main area of controversy is in the classification of the zoonoses and here we meet a confusing and at times incomprehensible terminology with the same terms having a completely different meaning in different countries (see Nelson, 1960 and Schwabe, 1969). Even the origin of the term zoonosis is in dispute (Fiennes, 1967). But the name has come to stay and there is no doubt that it serves an excellent function in focussing attention on the zoological aspects of disease transmission.

The concern of this symposium is with infections that are transmitted from animals to man and *vice versa* and with the consequence of this transmission in terms of animal and human health. In the past the main interest in the zoonoses has been with diseases producing obvious morbidity or mortality, for example rabies, yellow fever, plague, trypanosomiasis, bovine tuberculosis or hydatid disease. There are all zoonoses of considerable public health importance but in terms of man's survival and his general well-being they may be far less important than the more prevalent, less dramatic, or even occult zoonotic infections that stimulate man's immunological mechanisms so that he is able to resist the more pathogenic organisms in his environment. This is the phenomenon that we have called zooprophylaxis (Nelson *et al.*, 1962).

Zooprophylaxis was first demonstrated by the Devonshire farmer Benjamin Jesty 200 years ago in 1774 when he inoculated his wife with pox virus from one of his cows in an attempt to protect her against smallpox. But it was Jenner in 1796 who confirmed that cross immunity was a reality, when he inoculated an 8 year old boy with cowpox from a vesicle on the hand of a dairy-maid and then six weeks later proved that the boy was immune to smallpox. This experiment, which nowadays would be regarded as unethical, is perhaps the most important landmark in preventive medicine. Jenner's mother or his nursemaid should be given some of the credit for this discovery for they no doubt taught him to recite the nursery rhyme:

"Where are you going, my pretty maid?"
"I'm going a'milking, Sir" she said.
"What is your fortune, my pretty maid?"
"My face is my fortune, Sir" she said.

Jenner realised that her face was her fortune because, as a result of *natural* exposure to cowpox, she had escaped the disfiguring smallpox that affected so many other young ladies in the eighteenth century.

Although Jenner's experiment led to the development of a potent vaccine against a major infectious disease the epidemiological significance of the observation that the immunity resulted from natural exposure to a less pathogenic organism was lost sight of and even today there are very few microbiologists or parasitologists who are concerned with or even aware of this important aspect of immunology.

I have defined zooprophylaxis as "the prevention or amelioration of disease in man as a result of previous exposure to heterolgous infections of animal origin". Cross protection is not confined to cowpox versus smallpox but it is operative throughout the whole range of pathogenic organisms from viruses to helminths not only between closely related species but often between quite diverse groups of organisms.

This conference is concerned with parasitic zoonoses and I intend to illustrate zooprophylaxis by reference to schistosomiasis and filariasis but before we deal with these two diseases it is perhaps worth noting a few examples of natural cross immunity from other disciplines. There is evidence suggesting that heterologous immunity is of significance in limiting the distribution of some of the more virulent arboviruses. For example the Wesselsbron virus first isolated from sheep in South Africa by Weiss *et al.* (1956) is known to be widespread in man and animals in East Africa and Henderson *et al.* (1970) have shown that the virus can be used to immunise monkeys against yellow fever. It has been suggested that the Wesselsbron and other arboviruses may produce an immunological barrier preventing the spread of yellow fever in Africa and preventing its establishement in Asia in the same way as the Murray Valley virus is thought to prevent the introduction of Japanese encephalitis into northern

Australia (Andrews, 1967).

The best example of natural heterologous immunity in man is the protective effect of a previous infection with yaws against subsequent exposure to syphilis. This is a commonplace observation by everyone who has worked in areas where yaws is endemic but again the epidemiological implications have been neglected and there is no clear documentation of the public health significance of this cross protection. The same type of cross protection is thought to occur between bovine tuberculosis and human tuberculosis and leprosy. The effect of cross protection between tuberculosis and leprosy on the prevalence and distribution of leprosy has been argued extensively by Chaussinand (1948; 1950) and as a result of a detailed study of the epidemiology of leprosy in the West Nile District of Uganda I suggested that cross protection between the two organisms was the most likely explanation of the peculiar distribution pattern of leprosy in that area (Nelson, 1958). Subsequent attempts to apply the principle of cross protection for the control of leprosy by the use of B.C.G. vaccination by Brown *et al.* (1968) in Uganda, Bechelli *et al.* (1970) in Burma and Russel *et al.* (1968) in New Guinea have been disappointing but much better results have been obtained with B.C.G. in the control of Buruli ulcer which is caused by infection with *Mycobacterium ulcerans* (Uganda Buruli Group, 1969). The inferences from these observations is that zooprophylaxis may be of significance in reducing the prevalence of leprosy and Buruli ulcer in communities where there is a high exposure to bovine tuberculosis.

If we look briefly at the protozoa we will see that there is considerable experimental evidence for cross protection between different malaria parasites in both man and animals (see Cohen 1973 for a review of this subject) and also between different groups of organisms for example between *Eperythrozoon* and malaria (Peters, 1965) and between piroplasms and malaria (Cox, 1970). There is also evidence of zooprophylaxis affecting the distribution and prevalence of kala-azar in Kenya where cross protection results from previous exposure to non pathogenic leishmania of rodents or lizards (Southgate, 1967; Southgate and Oriedo, 1967) and Blair *et al.* (1968) have suggested that the relatively low incidence of sleeping sickness in the people resident in the endemic areas in Rhodesia compared with the high risk to immigrants is due to the constant exposure of the indigenous population to non pathogenic trypanosomes.

There is evidence that cross protection is equally important in many of the helminth infections of both man and his domestic animals. For example between different species of nematodes such as *Haemonchus* (Allen and Samson, 1961), *Dictyocaulus* (Sinclair, 1967) and hookworms (Miller, 1968) and between different species of cestodes e.g. *Hymenolepis* spp. (Heyneman, 1962) and *Taenia* spp. (Gemmel, 1964). In the following account the possible relevance of zooprophylaxis is illustrated by reference to schistosomiasis and filariasis.

SCHISTOSOMIASIS AND ZOOPROPHYLAXIS

My personal interest in the epidemiological significance of cross immunity began with a study of schistosomiasis in East Africa. To begin with I was concerned with the study of schistosome infections as zoonoses (Nelson, 1960). It was found that baboons played some rôle in transmission of *Schistosoma mansoni* and the discovery of schistosomes in rodents suggested that they might also be involved as reservoir hosts but soon it became obvious that other species of schistosomes were prevalent in livestock and wild animals and that man was constantly exposed to the cercariae of these zoonotic species. In the past the main interest in these "non human" schistosomes has been the rare appearance of patent infections in man or their rôle as the aetiological agents in swimmers' itch or cercarial dermatitis. There has also been some considerable interest in the effect of these abortive infections on serological diagnostic techniques since they are responsible for numerous false positive reactions. But very little consideration has been given to their rôle as natural immunising agents.

The concept of zooprophylaxis in schistosomiasis was introduced by Nelson *et al.* (1962) in their attempt to explain differences in the severity of schistosomiasis in the Lake Victoria and coastal areas of Kenya. In both areas there were communities where *S. haematobium* showed very high prevalence rates but the most severe complications were seen only in the coastal region. Similar differences in pathogenicity have been noted in other parts of the world and it is generally accepted the infections with *S. mansoni* are more severe in Egypt and Brazil than in most parts of tropical Africa. Many factors can explain these differences including genetic differences in the parasites and their hosts and differences in the pattern of transmission but from the point of view of the pathology in man the main differences are thought to be due to differences in the worm load and in the immune reaction. In our study in Kenya we found that in the Lake Victoria area the bulinid snail hosts of

S. haematobium were infected with both *S. haematobium* and *S. bovis* whereas in the Coast Province they contained only *S. haematobium* cercariae (Teesdale and Nelson, 1958). The Central Lakes area is the primaeval home of the African schistosomes. It is there where the parasites and their snail hosts show their greatest complexity. Apart from the so-called human schistosomes, *S. mansoni, S. haematobium and S. intercalatum,* there are a variety of other species in domestic and wild animals, for example *S. bovis, S. mattheei, S. leiperi* and *S. margerebowie* in cattle and sheep and wild ungulates, *S. rodhaini* in rodents and carnivores and *S. hippopotami* and *S. edwardiense* in the hippopotamus (Thurston, 1963, 1964). These parasites are often transmitted by the same snail host as the human parasites so that in many parts of Africa man is inevitably exposed to a variety of heterologous infections. It is perhaps significant that none of these schistosomes exist in Egypt or Brazil.

An interesting situation exists in Formosa where there is very little human schistosomiasis although *S. japonicum* is widespread in animals (Hsü *et al.*, 1954). It has been shown that this zoonotic strain fails to reach maturity in man (Hsü and Hsü, 1956) and it has been suggested that previous exposure to the non pathogenic strain may prevent the more virulent strains from mainland China and Japan from becoming established in Formosa.

With most helminth infections man develops some degree of immunity but the immunity is incomplete and one does not expect an all or nothing effect as with viruses of bacteria. The immunity in schistosomiasis is recognised as a resistance to superinfection with a decrease in the number of eggs deposited in the tissues. This explains the apparent paradox of a high level of immunity to schistosomiasis even in communities with a high prevalence rate. Immunity results in an amelioration of the disease and a resistance against reinfection not the absence of infection. Experimental studies suggest that the immunity to schistosomiasis is produced either (a) by adult worms which have undergone a process of antigenic disguise which enables them to produce antibodies against the invading schistosomular stages of the parasites whilst they themselves are unaffected or (b) by the earlier stages of the infection which are rejected before reaching maturity. The first type of immunity which depends on the development of the parasites to maturity has been studied extensively by Smithers and his colleagues (see Smithers 1972 for a review of this work). The second type of immunity has been demonstrated in experiments using irradiated vaccines by Villella *et al.* (1961), Hsü *et al.* (1962), Sadun *et al.* (1964) and many other workers and also in heterolgous infections by Kagan (1952), Meleney and Moore (1954), Hunter *et al.* (1961) and especially by Hsü and his colleagues (see Hsü and Hsü, 1961 and Eveland *et al.*, 1969). We have been particularly interested in heterologous immunity and in our experiments in mice and monkeys we have used a variety of animal schistosomes to produce protective immunity against challenge with the human schistosomes (Nelson *et al.*, 1968; Amin *et al.*, 1968; Amin and Nelson, 1969). We have also shown that it is possible to partially protect cattle and sheep against *Schistosoma bovis*, *S. mattheei* and *Ornithobilharzia turkestanicum* using the human parasites *Schistosoma mansoni* and *S. haematobium* as the immunising agents (Hussein *et al.*, 1970; Preston *et al.*, 1972; Massoud and Nelson, 1972). In almost every case we found that previous exposure of animals to one species of schistosome confers some degree of immunity against challenge with another species.

A further experimental approach has been to try and produce avirulent hybrids that are fully infective and immunogenic but not pathogenic because of their low egg production. A variety of hybrids have been produced by Taylor (1970) but so far they have shown less promise as immunising agents against *S. mansoni* in baboons than infection with the heterologous parent schistosomes *S. rodhaini* and *S. bovis* (Taylor *et al.*, in press). It is hoped that these studies will eventually lead to the development of a vaccine but this is a long way off and the main significance of these studies has been to confirm that the cross protection can occur suggesting that the principle of zooprophylaxis may be of some importance in understanding the epidemiology of the human disease and that reverse zooprophylaxis may in part explain the relatively low morbidity of schistosimiasis in livestock in areas where the human disease is prevalent

FILARIASIS AND ZOOPROPHYLAXIS

The significance of zooprophylaxis in filarial infections is much more speculative than with schistosomiasis because so far no attempts have been made to study the phenomenon in the laboratory. But we do know that in much the same way as man is constantly exposed to infection with a wide variety of schistosomes of animal origin he is also constantly exposed to a variety of infective larvae of "non-human" filarial parasites that are prevalent in man-biting arthropods especially mosquitoes and simuliids. The identification of the filarial species sharing the same vectors as the human parasites has been discussed in previous publications (Nelson, 1959; Nelson, 1964; Nelson and Pester, 1962). More recent studies by Brengues *et al.* (1968) in West Africa, by Brunhes *et al.* (1972) in Madagascar on filarial larvae in mosquitoes and by Duke (1967) and by Voelker and Garmes (1972) on larvae in simuliids have confirmed that many of the infective larvae in these man-biting insects are of non-human origin.

Immunological studies on the filarial parasites of man have been handicapped because the two most important species, *W. bancrofti* and *O. volvulus*, have not been established in normal laboratory animals. A good deal has been learnt about immunity to filarial infections as a result of the studies on rodent parasites particularly by Bertram (1966) and by Bagai and Subrahmanyam (1970) but the observations which may be more relevant to the human situation are those on *Brugia* species in monkeys and cats by Wong *et al.* (1969), Ramachandran (1970) and Denham *et al.* (1972a and b) and on *Loa loa* by Duke (1960). It has been shown that protective immunity can be established either by repeated infection with normal infective larvae or after inoculation of infective larvae that have been attenuated by irradiation. The successful results with this latter method suggest that as with the schistosomes heterologous infections might be used to see if they can ameliorate the effect of reinfection. If some degree of protection is established it would suggest that zooprophylaxis may be of significance in modifying filarial infections of man under natural conditions.

As with the schistosomes not all filarial parasites of animal origin are innocuous and some price may have to be paid for the development of immunity. Some animal species will occasionally reach maturity in man, for example *Dirofilaria immitis* from the dog which can produce rare pulmonary lesions (Yoshimura and Yokogawa, 1970), *D. tenius* from the raccoon which produces subcutaneous granulomas (Beaver and Orihel, 1965) and *D. repens* from cats and dogs which can involve the eye (Dissanaike, 1971). Other species from animals can produce hypersensitivity reactions resulting in tropical pulmonary eosinophilia (Buckley, 1958). But these pathological reactions are relatively rare and most of the abortive infections are non pathogenic. They result in numerous false positive reactions when immunolgoical tests are used for either individual diagnosis or for epidemiological studies (Smith *et al.*, 1971). It would be surprising if a closer study did not reveal some evidence of cross protection resulting from exposure to these abortive infections. Although we cannot test this hypothesis with *W. bancrofti* there are now a wide variety of filarial infections being maintained in laboratory animals and I have no doubt that studies similar to these carried out with different species of schistosomes will be equally rewarding.

DISCUSSION

The term zooprophylaxis like zoonosis is a Humpty-Dumpty-ism that will inevitably arouse the anger of the etymologists. But as Whitehead says in his "Introduction to Mathematics" - "The scientist shares with Humpty-Dumpty the privilege of paying words extra and making them mean what he likes." We require a peg on which epidemiologists can hang the concept of natural heterologous immunity; if there is no peg the subject will be neglected. Rather than introduce a new term for this type of cross protection I have resurrected an old term that was used by entomologists to describe the practice of protecting man from the bites of the vectors of human diesase by providing alternative animal hosts to attract the vectors and so prevent them from biting man. Since most entomologists prefer the term deviation for this phenomenon and since zooprophylaxis is not included in the World Health Organization (1963) handbook of "Terminology of Malaria and Malaria Eradication" I have borrowed the term zooprophylaxis and expanded the concept to include the protective effect of heterologous infections.

It is probably no exaggeration to say that zooprophylaxis is of vital importance in determining the survival and health of man especially in the tropics. If man's only defence against the vast numbers of virulent organisms in his environment was the development of homologous immunity to each in turn it is doubtful if he could survive in this pathogen polluted world. The same is probably true of his livestock and I would suggest that the phenomenon of reverse zooprophylaxis may be of importance in the livestock industry.

It is only in recent years that we have begun to realise that cross protection exists not only between closely related organisms but also between organisms as distinct as nematodes and bacteria or protozoa and fungi. Antigens may be shared and common antibodies may be produced but perhaps or more importance, as has been demonstrated with *Toxoplasma*, may be the general stimulation of the immune mechanisms by occult infections (Remington and Merigan, 1969; Ruskin *et al*., 1969; Gentry and Remington, 1971).

In most parasitic diseases cross protection will be evident from a reduction in intensity of the infection but this is not the only mechanism responsible for a reduction in the severity of the disease. In many parasitic diseases the pathological processes are themselves dependent on immunological mechanisms for example in schistosomiasis where the granuloma around the egg is primarily a cell mediated response which can be modified by interfering with the host's immune mechanism (Warren, 1972). It seems likely that many of the cross protective effects of heterologous infections operate by modifying the immunopathological response by interfering with the cell mediated immunity - a mechanism which has been demonstrated by Salaman (1970) with viruses and malaria, by Greenwood *et al.* (1971) with malaria, by Alt *et al.* (1971) and Goodwin *et al.* (1972) with trypanosomes, by Keller and Jones (1971) with *Nippostrongylus* and by Strickland *et al.* (1972; 1973) with *Toxoplasma.*

The immunological response is a two edged sword: in some cases the immunological effect may be to make the host more susceptible and less resistant to subsequent infections with other organisms, in other cases severe hypersensitivity reactions may occur but the general biolgoical purpose of cross reactions from heterologous infections is to reduce the severity of the infective processes to the mutual advantage of the host and the organisms themselves. What we require is more epidemiological evidence. This is an area of research which is of mutual interest to the biologist, the epidemiologist and the medical practitioner and yet it is almost entirely neglected. It will not be easy to get the epidemiological data but the effort will be worthwhile and the results are likely to be more rewarding than many more obvious studies on zoonotic diseases.

SUMMARY AND CONCLUSIONS

Zooprophylaxis is defined as "the prevention or amelioration of disease in man as the result of previous exposure to heterologous infections of animal origin." The classical example is the protective effect of cowpox against subsequent infection with smallpox but it is a much more widespread phenomenon. It is suggested that man's constant exposure to occult and mainly non-pathogenic zoonotic infections is of major importance in relation to his general well-being and of his survival, particularly in the tropics.

Surprisingly little attention has been given to the epidemiological significance of zooprophylaxis although there is experimental evidence of cross protection between many different viruses, bacteria, fungi, protozoa and helminths. Cross protection in parasitic disease is rarely complete and the effect is to limit the severity of the disease by reducing the intensity of the infection by preventing reinfection or by modifying the immunopathological response of the host. Although the immunolgoical response is a two edged sword which may actually aggravate the disease the general effect of exposure to occult heterologous infections of animal origin is thought to be beneficial. The phenomenon of zooprophylaxis is illustrated by reference to experimental studies on schistosomiasis, which indicate that previous exposure to "non pathogenic" schistosomes from livestock and wild animals will reduce the severity of subsequent infections with the human parasites *S. mansoni* and *S. haematobium*. It has also been shown that the reverse process occurs and sheep and cattle can be protected against the serious effect of *S. mattheei* and *S. bovis* infections by previous exposure to the human schistosomes - this phenomenon of "reverse zooprophylaxis" may be of significance in the livestock industry. Constant exposure to heterolgous infections that fail to reach maturity will act in the same way as irradiated vaccines but with the added advantage of repeated natural antigenic stimulus. It has been shown that in areas where filariasis or onchocercariasis is endemic that man is exposed to repeated infections with "non pathogenic filarial parasites of animal origin." It is likely that these heterologous infections may modify the disease in man in much the same way as exposure to animal schistosomes is thought to modify human schistosomiasis.

REFERENCES

Allen, R.W. and Samson, K.S. (1961). *J. Parasit.*, *47*, (Suppl.) 22.

Alt, G., Evans, E.M.E., Evans, D.H.L. and Targett, G.A.T. (1971). *Nature*, *233*, 197.

Amin, M.A. and Nelson, G.S. (1969). *Bull. Wld. Hlth. Org.*, *41*, 225.

Amin, M.A., Nelson, G.S. and Saoud, M.F.A. (1968). *Bull. Wld. Hlth. Org.*, *38*, 19.

Andrews, Sir C.H. (1967). *In* "The Natural History of Viruses" (R. Carrington, ed.). Weidenfeld and Nicolson: London.

Bagai, R.C. and Subrahmanyam, D. (1970). *Nature*, *228*, 682.

Beaver, P.C. and Orihel, T.C. (1965). *Am. J. Trop. Med. Hyg.*, *14*, 1010.

Bechelli, L.M., Garbajosa, G., Uemura, K., Engler, V., Dominguez, V.M., Paredes, L., Sundaresan, T., Koch, G. and Matejka, M. (1970). *Bull. Wld. Hlth. Org.*, *42*, 235.

Bertram, D.S. (1966). *In* "Advances in Parasitology" (B. Dawes, ed.), Vol. 4, 255-319. Academic Press, London and New York.

Blair, D.M., Burnett Smith, E. and Gelfand, M. (1968). *Cent. Afr. J. Med.* (Suppl), *14*, 1.

Brengues, J., Subra, R., Mouchet, J. and Nelson, G.S. (1968). *Bull. Wld. Hlth. Org.*, *38*, 595.

Brown, J.A.K., Stone, M.M. and Sutherland, I. (1968). *Brit. Med. J.*, 6 January, 24.

Brunhes, J., Rajaonarivelo, E. and Nelson, G.S. (1972). *Cah. O.R.S.T.O.M., Ser. Ent. Med. et Parasitol.*, *10*, 193.

Buckley, J.J.C. (1958). *E. Afr. Med. J.*, *35*, 493.

Chaussinand, R. (1948). *Int. J. Leprosy*, *16*, 431.

Chaussinand, R. (1950). La Lèpre. L'Expansion Scientifique Française, Paris.

Cohen, J.E. (1973). *Quarterly Review Biology*, *48*, 467.

Cox, F.E.G. (1970). *Bull. Wld. Hlth. Org.*, *43*, 325.

Duke, B.O.L. (1960). *Ann. Trop. Med. Parasit.*, *54*, 15.

Duke, B.O.L. (1967). *Ann. Trop. Med. Parasit.*, *61*, 200.

Denham, D.A., Ponnudurai, T., Nelson, G.S., Guy, F. and Rogers, R. (1972a). *Int. J. Parasit.*, *2*, 239.

Denham, D.A., Ponnudurai, T., Nelson, G.S., Rogers, R. and Guy, R. (1972b). *Int. J. Parasit.*, *2*, 401.

Dissanaike, A.S. (1971). *Ceylon Med. J.*, *16*, 91.

Eveland, L.K., Hsü, S.Y. Li and Hsü, H.F. (1969). *J. Parasit.*, *55*, 279.

Fiennes, R. (1967). "Zoonoses of Primates" (R. Carrington and L.H. Mathews, eds.). 193 pp. Weidenfeld and Nicholson, London.

Gemmel, M.A. (1964). *Nature*, *204*, 705.

Gentry, L.O. and Remington, J.S. (1971). *J. Inf. Dis.*, *123*, 22.

Goodwin, L.G., Green, D.G., Guy, M.W. and Voller, A. (1972). *Brit. J. Exp. Pathol.*, *53*, 40.

Greenwood, B.M., Brown, J.C., de Jesus, D.G. and Holborow, E.J. (1971). *Clin. Exp. Immunol.*, *9*, 345.

Henderson, B.E., Cheshire, P.P., Kirva, G.B. and Lule, M. (1970). *Am. J. Trop. Med. Hyg.*, *19*, 110.

Heyneman, D. (1962). *Expt. Parasit.*, *12*, 7.

Hsü, H.F. and Hsü, S.Y. Li (1956). *Am. J. Trop. Med. Hyg.*, *5*, 521.

Hsü, S.Y. Li and Hsü, H.F. (1961). *Science*, *133*, ~~776~~. 766

Hsü, H.F., Hsü, S.Y. Li, Chu, K.Y., Huang, T.C., Tsai, C.T. and Wang, Y.W. (1954). *Riv. Parassit. XV*, 461.

Hsü, H.F., Hsü, Y.L. and Osborne, J.W. (1962). *Nature*, *194*, 98.

Hunter, G. W., Weinman, C.J. and Hoffman, R.G. (1961). *Expt. Parasit.*, *11*, 133.

Hussein, M.F., Saeed, A.A. and Nelson, G.S. (1970). *Bull. Wld. Hlth. Org.*, *42*, 745.

Kagan, I.G. (1952). *J. Inf. Dis.*, *91*, 147.
Keller, R. and Jones, V.E. (1971). *Lancet*, *ii*, 847.
Massoud, J. and Nelson, G.S. (1972). *Bull. Wld. Hlth. Org.*, *47*, 591.
Meleney, H.E. and Moore, D.V. (1954). *Expt. Parasit.*, *3*, 128.
Miller, T.A. (1968). *Trans. Roy. Soc. Trop. Med. Hyg.*, *62*, 473.
Nelson, G.S. (1958). *Trans. Roy. Soc. Trop. Med. Hyg.*, *52*, 176.
Nelson, G. S. (1959). *J. Helminth.*, *33*, 233.
Nelson, G.S. (1960). *Trans. Roy. Soc. Trop. Med. Hyg.*, *54*, 301.
Nelson, G.S. (1964). *In* "Host-Parasite Relationships in Invertebrate Hosts". Second Symposium of the British Society for Parasitology. (A.E.R. Taylor, Ed.), pp. 75-119. Blackwell Scientific Publications, Oxford.
Nelson, G.S. (1965). *J. Helminth.*, *39*, 229.
Nelson, G.S. and Pester, F.R.N. (1962). *Bull. Wld. Hlth. Org.*, *27*, 473.
Nelson, G.S., Teesdale, C. and Highton, R.B. (1962). *In* Bilharziasis. Ciba Foundation Symposium". (G.E.W. Wolstenholme and M. O'Connor, eds.), pp. 127-149, J. A. Churchill Ltd.
Nelson, G.S., Amin, M.A., Saoud, M.F.A. and Teesdale, C. (1968). *Bull. Wld. Hlth. Org.*, *38*, 9.
Peters, W. (1965). *Expt. Parasit.*, *16*, 158.
Preston, J.M., Nelson, G.S. and Saeed, A.A. (1972). *Bull. Wld. Hlth. Org.*, *47*, 587.
Ramachandran, C.P. (1970). *S. E. Asian J. Trop. Med. Publ. Hlth.*, *1*, 78.
Remington, J.S. and Merigan, T. C. (1969). *Proc. Soc. Exp. Biol. Med.*, *131*, 1184.
Ruskin, J., McIntosh, J., Remington, J.S. (1969). *J. Immunol.*, *103*, 252.
Russell, D.A., Scott, G. C. and Wigley, S.C. (1968). *In* Abstracts of papers of the Ninth International Leprosy Congress 1968. London, p. 58.
Sadun, E.H., Bruce, J.I. and Macomber, P.B. (1964). *Am. J. Trop. Med. Hyg.*, *13*, 548.
Salaman, M.H. (1970). *Proc. Roy. Soc. Med.*, *63*, 11.
Schwabe, C.W. (1969). "Veterinary Medicine and Human Health". Bailliére, Tindall and Cassell, London. 713 pp.
Sinclaire, I.J. (1967). *Res. Vet. Sci.*, *8*, 14.
Smith, D.H., Wilton, T., Berezancev, Ju.A., Lykov, V., Myo Paing, Chari, M.V. and Davis, A. (1971). *Bull. Wld. Hlth. Org.*, *44*, 771.
Smithers, S.R. (1972). *Brit. Med. Bull.*, *28*, 49.

Southgate, B.A. (1967). *J. Trop. Med. Hyg.*, *70*, 33.
Southgate, B.A. and Oriedo, B.V.E. (1967). *J. Trop. Med. Hyg.*, *70*, 1.
Strickland, G.T., Voller, A., Pettit, L.E. and Fleck, D.G. (1972). *J. Inf. Dis.*, *126*, 54.
Strickland, G.T., Pettit, L.E. and Voller, A. (1973). *Am. J. Trop. Med. Hyg.*, *22*, 452.
Taylor, M.G. (1970). *J. Helminth.*, *44*, 253.
Taylor, M.G., Nelson, G.S. and Smith, M. (1974). *Bull. Wld. Wlth. Org.*, (In press).
Teesdale, C. and Nelson, G.S. (1958). *E. Afr. Med. J.*, *35*, 427.
Thurston, J.P. (1963). *Parasitology*, *53*, 49.
Thurston, J.P. (1964). *Parasitology*, *54*, 67.
Uganda Buruli Group (1969). *Lancet*, *i*, 111.
Villella, J.B., Gomberg, H.J. and Gould, S.E. (1961). *Science*, *134*, 1073.
Voelker, J. and Garms, R. (1972). *Z. Tropenmed. Parasit.*, *23*, 285.
Warren, K.S. (1972). *Trans. Roy. Soc. Trop. Med. Hyg.*, *66*, 417.
Weiss, K.E., Haig, D.A. and Alexander, R.A. (1956). *Onderstepoort J. Vet. Res.*, *27*, 183.
Wong, M.M., Fredericks, H.J. and Ramachandran, C.P. (1969). *Bull. Wld. Hlth. Org.*, *40*, 493.
World Health Organization (1963). "Terminology of Malaria and of Malaria Eradication". World Health Organization, Geneva, 127.
World Health Organization Technical Report Series (1967). No. 378, 1-127.
Yoshimura, H. and Yokogawa, M. (1970). *Am. J. Trop. Med. Hyg.*, *19*, 63.

FILARIASIS IN DOMESTIC ANIMALS IN NORTHERN NIGERIA AND ITS RELATION TO HUMAN HEALTH

Tj. Schillhorn van Veen

Department of Parasitology and Entomology, Faculty of Veterinary Medicine, Ahmadu Bello University, Zaria, Nigeria

INTRODUCTION

Human filariasis is common in Nigeria and has been reviewed by Cowper, (1966, 1967). *Onchocerca volvulus, Loa loa, Dracunculus medinensis,* and to a lesser extent, *Wuchereria bancrofti* and *Acanthocheilonema perstans,* cause serious health problems.

Little is known about the filariases of animals, or of their potential public health significance, in Nigeria. This paper reviews the filarial infections in Nigerian animals and presents additional data from investigations on filariasis conducted between 1970 and 1973.

MATERIALS AND METHODS

Data were obtained from surveys at the post-mortem room of the Veterinary Faculty, Ahmadu Bello University, at the abattoirs of Zaria, Kano and Bauchi and occasionally at bush slaughter points.

Microfilarial surveys were carried out at the Zaria slaughterhouse and at the clinic of the Veterinary Faculty. The microhaematocrit method (Schalm and Jain, 1966) was used for the detection of microfilariae in peripheral blood. Skin snips of 1 x 1 cm were kept overnight in saline and examined the following day for microfilariae. Measurements of microfilariae, fixed in 2% formalin, were performed with an ocular micrometer.

RESULTS AND DISCUSSION

FILARIAE OF LARGE DOMESTIC ANIMALS

Equines

Onchocerca cervicalis and *Onchocerca reticulata* were found to be common parasites of donkeys and horses. The nodules and swellings caused by these helminths are readily found at autopsy. They have not been reported to be of clinical importance in Nigeria. Depigmentation and fistulous withers do occur in Nigerian horses and donkeys but the aetiological relationship with filariasis has not yet been proven.

Setaria equina has been found in 40 to 75% of the equines examined at autopsy in Zaria (Bello, 1971). The worms are generally located in the abdominal cavity though in one exceptional case a female *Setaria* was found in the thoracic duct near the heart. The present study showed the prevalence of microfilariae in the peripheral blood to be much lower, in that microfilariae were found in 21 out of 62 blood samples.

Dromedaries

Bello (1972) found *Onchocerca* spp. in the thoracic aorta of dromedaries in Kano abattoir. The pathological changes in the aorta were similar to those in bovine aortic onchocerciasis. In the present study, unidentified microfilariae were found in 8 out of 124 blood samples of dromedaries. Parasitic ulcers were once observed in a dromedary in Zaria. The larvae isolated from the ulcers were morphologically identical with the larvae isolated from bovine parasitic ulcers caused by the genus *Agamofilaria*.

Bovines

The prevalence of filarial infections of cattle in Nigeria is given in Table 1.

Table 1

Prevalence and importance of filarial infection in Nigerian cattle.

Filarial species	Prevalence	Importance
Onchocerca armillata	high: 80-100%	Sclerosis of aorta.
Onchocerca gutturosa	high: 40-70%	No lesions observed.
Onchocerca gibsoni (like?)	low: 10-20%	Nodules in connective tissue.
Onchocerca spp.	once observed in nodules on penis.	
Parafilaria bovicola	low: 1-10%	Chronic skin lesions.
Stephanofilaria spp.	low: 1-5%	Chronic skin lesions.
Agamofilaria spp. (?)	low: 1-5%	Cutaneous ulcers.
Setaria labiato-papillosa	high: 20-60%	No lesions observed.

These findings correspond to the surveys in neighbouring countries (Graber, Fernagut and Oumatie, 1966; Graber 1969). The findings also relate to the fact that many of the cattle slaughtered in Nigeria originate from Chad, Niger or the Cameroon.

Onchocerca armillata was found to be the most common filarial parasite of cattle, even though its occurrence has only occasionally been reported (Mohammed, 1931; Cowper, 1967). The parasite causes a chronic aortitis characterised by sclerosis, calcification and corrugation of the thoracic aorta. Less commonly the abdominal aorta and the carotid arteries are affected. Caseous nodules, in which the male is found, occur in the adventitia. Chronic infection reduces the elasticity of the aortic wall (Schillhorn and Robl, in preparation), but apparently, it has little influence on the general health of the animal.

Eye infections, as described by Patnaik (1962), were not observed.

Onchocerca gutturosa, which is found in the cervical ligaments, was common. These results are similar to those of Wouda (1972) who found microfilariae in 53% of the skin snips from cattle in the Zaria slaughterhouse. In 40% of the positive cases, the microfilariae showed morphological similarity to those of *O. gutturosa*.

Amariki (1973) in Ibadan described microfilariae in skin biopsies of cattle and suggested *O. gutturosa* as the helminth species involved. Histologically, he observed an inflammatory reaction around the microfilariae in the lower dermis. However, clinical dermatitis, or other lesions due to this infection, have not been reported.

Onchocerca gibsoni is more common in the north-eastern parts of Nigeria. The encapsulated nodules, characteristic for this infection in cattle, were mainly found in the subcutaneous and intramuscular connective tissues of the thorax. The morphological characteristics of this filarid do not completely correspond with the original description of *O. gibsoni* and some specimens show similarity with *O. volvulus*. This is probably the reason why it has been confused with the human parasite (Nigeria, 1958; Cowper, 1967). Confusion about speciation of the cattle form occurs in other parts of West Africa (Cameron, 1928; Bussieras, 1973). It is possible that this *Onchocerca* species is different from those hitherto reported from cattle. As far as can be determined, the parasite is not of public health importance.

Parafilaria bovicola occurred mainly in the subcutaneous tissue of the shoulder region. The haemorrhagic eruptions caused by this infection are very noticeable, but they do not seem to be of major importance to the health of the animal.

Stephanofilaria spp., causing a chronic dermatitis on the rump, have been reported by Oduye (1971) in Kano State. The lesions varied in diameter from 2 to 12 cm. and were characterised by loss of hair, crust formation and by a raised reddened periphery.

Chronic circumscribed skin ulcers, characterised by eosinophilic infiltration and similar to those caused by *Agamofilaria* larvae, as described by Fain and Herin (1955) in Ruanda Urundi, have been observed in northern Nigerian cattle. Larvae morphologically similar to *Agamofilaria* have been recovered from these lesions. Ulceration is observed just before and during the rainy season. Ulcers dry up during the dry season, but often reappear during the following rainy season.

Setaria (Artionema) labiato-papillosa was a common parasite in the abdominal cavity of cattle. Occasionally it causes a mild peritonitis consisting of a fibrous reaction around dead helminths.

Small ruminants

Sheep and goats were rarely infected with filariae, but more extensive surveys are needed on these animals. On one occasion adult *Seteria* spp. were found in the abdominal cavity.

Relationship of Equine and Ruminant filarids to human health

None of the filarids of horses or ruminants, reported above, have been incriminated as zoonotic entities in Nigeria.

FILARIAE OF PET ANIMALS

Dirofilaria immitis has not been demonstrated in Nigerian dogs, although veterinary field officers in Nigeria (as elsewhere, Nelson, 1966) often assume that dogs with microfilariae in their peripheral blood are infected with this heartworm. Routine post-mortem examinations of approximately 400 dogs at the Veterinary Faculty failed to detect *D. immitis*. In other parts of West Africa little is known about the prevalence of heartworm infections in dogs. Tendeiro (1947) mentioned *D. immitis* in a checklist of parasites in Guinea-Bissau and Gretillat and Gaillard (1965) reported a case of *D. immitis* infection in wild carnivores. Zielke (1972) found that *Anopholes gambiae* recovered from Kano were not susceptible to infections with *D. immitis* larvae. It is possible that *D. immitis* infections are restricted to the coastal region, as is the case in East Africa (Bwangamoi and Frank, 1970), but there are no reports available to verify this suggestion.

The most common filaria in Nigerian dogs and cats is *Dirofilaria repens*, which is found mainly in the subcutaneous connective tissue without causing any marked pathological changes. Adult specimens of *D. repens* are difficult to detect, but they have been demonstrated in three dogs and in one cat at autopsy in Zaria. *Dirofilaria repens* has not previously been reported in West Africa, although Bayliss (1928) described a closely related species, *Dirofilaria genettae*, in a genet from Nigeria.

In a survey of filarial infections in dogs in the Zaria area, using the microhaematocrit and saponin concentration methods, 9.4% of the dogs examined showed microfilariae of *D. repens* in their peripheral blood (Table 2).

Table 2

Incidence and types of microfilariae observed in the blood of 188 dogs in the clinic of the Veterinary Faculty, Zaria in 1972.*

Type of microfilariae	Size range (μ)	Incidence
D. repens	300-369	9.4%
Mf. I (not identified)	234-264	4.4%
Mf. II (not identified)	185	once recorded.

**Measurements made on brilliant cresyl-blue stained microfilariae; by this method the microfilariae were 5-10% longer than those fixed in 2% formalin and stained with methylene blue.*

Adult forms of other filarid species have not been recovered from dogs or cats in Nigeria. However, blood examination revealed two other types of microfilariae. The measurements and the G-cell pattern of the "mf. I" type of microfilariae noted in Table 2 suggest they are microfilariae of *Dipetalonema dracunculoides* (Schillhorn and Blotkamp, In Preparation). This filarid has been reported from other parts of West Africa (Leger, 1911; Neveu-Lemaire, 1936).

Microfilariae of *Dipetalonema reconditum* have not been observed. None of the microfilariae detected in the samples showed the typical acid-phosphatase staining as described by Chalifoux and Hunt (1971).

ANIMAL FILARIAE IN HUMAN HOSTS

Little is known about the occurrence of human infections with animal filariae in Nigeria. Pulmonary lesions, as described in other parts of the world (Buckley, 1958; Beaver and Orihel, 1965; Attygale and Dissanaike, 1970; Moorhouse, Abrahams and Stephens, 1971) have not been noted (Edington, 1973). Tropical eosinophilia is not uncommon in Nigeria (Hunter, 1946; MacFadzean, 1955; Monkosso, 1972) but generally is due to parasitic infections other than the filariases of animal origin (Monkosso, 1972).

Records of filarial infections of 24 dogs were available in the clinic of the Veterinary Faculty in Zaria. The medical records of persons in 17 households in which these dogs were or had been kept, were obtained in cooperation with the University Health Service during the last 2 years. None of the household members had any record of eosinophilia, pulmonary lesions or subcutaneous cysts. At least four households had been in regular contact with dogs which showed *D. repens* microfilariae in their peripheral blood on repeated examinations over two years. Thus human infections with *D. repens* are considered to be exceptional in Nigeria.

The present results suggest that animal filariae are not of major zoonotic importance in northern Nigeria.

SUMMARY

Filarial infections are common in domestic animals in northern Nigeria. *Onchocerca armillata, O. gibsoni* (or a related species), *O. gutturosa, Setaria labiato-papillosa* and *Stephanofilaria* spp. are the main species found in cattle, while *O. cervicalis* and *Setaria equina* are common in equines. *Onchocerca* spp. were also found in the aorta of dromedaries; *Setaria* spp. were detected once in the abdominal cavity of a sheep. None of these filariae are considered to be of zoonotic importance.

Dirofilaria repens was the most common filaria species in dogs and cats, whereas *D. immitis* has never been found. Surveys of the prevalence of microfilariae in the peripheral blood of dogs, revealed that 9.4% showed microfilarial of *D. repens*. Two other types of microfilariae were observed, the adult parasite of which have not yet been recovered.

Human infections with caine filariae have not been reported in Nigeria. Persons in households in which close contact with infected dogs occurred showed no evidence of infection.

ACKNOWLEDGEMENT

I am pleased to express my gratitude to Dr. I. Bhambri for her help to obtain the medical information, and to Prof. Dr. D. Zwart and Dr. H. J. Barnes for their advice and suggestions.

REFERENCES

Amakiri, S.F. (1973). *Bull. epizoot. Dis. Afr.*, *21*, 123.
Attygalle, D. and Dissanaike, A.S. (1972). *H.D. Srivastava Comm. Vol.*, 453.
Bayliss, H.A. (1928). *Parasitology*, *20*, 280.
Beaver, P.C. and Orihel, T.C. (1965). *Am. J. Trop. Med. Hyg.*, *14*, 1010.
Bello, S.I. (1971). (Pers. Communication)
Bello, S.I. (1972). Paper at *Ann. Meeting Nig. Vet. Ass. Enugu.*
Buckley, J.J.C. (1958). *E. Afr. Med. J.*, *35*, 493.
Bussieras, J. (1973). (Pers. Communication)
Bwangamoi, O. and Frank, H. (1970). *Small Anim. Pract.*, *11*, 273.
Cameron, T.W.M. (1928). *J. Helminth.*, *6*, 161.
Chalifoux, L. and Hunt, R.D. (1971). *J. Am. Vet. Med. Ass.*, *158*, 601.
Cowper, S.G. (1966). *West Afr. Med. J.*, *15*, 203.
Cowper, S.G. (1967). *West Afr. Med. J.*, *16*, 3.
Edington, G.M. (1973). (Pers. Communication)
Fain, A. and Herin, V. (1955). *Ann. Soc. Belge Méd. Trop.*, *35*, 535.
Graber, M. (1969). *Bull. epizoot. Dis. Afr.*, *17*, 403.
Graber, M., Fernagut, R. and Oumatie, O. (1966). *Rev. Elev. Med. vêt. Pays Trop.*, *19*, 149.
Gretillat, S. and Gaillard, M. (1965). *Rev. Elev. Med. vêt. Pays Trop.*, *18*, 395.
Hunter, E.A. (1946). *Brit. Med. J.*, *I*, 877.
Leger, D. (1911). *Bull. Soc. Path. exoth.*, *4*, 629.
McFadzean, J.A. (1955). *Brit. Med. J.*, *II*, 772.
Mohammed, A.S. (1931). *Ann. Trop. Med. Parasit.*, *25*, 509.
Monokosso, G.L. (1972). *J. Trop. Med. Hyg.*, *65*, 233.
Moorhouse, D.E., Abrahams, E.W. and Stephens, B.J. (1971). *Med. J. Aust.*, *2*, 1230.
Nelson, G.S. (1966). *Helm. Abstr.*, *35*, 311.
Neveu-Lamaire, M. (1936). *Traité de Helminthologie medicine et veterinaire.*, Vigot Fr. Paris.
Nigeria (1958). *Ann. Rep. Dept. Vet. Res. Nig.*, 1956-1957. Govt. Printer, Lagos.
Nigeria (1965). *Ann. Rep. Vet. Div. Min. Agric. For. Res. N. Nig.*, 1962-1963. Govt. Printer, Kaduna.
Oduye, O.O. (1972). *J. Comp. Path.*, *81*, 581.
Patnaik, B. (1962). *J. Helminth.*, *36*, 313.
Schalm, D.W. & Jain, C. (1966). *Calif. Vet.*, *20*, 14.
Tendiero, J. (1947). *Bol. cult. Guinê Port.*, *11*, 639.
Wouda, W. (1972). (Pers. Communication)
Zielke, E. (1972). *Angew. Zool.*, *59*, 419.

LARVA MIGRANS

Henri Galliard

Honorary Professor, Member of the "Académie de Médecine".
Faculty of Medicine, Paris.

INTRODUCTION AND DEFINITION

The larvae of numerous species of helminths, according to their host specificity, migrate in man or animals and reach sexual maturity in these hosts. As far as the nematodes are concerned, only few symptoms are associated with such normal migration. However, if such larvae are found in a non-specific, "abnormal", or unusual hosts, the symptoms are more severe. The developmental cycle may be interrupted at the larval stage or at the adult stage with abortive sexual development (e.g. *Gnathostoma, Angiostrongylus, Dirofilaria, Oesophagostomum*).

"Larva migrans" has been known since the 19th century, when Robert Lee (1874) in London described a syndrome of cutaneous lesions, due to larvae of *Ancylostoma*, under the name of "Creeping eruption". The recent interest in the condition was stimulated by Beaver *et al.*, (1952) when they identified the larva of *Toxocara canis* as the cause of visceral larva migrans.

It is well known that predator or carnivorous birds and mammals, may get infected with nematode larvae, such as the Ascaridae, either by the ingestion of embryonated eggs or by eating small animals or even arthropods, bearing second stage larvae in their tissues. Such second stage larvae pass from the digestive tract to the viscera each time they are eaten by an unfavorable "waiting host" until they are acquired by the specific host, in which development to sexual maturity occurs. Baer (1951) gave the name "paratenic host" to such "waiting hosts". This term was redefined by Beaver and applied by him in 1956 to humans bearing second stage larvae of *Toxocara canis*.

In man, infection is caused by the ingestion of eggs, which liberate the second stage larvae in the intestine. These migrate in the body without undergoing further development and are found in the liver, lungs, brain and eyes. Consequently, man can be considered as a paratenic host for *T. canis*.

With the *Ancylostoma* spp. larvae, which cause cutaneous larva migrans in man, the existence of paratenic hosts, which may contribute to the maintenance of the species in nature, is still an open question. In the case of *Ancylostoma caninum*, it is known that small mammals and insects can serve as experimental paratenic hosts (Nichols, 1956).

In general, the term "larva migrans" is strictly applied to the migrations in the human skin of larvae of dog *Ancylostoma* spp. and of *Strongyloides* sp. (cutaneous larva migrans, linear dermatitis, creeping eruption, larbish, larva currens), and the migration in the viscera of larvae of *Toxocara canis* (visceral larva migrans).

VISCERAL LARVA MIGRANS

Some allergic syndromes, of uncertain origin, and in which the lungs are affected, may be due to visceral parasitism of man by parasitic nematodes of animals. Examples of such are "Familial eosinophilia", "Weingarten" or "Frimodt Moller" syndromes, "pseudo eosinophilic leukemia", and "Loeffler's syndrome". In some instances, larvae are found in the liver, but these are usually those of *A. lumbricoides* since an association with intestinal parasitism is generally seen.

In 1952 Beaver *et al.*, in New Orleans, proved that the visceral syndrome with hepatomegaly and eosinophilia was due to larvae of *Toxocara canis*, a common parasite of the dog and of cosmopolitan distribution.

Toxocara canis *in dog.*

Toxocara canis is a common parasite of the dog and it is the major cause of visceral larva migrans in man. Its prevalence in dogs varies from 12 to 83% (mean 20%) on a global basis, and it is also found in foxes and numerous other species of the Canidae. *Toxocara cati* has been found occasionally in the intestine of man, but it is seldom found in the viscera. It is also cosmopolitan in distribution. *Toxascaris leonina* is less common in dogs and cats and is not incriminated in the visceral larva migrans syndrome.

Life cycle in the dog.

Sprent (1955, 1958) and Sprent and English (1958) showed that the life cycles of *T. canis* and *T. cati* were different and that each life cycle varied according to host species, and the age and sex of the host.

Dogs may be infected with *T. canis* in several ways. Direct infection may occur by the ingestion of eggs in the soil, or indirectly, by eating paratenic hosts bearing second stage larvae. As a dog increases in age, it becomes increasingly refractory to infection and increasing serves as a host for the infection. Prenatal transmission from the mother to the foetus occurs during this paratenic state. Nursing bitches may ingest third stage larvae shed by prenatally infected pups, and such larvae may develop directly to the adult stage in the intestine of the nursing bitch. It is probable that a similar development occurred to produce an adult specimen of *T. canis* in a child aged 16 months, in London (Bisseru, *et al.*, 1966).

Animal paratenic hosts of T. canis

In mice, larvae of *T. canis* remain in the liver for a few days and then migrate in the brain and muscles where they may be found several months after. Larvae of *T. cati* are never found in the brain of mice. In rats, hamsters and guinea pigs migration to the brain is common and numerous larvae may be found there. In rabbits and monkeys the majority of larvae are found in the liver and few occur in the brain. Beaver (1956) has observed that, seven years after infection of two monkeys, liver biopsies contained numerous viable larvae.

In adult sheep Schaeffler (1960) demonstrated that larvae did not pass beyond the liver, but in young lambs, larvae were found in the mesenteric nodes, pancreas, heart, lungs, kidneys and brain from the fourth day onwards. In pigs, larvae migrate to all organs. They are detectable in the liver, kidneys and heart and numerous granulomas may be formed in the posterior lobe of the cerebellum. The last named may cause nervous disorders.

Larva migrans in man.

According to Beaver (1969) more than 200 cases have been recorded since the first description of visceral larva migrans. Sixty of these cases were concerned with infection of the eye. In 36 cases, larve of *T. canis* were identified in biopsies of the liver (15), at autopsy (6), or in enucleated eyes (15). In England, 33 cases of ocular lesions have been recorded, of which 18 were confirmed histologically. While most of the recorded cases have occurred in the United States or Great Britain, the condition has been recorded from all parts of the world. However, it is unlikely that the recorded cases of visceral larva migrans represents the prevalence of the condition.

General symptoms.

The syndrome is observed in children from one to four years of age. Such children often suffer from "pica", a term used in the United States to describe abnormal geophagy or coprophagy.

The principal symptom is eosinophilia. In 80% of cases, eosinophilia may reach 50% and in some cases it can reach 90%. With an eosinophilia of under 30% the diagnosis is doubtful.

A notable feature of the eosinophilia is its chronicity in that it can last for more than 2 years. In addition to the eosinophilia, there is a leukocytosis, usually higher than 20,000 w.b.c. per $m.m^3$.

There is an increase of globulins and gamma globulins in the serum. This reaches a maximum at the acute period and decreases afterwards.

Hepatomegaly is a typical symptom. However it may be absent in light infections. In severe cases the liver may extend to the umbilicus. On laparotomy, miliary, whitish nodules are found which are eosinophilic granulomas. Llanio and Sotto (1972) in Havana, performed laparotomy on 22 cases and found prominent white strings or round spots on the surface of hypertrophied livers. On biopsy these lesions showed granulomas and micro-abscesses rich in eosinophils and fragments of larvae.

Pulmonary signs, such as broncho-pulmonary infiltration, are often seen in visceral larva migrans.

Experimental infection of man.

Smith and Beaver (1953), Chaudhuri and Saha (1959) infected volunteers with eggs of *T. canis*. A slight enlargement of the liver with eosinophilia occurred.

Evolution of the condition.

Generally, patients are seen when symptoms are maximal and little is known of the clinical manifestion during the evolution of visceral larva migrans. Physical signs of the disease and hematologic changes begin to regress about one month after the acute phase. The liver may return to normal size, but eosinophils persists at a high level. Sometimes hepatomegaly persists for several months, up to a year or more. In such cases eosinophilia persists in excess of 2 years.

Autopsy and histopathology.

Brill, Churg and Beaver (1953) reported the autopsy of a 2 year old child with fever, hepatomegaly and 40% eosinophila and who had died in a comatose state. Numerous nodules were found in the lungs, heart and liver. Dent *et al.*, (1956) reported the case of a child, aged 19 months, with marked hepatomegaly and 60% eosinophila. Numerous granulomas were found on liver biopsy. Peptic digestion of liver samples revealed a larval burden of 60 viable larvae per gram. In the muscles and nervous system, there were 5 and 5 larvae per gram of tissue respectively, given a total burden of more than 50,000 larvae.

In recent lesions, in which larvae tunnel through the hepatic parenchyma, the center of the lesion consists of necrotic cells, degenerating eosinophils and connective tissue fibres. The adjacent tissues are heavily infiltrated with eosinophils, histiocytes and plasmocytes. In older lesions the larva are degenerated and an eosinophilic allergic granuloma is produced (Churg and Strauss, 1951). Severe neurological symptoms have been attributed to granulomas and larvae in the nervous system.

Ocular lesions.

Eosinophilic granulomas have been found in ocular lesions. The clinical signs usually occur after 4 years of age or in adults. The ocular manifestations are usually isolated and frequently occur without generalized eosinophilia, hyperglobulinemia or liver hypertrophy. Etiologic diagnosis is difficult unless the eye is enucleated.

There are three major ocular signs: chronic endophthalmy retinal granuloma and peripheral retinitis. Tumefaction of the posterior segment is suggestive of retinoblastoma.

Diagnosis.

Woodruff (1970) considers that visceral larva migrans is widespread in the world, even though only about 200 cases have been detected with certainty in man. The only certain evidence for the infection is the identification of the larva in the tissues either by liver biopsy or eye enucleation.

The two signs of major importance in clinical diagnosis are eosinophilia of a persistant nature and hepatomegaly.

Beaver (1962) notes the necessity to differentiate between pulmonary tropical eosinophilia and larva migrans. In the first, the liver is normal and the action of diethyl carbamazine or arsenic compounds is prompt and decisive on the clinical signs and eosinophilia. Visceral larva migrans is observed in children under 4 years of age and rarely or never in adults. The eosinophila is higher (30,000 v. 10,000) and more persistant in visceral larva migrans.

Arsenical compounds have no action of larvae of *T. canis* and while diethyl carbamazine treatment improves the condition of the patient and lowers the eosinophilia, the latter returns to pretreatment levels when the drug is discontinued.

In the event that larvae cannot be detected by tissue biopsy, diagnosis must be based on clinical signs and serodiagnosis, for the latter intradermal tests and immunofluorescent tests have been used.

Therapy.

Beaver (1962) observed that diethycarbamazine was the drug

of choice for visceral larva migrans, even though its action was somewhat limited. It has no effect on eosinophilia but fever, cough, general malaise and liver enlargement respond rapidly to treatment.

In patients with larvae in the liver, diethycarbamazine given at the rate of 150 mg/kg. for 3 weeks lowered the level of antibodies over a 14 to 24 months period (Wiseman *et al.*, 1970).

Dent *et al.*, (1956) and Snyder (1961) observed that cortisone may be used in severe cases with pulmonary disorders.

CUTANEOUS LARVA MIGRANS

The syndrom of cutaneous larva migrans was described first by Robert Lee in London in 1874. Since then, it has been observed frequently in many parts of the world and is attributed to multiple causes.

Kirby-Smith, Dove and White (1926) in Florida found nematode larvae three times in 200 biopsies of cases of creeping eruption. Their subsequent research with experimental infections led them to identify such larvae as those of *Ancylostoma braziliense* a common species of dogs. This has since been confirmed by numerous authors.

Other species are known to cause "creeping eruption" but larva of these species have not been identified in spontaneous infections.

Lesions due to Ancylostoma *larvae.*

The fate of larvae which penetrate the skin has not been fully determined. Some may die in the skin, but others may migrate to the lungs. Dove (1928) reported a case of cutaneous and intestinal infection by *A. ceylanicum* (Biocca, 1951).

Muhleisen (1953) observed numerous larvae in bronchial excretions of a patient presenting severe and extensive dermatitis. The larvae were not identified, but no intestinal infection existed nor developed subsequently.

Symptomatology.

Lesions are first evident in the epidermis. A papule and then a vesicular lesion appears at the site of penetration. Later the track of the larva is marked by an irregular, serpentine line, which after a few hours becomes intensily pruritic especially at night. The lesion progresses at about 3 cm. per day. Sometimes the lesions are multiple and diffuse the whole of the body. However, larvae do not appear to penetrate the vaginal or anal mucosa (Homez, 1967). Pruritis may be so intense as to prevent sleep.

The level of eosinophils is variable being high in the cases with multiple lesions. Homez (1967) reported an eosinophilia of 65% in one case.

Histopathology.

The lesions have been described by Kirby-Smith, *et al.*, (1926). Larvae are found in tunnels in the malpiphian layer, surrounded by degenerated epithelial cells and numerous eosinophils. Superficially, the lesions are string-like and are readily palpable.

Lesions due to Strongyloides *sp. larvae.*

Though the presence of *Strongyloides* sp. larvae has never been identified positively in the skin, it is admitted that the clinical signs appear specific. They are characterized by a wide urticarial area which shows extraordinarily rapid progression, for which reason they were named "larva currens" by Arthur and Shelley (1958).

Fülleborn (1926) gave the first description of 8 cases including his own, which he thought was due to auto infection beginning by the perianal region. Caplan (1949) in a study of several hundred patients in Birmania, Thailand and Java, found an intestinal infection with *Strongyloides* in 98% of cases. In these, eosinophils varied from 10 to 25%.

Sandosham (1952) suggested several hypothesis to explain the various manifestions of *Strongyloides* infection. For example, he considered that skin migrating larvae might be of feline origin and that on immune response in man prevented normal migration. Alternatively, there may be a loss of virulence in a strain due to its age and repeated auto-infection. For example, the strain from a patient who had been infected for 4 years, failed, on two occasions to infect volunteers.

Galliard and Chabaud (1952) studied a strain of *Strongyloides* from a case of creeping eruption from North Vietnam. The strain appeared to be of canine origin and in Hanoi the infection was purely intestinal but the cutaneous syndrom appeared when the patient returned to France. Similarly, Sandosham (1952) reported on a patient who, in Malaya, had an infection which was exclusively intestinal, which became cutaneous in England and reverted to the intestinal form on his return to Malaya.

Nitzulescu (1967) studied a case where there was creeping linear dermatitis. Multiple points of emergence were present and the speed of progression was as much as 10 to 12 cm. per hour. An intradermal injection of "Resoquin" at the anterior extremity of the lesion made the track turn immediately 180° to retrace the previous migration path. This indicated that the creeping eruption lesion contained a larva.

L.C. Brumpt and Ho Thi Sang (1973) reported a case of "larva currens" from Gabon, which lasted 40 years after the return to France. The dermal lesion was the only evidence of strongyloidosis in the patient.

Diagnosis.

Diagnosis of cutaneous larva migrans is relatively easy. Some authors consider that parasitism by *Gnathostoma spinigerum* should be included in this condition, believing that man serves as a paratenic host for that parasite. However, it is an error to confuse cutaneous larva migrans with those migrating oedemas (Daengsvang, 1949) which contain voluminous "cord like masses" and from which the adult worms either escape spontaneously, or are extracted with a pin by the patient. Diagnosis is related to the numerous locations and the size of the lesion which occur in the ocular, cephalo-rachidian and abdominal regions.

Treatment.

A variety of physical and chemical treatments have been used. Thiabendazole is now the drug of choice. A single dose of 50 mg/kg. cures patients with multiple lesions. In a case with 300 lesions, a complete cure was obtained in one week with 2 g of thiabendazole per day for 5 days (Baranski and Carneiro 1966).

"Larva currens" due to *Strongyloides* has been treated by diverse methods. Arthur and Shelley (1958) used trypsin which had a "destructive action on proteolytic enzymes in nematode intestinal infections". In their case, the larva was killed by a single injection made at the extremity of the tract.

However, thiabendazole is the drug of choice, and is effective even as an aqueous solution applied on the skin.

SUMMARY AND CONCLUSIONS

The term "larva migrans" was used first to design a cutaneous disease entity caused by infective larvae of *Ancylostoma* parasite of dogs. In 1952, the visceral syndrom was related to the migration of larvae of *Toxocara canis* in man.

Toxocara canis in dogs is cosmopolitan in distribution. On ingestion of infective eggs by man, larvae are distributed to the liver, lungs, muscles, eye and brain. Larvae may survive indefinitely in the tissues (7 years in the monkey). Man and other animals are paratenic hosts for *T. canis*.

The adult dog is refractory to infection, but serves as a paratenic host. Epidemiologically, it is the new born pup, infected as foetus by larvae in the mother, which perpetuates infection.

In man the visceral syndrome is seen in children from about one to four years of age, which show geophagy (pica). The major clinical signs is a hypereosinophilia of long persistance. Hepatomegaly is common. Histologically, "allergic eosinophilic granulomas" are found containing larvae. The prognosis depends of the intensity of the infection and on the frequency of re-infection.

Diagnosis is based on the persistant hypereosinophilia, the presence of granulomas, and the detection of larva in liver biopsies. The syndrome is different from tropical eosinophilia which occurs in adults and in which pulmonary symptoms are always present and intense. Tropical eosinophilia is cured by diethylcarbamazine and arsenical compounds while the latter are ineffective in "larva migrans".

Ocular lesions due to larvae of *T. canis* are observed in older persons. The formation of eosinophilic granulomas produces an endophthalmitis. Frequently patients have no other clinical signs, such as eosinophilia.

The syndrome of "cutaneous larva migrans" is caused by the infective larvae of *Ancylostoma* spp. of dog. The linear, creeping eruption, the inflammation and the intense pruritis are characteristic signs of the syndrome. The larvae occur in the malpighian layer of the skin, surrounded by epithelioid and eosinophilic cells and form a thick cord which migrates progressively.

Larvae of *Strongyloides stercoralis,* though they have never been identified in human skin are also considered to be the cause of the disease. Intestinal infection often coexists. The extremely rapid progression of the lesion (larva currens) gives to the syndrome a specific diagnostic character.

Thiabendazole is the drug of choice and is remarkedly effective in creeping eruption.

REFERENCES

Arthur, R.P. and Shelley, W.B. (1958). *Arch. Dermat. 78,* 186.
Baer, J.G. (1951). *Ecology of parasites*, Univ. of Illinois Press, Urbana.
Baranski, M.C. and Carneiro, M. Jr. (1966). *Rev. Brazil. Med. 23,* 233.
Beaver, P.C. Snyder, H., Carrera, G., Dent, J. and Lafferty, J. (1952). *Pediatrics. 9,* 7.
Beaver, P.C. (1956). *Expt. Parasit. 5,* 587.
Beaver, P.C. (1962). *Bull. Soc. Path. Exot. 55,* 555.
Beaver, P.C. (1969). *J. Parasit. 55,* 3.

Biocca, E. (1951). *J. Helminth.* *25*, 1.
Bisseru, B. and Woodruff, A.W. (1968). *J. Clin. Path.* *21*, 449.
Brill, R., Churg, J. and Beaver, P.C. (1953). *Amer. J. Clin. Path.* *23*, 1208.
Brumpt, L.C. and Ho Thi Sang. (1973). *Ann. Parasit. Hum. Comp.* *48*, 92.
Caplan, J.P. (1949). *Brit. Med. J.* *I*, 396.
Chaudhuri, R.N. and Saha, T.K. (1959). *Lancet*, *2*, 493.
Churg, J. and Strauss, L. (1951). *Amer. J. Path.* *27*, 277.
Daengsvang, S. (1949). *J. Parasit.* *35*, 116.
Dover, W.E. (1928). *J. Parasit*, *14*, 199.
Dent, J.H., Nichols, R., Beaver, P.C., Carrera, G.M. and Staggers, R. (1956). *Amer. J. Path.* *32*, 777.
Fülleborn, F. (1926). *Arch. Schiffs Trophyg.* *30*, 821.
Galliard, H. and Chabaud, A.G. (1952). *Ann. Parasit. Hum. Comp.* *27*, 588.
Homez, J. (1967). *Med. Cutanea*, *2*, 263.
Kirby-Smith, J.L. Dove, W.E. and White, G.F. (1926). *Arch. Dermat. Syph.*, *13*, 137.
Lee, R. (1874). *London Clin. Trans.* *8*, 44.
Llanio, R. and Sotto, A. (1972). *Sem. Hop. Paris*, *48*, 1223.
Muhleisen, J.P. (1953). *Ann. Intern. Med.* *38*, 595.
Nichols, R.L. (1956). *J. Parasit.* *42*, 349.
Nitzulescu, V. (1967). *Bull. Soc. Path. Exot.* *60*, 653.
Sandground, J.H. (1939). *Geneesk Tidjschr. Nederl. Indies.* *79*, 895.
Sandosham, A.A. (1952). *J. Helmint.* *26*, 1.
Schaeffler, W.F. (1960). *Ill. Vet.* *3*, 99.
Smith, M.M.D. and Beaver, P.C. (1953). *Pediatrica.* *12*, 491.
Snyder, C.H. (1961). *Pediatrics.* *28*, 85.
Sprent, J.F.A. (1955). *Parasitology*, *45*, 31.
Sprent, J.F.A. and English, P.B. (1958). *Aust. Vet. J.* *34*, 161.
Wiseman, R.A., Fleck, D.G. and Woodruff, A.W. (1970). *Brit. Med. J.* *I*, 152.
Woodruff, A.W. (1966). *Brit. Med. J.*
Woodruff, A.W., Bisseru, B. and Bowe, J.C. (1966). *Brit. Med. J.* *I*, 1576.
Woodruff, A.W. (1970). *Brit. Med. J.* *3*, 663.

IMMUNODIAGNOSIS OF VISCERAL LARVA MIGRANS IN MAN

J. Lamina

Abtlg. für Parasitologie und Zoologie der TU - München
Federal Republic of Germany.

INTRODUCTION

"Larva migrans", also described as "immature nematodiasis" includes the following terms, which are found frequently in literature: Weingarten's disease, Frimodt-Möller's syndrome, cutaneous larva migrans, creeping eruption, larval gnathostomiasis and larval filariasis including tropical eosinophilia. Such conditions are caused by nematode larvae, some specific and others not specific for man. The following families of nematodes may be concerned in the larva migrans syndrome: Ancylostomatidae, Strongyloididae, Ascaridae, Anisakidae, Gnathostomidae, other Spiruroidea, Metastrongylidae and Filaridae.

In Central Europe, ascarids, especially those of the genus *Toxocara*, have great significance as the cause of larva migrans. The prevalence of *Toxocara* spp. in dogs and cats in various countries is estimated at 20% (Lamina 1970, Kozlovska 1953, Stoimenov 1959, Lis und Schanzel 1961, Gräfner und Danailov 1964, Plass 1965). It is suspected that the prevalence is increasing and Buchwalder (1973) and Williams and Menning (1961) believe that a prevalence in excess of 7% for *Toxocara* infection in dogs is indicative of a health hazard to man. Based on such estimates it is fairly certain that human infections with *Toxocara* are common in areas where the prevalence of canine infection is high.

The development of *Toxocara canis* varies according to the age of a dog (Sprent 1958, Lamina 1964, 1966, 1970). In a dog under 6 months of age, the tracheal route of migration occurs, while somatic migration occurs in the older dogs, and larvae migrate into all organs of the body. Such larvae are responsible for prenatal infection of the foetus. Infection of an unnatural host (e.g. rodent or man) results in a similar migration of larvae as in the older dog. In an unnatural host larvae demonstrate an affinity for the central nervous system and the eye. In these locations they may survive for weeks or months without being encapsulated (Fig. 1).

The clinical diagnosis of *T. canis* infection in man is not easy. Characteristic findings may be present in the eye and larvae may be observed with an ophthalmoscope, but usually symptoms of central nervous disorders a high eosinophilia and a history of contact with dogs and cats are those which suggest *T. canis* infection.

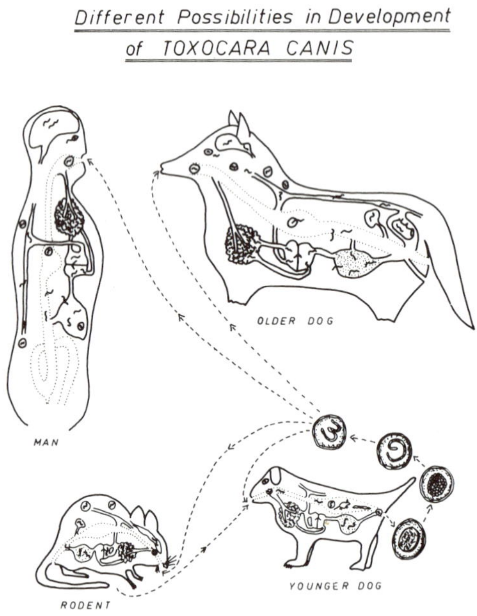

←*Fig. 1. Migration characteristics of* Toxocara canis *in various hosts.*

Histological diagnosis (Lamina, 1964) has variable effectiveness and increasingly attention is being paid to the diagnosis of visceral larva migrans by immunobiological methods. Various techniques have been used (Francis and Fellers 1953, Heiner and Kevy 1956, Kagan 1957, Olson 1960, Jung and Pacheco 1960, Barna *et al.*, 1962, Huntly and Moreland 1963, Mitchell 1964, Remky and Kraft 1965, Wood 1965, Hogarth-Scott 1966, 1969, Woodruff 1966, Bisseru and Woodruff 1968, Perlmutter *et al.*, 1968, Rifaat *et al.*, 1968, 1970, Wisemann 1968, 1970, 1971, Reichenmüller 1969, Reekie and Miller 1969, Bradford 1970, Lamina 1970, Ball 1971, Baufine-Ducrocq *et al.*, 1971, Engel *et al.*, 1971, Khalil *et al.*, 1971, Moreau *et al.*, 1971, Laqua 1972, Lee and Danaraj 1972 and Müller-Jensen *et al.*, 1973), but these, in general, have demonstrated lack of specificity and cross reactions occurred when sensitization to other helminth infections was present. However, the micropricipitation test using living larvae of ascarids may offer a useful means to identify *Toxocara* spp. infections in man. This technique was first used by Oliver-González (1940) and Roth (1941) for the diagnosis of *Trichinella spiralis*.

MATERIALS AND METHODS

For the present study larvae were obtained from the livers and lungs of mice on the 2nd and 3rd day after infection with infective eggs of *T. canis* larvae were allowed to migrate from the minced tissue and were cleared of tissue debris by sedimentation in saline. A suspension of larvae (10) was then mixed with 1 ml of test serum in a "well slide" and this after sealing was incubated in a moist chamber for 24 hours at 37°C. In the presence of antibodies in the serum, small precipitates occurred at the external openings of the larvae, such as the mouth, excretory pore and anus. These precipitates were evident as early as after 4 to 6 hours of incubation. On continued incubation, the precipitates increased in size until the larvae died.

Additionally, sera were examined by the agar-gel precipitation technique using saline extracts of fresh or lyophilized adult *Ascaris*, *Toxocara*, *Trichinella spiralis*, *Dirofilaria immitis*, *Strongyloides ransomi*, *Taenia saginata*, *Fasciola hepatica* and the fluid from hydatid cysts.

RESULTS

Over the last 3 years, 707 samples of serum from suspected cases of visceral larva migrans were examined from the Federal Republic of Germany and occasionally from neighbouring countries. All sera were examined by the microprecipitation technique with living larvae and by gel precipitation.

Gel precipitin reactions were observed with 149 sera with at least one of the *T. canis* antigens. The microprecipitation test with living *T. canis* larvae was positive with 73 sera. These sera also produced a gel-precipitin reaction, though at times faint, with at least one of the *T. canis* antigens (fresh or lyophilized). Sixteen of the 73 sera produced gel-precipitin reactions with the other helminth antigens. The clinical history of these 16 patients was such that it was not possible to decide whether the reactions were cross reactions or whether they were reactions due to multiple infections with parasites.

With 76 sera, gel-precipitin reactions occurred with antigens other than those of *T. canis*. It is of interest, that of serum samples sent in from patients suspected of helminth infections other than *T. canis* 10 samples showed positive reactions with the *T. canis* antigens. However the sera from 5 of these patients contained antibodies against other helminths and it was not possible to determine whether this was due to cross reactions or double or multiple infections. The results are summarized in Table 1.

Table 1

Serological reactions with sera of patients with suspected visceral larva migrans (707 samples examined).

Distribution of reactivity of 149 serum samples which reacted either in the microprecipitin test (MPT) with living *T. canis* larvae or gel precipitation (GP) with *T. canis* adult worm antigen.

No Positive on MPT and GP with *T. canis* antigens	No. Positive on GP with *T. canis* alone	No Positive on GP with *T. canis* and *Ascaris*	No Positive on GP with *T. canis*, *Ascaris* and other helminths
73*	11	36	29

(*of these 16 reacted in GP with other helminth antigens)

DISCUSSION

Our examinations showed that of 707 serum-samples examined 73 (8.7%) contained antibodies against *T. canis* detectable by the microprecipitation technique using living larvae and by precipitation in agar gel. It is considered that such reactions were specific for *T. canis* infection. The clinical history of the donor patients was, in nearly all cases, a relatively high peripheral blood eosinophilia, eosinophic infiltrations in various organs, central nervous disorders or pathological conditions of the eyes. Often a close contact with dogs or cats was noted, though under good hygenic conditions. Many patients had taken a vacation or had spent time in a Southern European country or in a tropical area. Thus it cannot be excluded that the condition might have been acquired abroad.

Because of these studies it is concluded that human *Toxocara*-infections exist in the Federal Republic of Germany. However, it is not clear, whether the majority of these infections were acquired at home or abroad.

The results indicate that the microprecipitin test using

living larvae of *T. canis* may be a very specific means of detecting human visceral larva migrans. The technical efforts necessary to conduct this test are considered worthwhile because of the specificity of the test.

Since other helminth infections may be the cause of illnesses similar to visceral larva migrans, it is recommended that other helminth antigens be included in the immunodiagnostic procedures.

SUMMARY

In the last 3 years (1969-1972) 707 serum samples from patients from different parts of Germany and from neighbouring countries were submitted for serodiagnosis for *Toxocara* infection.

Using the micro-precipitation test with living larvae and the Ouchterlony gel-precipitin test with *Toxocara* antigens, 73 serum samples were found to be positive. In 16 of these samples a positive gel precipitin reaction was seen with other helminth antigens. In samples submitted with suspicion of other parasite infections, 10 further patients showed positive results. In 5 of these, sera reacted additionally with other helminth antigens.

The micro-precipitations test on living larvae is considered to be a very sensitive and specific method of diagnosis. It is concluded that these patients were suffering from *Toxocara* infection. Indeed, in most cases, these patients showed clinical signs of visceral larva migrans. Some had been abroad and infection may have taken place there.

REFERENCES

Ball, P.A.J., Voller, A. and Taffs, L.F. (1971). *Brit. Med. J. i*, 210.

Barna Richards, Oson, L.J. and Box, Q.T. (1962). *J. Parasit. 48*, 3.

Baufine-Ducrocq, Couzineau, H.P., Beauvais, B. and Lariviere, M. (1971). *C. R. Soc. Biol. 165*, 273.

Bisseru, B. and Woodruff, A.W. (1968). *J. Clin. Path. 21*, 449.

Bradford, D.E. (1970). *J. Roy. Army. Med. Cps. 116*, 89.

Buchwalder, R. (1973). *Monat. Vet. Med. 28*, 98.

Engel, H., Spiekermann, D.A., Tismer, R. and Möbius, W. (1971). *Dtsch. Med. Wschr. 96*, 1498.

Francis, M.X. and Fellers, M.C. (1953). *Amer. J. Dis. Child. 86*, 767.

Gräfner, G. and Danailov, J. (1964). *Mh. Vet. Med. 19*, 869.

Heiner, D.C. and Kevy, S.V. (1956). *New Eng. J. Med. 254*, 629.
Hogarth-Scott, R.S. (1966). *Immunology, 10*, 217.
Hogarth-Scott, R.S., Johannsson, S.G.O. and Bennich, H. (1969) *Clin. Expl. Immunol. 5*, 619.
Huntley, C. and Moreland, A. (1963). *Amer. J. Trop. Med. Hyg. 12*, 204.
Jung, R.C. and Pacheco, G. (1960). *Amer. J. Trop. Med. Hyg. 9*, 185.
Kagan, I.G., Normann, L. and Allain, D.S. (1957). *J. Immunol. 83*, 297.
Khalil, H.M., Khattab, A.K., El-Fattah, S.M.A., Khalid, M.L., Awaad, S. and Riffat, M.A. (1971). *Trans. Roy. Soc. Trop. Med. Hyg. 65*, 599.
Kozlovska, J. (1953). *Acta Parasit. Polon. 1*, 403.
Lamina, J. (1964). *Z. Parasitenk. 24*, 600.
Lamina, J. (1964). *Z. Parasitenk. 25*, 52-67.
Lamina, J. (1966). *Dtsch. Tierärztl. Wschr. 73*, 208.
Lamina, J. (1970). *Kleintier-Praxis, 15*, 105.
Lamina, J. (1970). *Z. Bakt.* (1. Orig) *215*, 259.
Lamina, J. (1970). *Z. Bakt.* (1. Orig) *215*, 386.
Laqua, H. (1972). *Klin. Mbl. Augenheilk. 161*, 215.
Lee, H.F. and Danaraj, T.J. (1972). *Amer. J. Trop. Med. Hyg. 21*, 174.
Lis, M. Schanzel, H. (1961). *Angew. Parasit. 2*, 23.
Mitchell, I.R. (1964). *Proc. Soc. Exp. Biol. Med. 117*, 267.
Moreau, A.F. Mary, R. and Junod, C. (1971). *Rev. Fran. Allergol. 11*, 271.
Müller-Jensen, A., Schall, J., Weisner, B. and Lamina, J. (1973). *Dtsch. Med. Wschr. 98*, 1175.
Oliver-González, J. (1940). *J. Infect. Dis. 67*, 292.
Perlmutter, A.D., Edlow, J.B. and Kevy, S.V. (1968). *J. Pediatr. 73*, 340.
Plass, H. (1965). *Diss. med. vet. Berlin,* Humbold University.
Reekie, A., Miller, C.G. (1969). *Trans. Roy. Soc. Trop. Med. Hyg. 63*, 547.
Reichenmüller, H.E. (1969). *Med. Klinik, 64*, 30.
Remky, H., Kraft, H. (1965). *Klin. Mschr. Augenheilk. 147*, 692.
Rifaat, M.A., Salem, S.A. and Khaled, M.C. (1968). *Proc. Int. Congr. trop. Med. Malar.* (8th) Teheran, Sept. 7-15, 1968.
Rifaat, M.A. (1970). *J. Parasitol. 56*, (Sect. II) (Part 1), 283.
Roth, I. (1941). *Acta path. microbiol. Scand. 18*, 160.
Schoop, G. and Lamina, J. (1966). *Dtsch. Med. Wschr. 91*, 848.
Sprent, J.F.A. (1958). *Parasitol. 48*, 184.

Stoimenov, K. (1959). (Cited by Plass, 1965).
Williams, R.W. and Menning, E.L. (1961). *J. Parasitol.* *47*, 947.
Wiseman, R.A. and Woodruff, A.W. (1968). *Br. med. J.* (March) *i*, 677-678.
Wiseman, R.A. and Woodruff, A.W. (1970). *Trans. Roy. Soc. Trop. Med. Hyg.* *64*, 239.
Wiseman, R.A. and Woodruff, A.W. (1971). *Trans. Roy. Soc. Trop. Med. Hyg.* *65*, 439.
Wood, R.M., Ellison, A.C., Kelley, K.C. and Kaufman, H.E. (1965). *Arch. Ophthal.* *73*. 482.
Woodruff, A.W. (1966). *Brit. Med. J.*, *i*, 1576.

THE TISSUE REACTION TO MIGRATING LARVAE OF *ASCARIS SUUM*

Erling Bindseil

Department of Pathology, the Royal Veterinary and Agricultural University, Copenhagen, Denmark

INTRODUCTION

Larvae of *Ascaris suum* - the large roundworm of pigs - are generally not considered to be of any significance for larva migrans in man. Considering the large percentage of pigs infected with *Ascaris suum* (often more than 50%), the ability of the larvae to migrate in alternate hosts, and the resistance of the eggs to the environment, one might expect infections in man, particularly in farmers and in other rural dwellers.

As far as is known, nothing has been published on the lesions in man caused by migrating larvae of *A. suum*. Lesions have been described for infections in pigs, rabbits, guinea pigs, and mice in which the main organs involved in the migratory phase are the liver and the lungs.

The present communication describes the characteristic features of larval infection of these organs.

MATERIALS AND METHODS

Pigs

Two litters from 2 different sows were used. One litter consisted of 10 pigs and was divided into 2 groups of 5 pigs each, an experimental group and non-infected group as controls. The second litter consisted of 8 pigs and was similarly divided into 2 groups of 4 pigs each. The experimental group of the first litter was infected with *A. suum* when 2 days old, and the experimental group of the second litter was infected when 30 days old.

Mice

Twenty male, white, mice aged 4 weeks were used in the experiments.

Infective Eggs of A. suum

The eggs were obtained as described previously (Bindseil, 1969a). An infective dose of 2,000 eggs was given per os to each pig and to each mouse by a stomach tube. Some mice were re-infected 1, 2 or 3 times, and some remained as uninfected controls.

Hatched second stage larvae were obtained earlier (Bindseil, 1970).

Post Mortem Examination

Eight days after infection the experimental animals and the controls were sacrificed. Livers and lungs were removed and their gross appearance was recorded. Samples of tissue were taken for histological examination following the procedures previously mentioned (Bindseil, 1969b).

RESULTS

Liver

Pigs

Animals infected 30 days old. The livers of the infected group displayed a varying number of "milk spots" (Fig. 1).

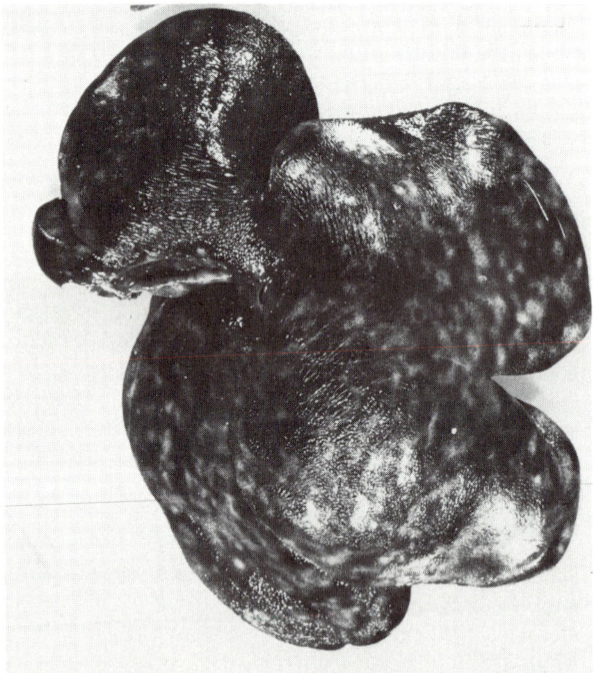

Fig. 1. Gross appearance of pig liver 8 days after infection with 2,000 eggs of A. suum *at 30 days of age.*

"Milk spots" consist of an interstitial hepatitis and have been described in the literature.

Histopathologically the livers showed oedematous septa with proliferation of connective tissue and heavy infiltration with eosinophils and with lymphocytes with pale nuclei (Fig. 2).

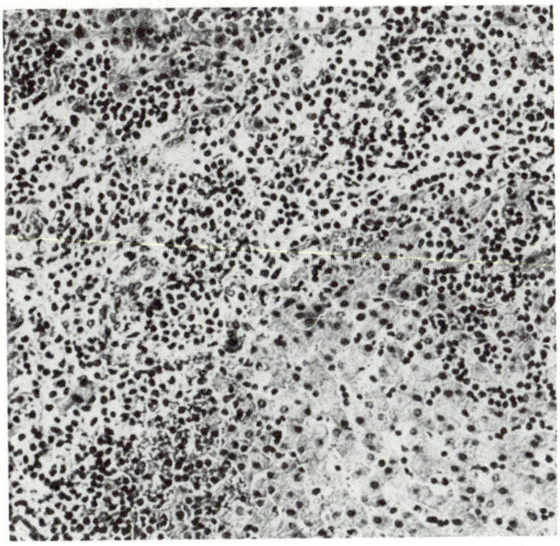

Fig. 2. Histological section of the liver shown in Fig. 1. Note the marked edema of the interstitial connective tissue and of a portal tract. The heavy cellular infiltration is not confined to these areas but is also detected in the parenchyma. Haematoxylin eosin. 125 x

Adjacent parts of the parenchyma were infiltrated with these cells. Some acini showed severe haemorrhage which disrupted the normal structure of the acini.

The non-infected control animals had no signs of "milk spots". A few minute grey foci were observed, consisting of accumulations with lymphocytes.

Animals infected at 2 days of age. None of the livers of the infected group displayed milk spots. Only few minute greyish lesions were seen reflecting small areas of cellular infiltration of lymphocytes and macrophages in the parenchyma.

Mice

In mice infected with eggs of *A. suum* there was no development of milk spots on the liver. Only faintly visible haemorrhages were detected on the surface of the liver but its colour was greyish mottled. Histologically these findings were reflected in large areas of parenchymatous necrosis and scattered haemorrhage (Fig. 3). Infiltration with macrophages, heterophils, and lymphocytes was not marked at the beginning, but increased later. Eosinophils were very few. The pathological picture did not change markedly following re-infection.

In mice subjected to intraperitoneal injection of hatched second stage larvae similar lesions were observed in the liver as described in mice infected orally with eggs.

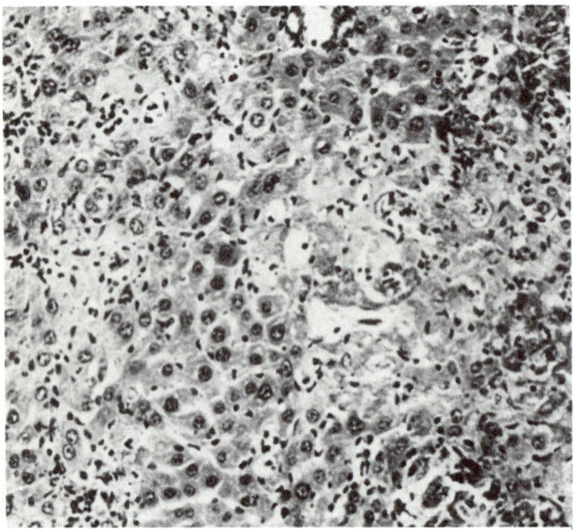

Fig. 3. Liver of 5 week old mouse infected 8 days earlier with 2,000 eggs of Ascaris suum. *Irregular areas of necrosis partially infiltrated with cells are seen. Haematoxylin eosin, 125X.*

Lung

The pathological lesions in the lungs of infected pigs and mice were identical. The lungs were not well collapsed due to emphysema. Petechiae, focal pneumonia and exudative bronchitis were present throughout the lungs. The cell picture was a mixture of many eosinophils, heterophils, lymphocytes, plasma cells and histiocytes.

DISCUSSION

The difference in the pathological pictures between 2 day old pigs and the 30 day old ones may be due to the lack of a distinct network of connective tissue in the livers of the younger pigs. However, in SPF-pigs, aged 8 weeks or more, typical "milk spot" lesions develop only after re-infection with *A. suum* (Ferguson *et al.*, 1968) and primary infections of SPF-pigs results in lesions similar to the lesions seen in conventional pigs infected at 2 days of age. Hence the status of the connective tissue in older pigs is not of primary importance for the development of milk spots. Immune reactions are more likely to be involved, and this is strongly suggested by the histological findings.

The pathogenesis of the liver damage in mice seems to be quite different. Here the picture is dominated by the large confluent areas of parenchymatous necrosis, a feature which is rarely seen in pigs. Furthermore, the cellular infiltrations in these areas is dominated by heterophils and not eosinophils, which are rarely seen. The fact that the picture does not change following re-infection is strongly indicative of a physical cause for the liver damage. The confluent areas of necrotic parenchyma in the liver of mice suggest an anaemic necrosis, and it may be provoked by thrombosis of the small blood vessels by larvae. However, intraperitoneally injected second stage larvae produce similar lesions of necrosis. Since such larvae are presumed to penetrate the liver capsule and then migrate at random in the hepatic tissue, thrombosis of blood vessels by them would seem unlikely.

This response in mice is not in accord with findings of Taffs (1965), who found an increasing degree of damage and cell infiltration in the liver of rabbits and guinea pigs following re-infection. Similar observations were made in guinea pigs by Kerr (1938) and in mice by Sprent and Chen (1949). Taffs (1965) also reported more widespread areas of parenchymatous degeneration in rabbits and guinea pigs than in pigs.

Thus the pathogenesis of the liver lesions in small laboratory animals caused by *A. suum* larvae still requires clarification. Much of the discrepancy in opinions may be due to (1) variation in infective doses, (2) the use of animals of different ages, and (3) variations in the interval between reinfection.

However, there seems little doubt that "milk spots" in pig livers caused by migrating larvae of *A. suum* are due to a hypersensitivity reaction. The most conclusive evidence for this is the work on SPF-animals. The lung damage caused by larvae of *A. suum* seems to be independent of the host species.

The primary lesions consisting of small haemorrhages are followed by focal pneumonia and exudative bronchitis. The cellular picture is similar for all species.

The reaction of the human to larvae of *A. suum* is unknown, but might be hypothesized from the reactions to infections in other hosts. It is likely that the hepatic response is different from that of the pig, since if lesions similar to the "white spot" response of pigs occurred in man, it is probable they would have been reported in the literature. It is hypothesized that migrating larvae of *A. suum* in the liver of man will give rise to minute white or greyish foci on the surface which will be reflected histologically as discrete necrosis with infiltrations of macrophages and lymphocytes and possibly granulocytes. Perhaps granulomatous lesions may occur, but the lesions will probably disappear in 1-2 weeks leaving small areas of fibrous tissue.

On the other hand it is justified to believe that the lung damage in man will be much like the damage mentioned above.

Emphysema, small haemorrhages in the tissue, bronchitis and probably minute granulomas are to be expected. The picture is presumed to be similar to "Eosinophilic lung" and other situations of larva migrans in the lungs.

SUMMARY

Lesions in man caused by migrating larvae of *Ascaris suum* are not known. The hypothesis is put forward that the human reaction to the larvae in the liver is not likely to be an immune reaction as seen in pigs after re-infection. Rather a more local and confined tissue reaction is expected as is seen in primary infections in SPF-pigs, in conventional baby pigs, and in small laboratory animals.

It is considered that the lung lesions will be desseminated and granulomatous in nature, with marked eosinophilia and emphysema.

REFERENCES

Bindseil, E. (1969a). *Acta Path. Microbiol. Scand*, *77*, 218.
Bindseil, E. (1969b). *Acta Path. Microbiol. Scand*, *77*, 223.
Bindseil, E. (1970). *Acta Path. Microbiol. Scand*, *77*, 183.
Ferguson, D.L., C.A. Mebus and Twiehaus, M.J. (1968). *Am. J. Vet. Res.*, *29*, 233.
Kerr, K.B. (1938). *Am. J. Hyg.*, *27*, 28.
Sprent, J.F.A. and H.H. Chen. (1949). *J. Inf. Dis.*, *84*, 111.
Taffs, L.F. (1965). *J. Helminth*, *39*, 297.

THE INTESTINAL PHASE OF *TRICHINELLA SPIRALIS* INFECTION

E.J. Ruitenberg, J.S. Teppema and P.A. Steerenberg

Rijks Instituut voor de Volksgezondheid, Bilthoven, Netherlands.

INTRODUCTION

In *Trichinella spiralis* infection both a humoral and a cell-mediated immunity is provoked (Catty, 1969). From studies in which the course of infection in the rat was examined, it was concluded that the humoral type is more marked (Ruitenberg and Duyzings, 1972). However, this does not necessarily imply that this type of immunity is more important for host protection.

It might be assumed that at least a part of the immunological response is functional, i.e. directed towards one or more stages of the parasite. Previous studies have shown that the immunity is not directed against the muscle phase, since the muscle larva is probably efficiently protected against the immunity by the capsule (Ruitenberg, in press). The intestinal phase is, however, subject to the influence of host immunity (Gore *et al.*, 1970).

In our rat strain (SPF, Wistar) the majority of the adult worms leave the intestinal tract at 12 days after infection (Ruitenberg, in press). The worms are forced to leave for immunological reasons, and not because of a limited viability. This conclusion is based on the fact that treatment with ATS (anti rat thymus cells serum) prolongs the intestinal phase, and this also results in a higher yield of muscle larvae. This indicates that the reproductive capacities of the worms remain intact.

Various aspects of the effect of host immunity on the intestinal phase of the infection will be described in this communication.

EFFECT OF IMMUNITY ON ENZYME HISTOCHEMICAL PROFILE OF ADULT WORMS

Following the studies with *Nippostrongylus brasiliensis* (Edwards *et al.*, 1971), we have examined whether the effects of immunity would be reflected by histochemical changes in the adult worms, during the course of the infection.

For histochemical studies cryostat sections (10 μ thick) of pieces of the small intestine from *T. spiralis* infected rats (non-treated and ATS-treated) were cut and stained with haematoxylin and eosin (H and E) and the periodic acid-Schiff (PAS) stain for the demonstration of neutral mucopolysaccharides and glycoproteins.

The following enzymatic reactions were studied: alkaline phosphatase (Burstone, 1958); acid phosphatase (Barka and Anderson, 1965); glucose-6-phosphatase (Wachstein and Meisel, 1957); adenosine triphosphatase (Wachstein and Meisel, 1957); succinate dehydrogenase (Nachlas *et al.*, 1957); nicotinamide adenine dinucleotide (NADH) oxidoreductase (Barka and Anderson, 1965); lactate dehydrogenase (Pearse, 1961); non-specific esterase, Naphtol AS-D acetate method (Gössner, 1958) and leucine aminopeptidase (Pearse, 1961). Various enzyme activities and the PAS reaction were compared semi-quantitatively at 1 and 6 days after infection, the results of which are summarized in Table 1.

Table 1

(Enzyme) histochemistry of T. spiralis *adult worms (1 and 6 days after infection).*

	reaction	
	1 day p.i.	6 days p.i.
PAS	+	+
AlPase	-	-
AcPase	++	++
G-6-Pase	-	-
ATPase	+	+
SDHase	+++	++
NADHox.red.ase	++	++
NSEase	+	+
LAPase	+	±

There was a complete absence of activity of alkaline phosphatase and glucose-6-phosphatase (G-6-Pase) but some ATP-ase and acid phosphatase activity was present. Oxidative enzymes such as succinate dehydrogenase (SDHase) and NADH oxidoreductase showed moderate activity. Non-specific esterase (NSE) and leucine-amino peptidase (LAPase) showed some activity, and this was mainly localized in the gut of the worms. When compared at 1 and 6 days post infection, the activities of most enzymes were not changed, with exception of the succinate dehydrogenase and the leucine aminopeptidase activities, in which some decrease were observed. A decrease in SDH-ase activity was observed only in the hypodermis and the musculature of the worm LAP-ase activity in the gut was diminished at 6 days post infection (Table 2).

Table 2.

Comparison of LAPase activity in T. spiralis *adult worms at 1 and 6 days after infection.*

	activity	
	1 day p.i.	6 days p.i.
cuticle	-	-
hypodermis and musculature	-	-
lines		
dorsal, ventral	-	-
lateral	-	-
alimentary canal		
oesophagus	-	-
gut	+	±
stichosome cells	-	-

This last observation is of some interest since *T. spiralis* adult worms lack other enzymes for the resorption of nutrients (e.g. alkaline and acid phosphatases). The decrease of leucine aminopeptidase activity may indicate that the adult worms are less equipped to survive in the intestinal tract of the host.

Studies were then undertaken to determine whether the observed decreases of enzyme activity were immunity-induced. Table 3 presents data on the effect of ATS treatment on three oxidative enzymes in *Trichinella spiralis* adult worms studied at 1, 6 and 9 days after infection. From these results it is evident that no changes in the enzymatic staining reaction were observed at the various post infection days, either in the non-treated, or in the ATS-treated animals.

Table 3

Effect of ATS on SDHase, NADHox.red.ase and LDHase activity in T. spiralis *adult worms (1, 6 and 9 days after infection).*

Enzyme	Treatment	
	none	ATS
SDHase	+++	+++
NADHox.red.ase	++	++
LDHase	++++	++++

In Table 4 studies of the effect of ATS treatment on LAP-ase activity in *T. spiralis* adult worms are presented. Both in the treated and non-treated animals a decrease in enzyme activity was observed at 6 and 9 days after infection. From these results it might be concluded that there is no conclusive evidence for immunity-induced alterations in the enzyme histochemical staining pattern of *T. spiralis* adult worms.

Table 4

Effect of ATS on LAPase activity in T. spiralis *adult worms (1, 6 and 9 days after infection).*

Days p.i.	Treatment	
	none	ATS
1	++	++
6	+	+
9	+	+

In explaining these negative results the following arguments should be borne in mind. The enzyme histochemical approach is probably not sufficiently sensitive to guarantee the observation of a possibly slight alteration in enzyme activity. Further, the enzyme histochemical approach is of a semi-quantitative nature. In order to obtain more precise information about a possible change in enzyme activity a more quantitative technique should be used, e.g. the quantification of isoenzyme patterns. In the present experiments we have only studied the adult worms which have penetrated in the intestinal tract. It is possible that in these worms the enzyme activity does not change very dramatically, since it might be assumed that these worms are the most vital ones. It is conceivable that by studying the worms present within the lumen some changes might have been observed, as have been described for *N. brasiliensis* (Edwards *et al.*, 1971).

EFFECT OF IMMUNITY OF THE ANTIGENIC PROPERTIES OF ADULT WORMS

An attempt was made to study whether the antigenic make-up of the worms would change during infection and whether such a change would be prevented by ATS treatment. For this purpose the bridge immuno-peroxidase anti-peroxidase (BIPAP) technique was applied on cryostat sections (10 μ thick) of pieces of the small intestine of *T. spiralis* infected rats (non-treated and ATS-treated). The principle of this technique is that antigens are visualised by means of the enzyme peroxidase (Fig. 1) (Mason *et al.*, 1969).

Graham and Karnovsky stain
↓ ↓
Peroxidase
↓ ↓
Anti-peroxidase rabbit serum
↑ ↑ ↑ ↑
Anti-rabbit 7 S γ-globulin goat serum
↓ ↓ ↓ ↓
Anti-*T. spiralis* rabbit serum
↓ ↓ ↓ ↓

T. spiralis antigen

Fig. 1. Bridge immuno peroxidase-anti-peroxidase (BIPAP) technique for the detection of T. spiralis *antigen.*

With the aid of this technique, it was possible to detect *T. spiralis* antigens by using a specific anti *T. spiralis* serum. Antigenic sites displayed a brown colour.

In experiments performed to detect antigens in worms at 1, 6 and 9 days post infection, in non-treated and ATS-treated animals, no specific brown precipitate was observed at the cuticle, which is known to be antigenic in nature (Ruitenberg *et al.*, 1968). The brownish colour observed in the internal structures of the worm was non-specific and possibly due to endogenous peroxidase. It is conceivable that the reason for these negative results is that immunoglobulins produced by the host were already present at the antigenic sites of the worms, and if so, visualization of antigens would be impossible. However, if it is assumed that antibodies are already present at the antigenic sites, it should be possible to detect these antigen/antibody complexes with a modification of the same technique (Fig. 2). Table 5 presents a summary of the results of studies in which antigen/antibody complexes were detected. It is evident that at all post infection days immunoglobulins could be detected around the cuticle of the adult worms, both in non-treated and ATS-treated animals. To explain these observations it could be postulated that *T. spiralis* produces two categories of antigens. First, T-cell dependent antigens are produced. These antigens are the functional antigens which provoke host protection (Ruitenberg, in press). Next, T-cell independent antigens are produced. These are not host-protective. The fact that T-cell independent antigens are produced was found recently in studying the course of a *T. spiralis* infection in thymectomized, irradiated and bone-marrow reconstituted mice. In this case, the host reacted with humoral immunity in the absence of T-cells (Ljungström and Ruitenberg, in preparation).

Graham and Karnovsky stain
↓ ↓
Peroxidase
↓ ↓
Anti-peroxidase rabbit serum
↑ ↑ ↑ ↑
Anti-rabbit 7 S γ-globulin goat serum
↓ ↓ ↓ ↓
Anti-rat 7 S γ-globulin rabbit serum
↓ ↓ ↓ ↓

Anti-*T. spiralis* rat immunoglobulin
T. spiralis antigen

Fig. 2. Bridge immuno peroxidase-anti-peroxidase (BIPAP) technique for the detection of T. spiralis *antigen-antibody complexes.*

Table 5

Detection of T. spiralis *antigen/antibody complexes in non-treated and ATS-treated* T. spiralis-*infected rats at 1, 6 and 9 days after infection.*

Days p.i.	Treatment none	Treatment ATS
1	+	+
6	+	+
9	+	+

In ATS-treated animals, in which the circulating pool of T-cells is eliminated, no host-protective immunity is observed. Under these conditions a prolongation of the intestinal phase and a higher yield of muscle larvae is seen. From our present studies we know that immunoglobulins are present on the cuticle of the adult worms even in ATS-treated animals. These immunoglobulins are probably the result of an immunological response of the host against T-cell independent (non host-protective) antigens. It is conceivable that the immunoglobulins provoked by T-cell independent antigens might act as blocking antibodies and interfere with the immune expulsion of adult worms. This would mean that in analogy with the situation in tumor immunology and transplantation immunology (Feldman, 1973) immunological enhancement might be present in the *T. spiralis* host relationship.

Of the two categories of antigens produced by *T. spiralis* adult worms, the T-cell dependent antigens would be the ones which would induce host protection, while the T-cell independent antigens could provoke parasite protection. If this were to be true an explanation might be available in the immunosuppressive effect of *Corynebacterium parvum* on the immune expulsion of adult worms, found previously by Ruitenberg and Steerenberg (1973). It has been shown that *C. parvum* exerts a marked adjuvant effect on T-cell independent antigens (Howard *et al.*, 1973). It is conceivable, therefore, that *C. parvum* exerts an adjuvant effect on the T-cell independent antigens of *T. spiralis* producing an increase of blocking antibodies, which could then interfere with the T-cell dependent host-protective immune response.

SUMMARY

The intestinal phase of *T. spiralis* is subject to host immunity. No evidence was found for immunity-induced changes in the enzyme histochemical staining pattern of the adult worms. This might be due to the lack of sensitivity of the technique used. Immunoglobulins were found around the cuticle of adult worms, even in ATS-treated animals. The hypothesis was put forward, that in a *Trichinella spiralis* infection in the rat, immunological enhancement may play a role.

REFERENCES

Barka, T. and Anderson, P.J. (1965). *Histochemistry. Theory, practice and bibliography*. Harper and Row, New York, Evanston and London.

Burstone, M.S. (1958). *J. Histochem. Cytochem. 6*, 322.

Catty, D. (1969). *The immunology of nematode infections. Trichinosis in guinea pigs as a model. Monogr. Allergy 5*, S. Karger, Basel.

Edwards, A.J., Burt, J.S. and Ogilvie, B.M. (1971). *Parasitology 62*, 339.

Feldman, J.D. (1973). *Adv. Immunol. 16*, 167.

Gore, R.W., Burger, H.J. and Sadun, E.H. (1970). *J. Parasit. 56*, 122.

Gössner, W. (1958). *Histochem. 1*, 48.

Howard, J.G., Christie, G.H. and Scott, M.T. (1973). *Cell. Immunol. 7*, 290.

Mason, T.E., Phifer, R.F., Spicer, S.S., Swallow, R.A. and Dresking, R.B. (1969). *J. Histochem. Cytochem. 17*, 563.
Nachlas, M.M., Tsou, K.C., Souza, E.de, Chang, S.S. and Seligman, A.M. (1957). *J. Histochem. Cytochem. 5*, 420.
Pearse, A.G.E. (1961). *Histochemistry, theoretical and applied (2nd ed.)*. J. and A. Churchill, London.
Ruitenberg, E.J. and Duyzings, M.J.M. (1972). An immuno-histological study of the immunological response of the rat to infection with *Trichinella spiralis*. *J. Comp. Path. 82*, 401.
Ruitenberg, E.J. (1972). *Proc. 3rd Int. Conf. Trichinellosis, Miami*, U.S.A., (In Press).
Ruitenberg, E.J., Kampelmacher, E.H. and Berkvens, J.M. (1968) *Neth. J. vet. Sci. 2*, 143.
Ruitenberg, E.J. and Steerenberg, P.A. (1973). *Nature. New Biology 242*, 149.
Wachstein, M. and Meisel, E. (1957). *Amer. J. clin. Path. 27*, 13.

EGG PRODUCTION AND HOST REACTION IN *CAPILLARIA HEPATICA* INFECTION OF *MASTOMYS NATALENSIS**

G. Lämmler, H. Zahner, R. Vollerthun and R. Rudolph

Institute of Parasitology and Parasitic Diseases of Animals and Institute of Veterinary Pathology, Justus Liebig University, Giessen, Federal Republic of Germany.

INTRODUCTION

The liver hairworm *Capillaria hepatica* (Order: Trichocephalida) is a world wide distributed parasite which has a broad spectrum of hosts. The worm is mainly described as a parasite of rodents (see Bruckmann, 1972).

The zoonotic implication of *Capillaria hepatica* is impossible to estimate clearly at the present time. Following the earliest report, a case of a 20-year old man in India (Dive *et al.*, 1924), the literature for the years 1950-1973 shows 12 further reports of human infections in which patent stages occurred (see Vollerthun, 1972; Silverman *et al.*, 1973). However, findings in the last few years could indicate that *C. hepatica* is more common in humans than it has been supposed. Šlais and Štěrba (1972) observed specific liver lesions in 10 persons during routine autopsies in a period of 10 years and attributed the findings to non-patent infections with *C. hepatica.* The report of Odunjo (1970), who described "dead *Trichuris* worms and ova in the liver" in autopsied children "with convulsion of sudden onset" as "prominent features" should be specially considered. There is the possibility that the similarity between eggs of *Trichuris spp.* and *Capillaria spp.* led to a false diagnosis of capillariasis as trichuriasis.

In this disease, the presence of a large number of unrecognized cases would not be unexpected. Because of the life cycle of the parasite, diagnosis, hitherto, has been based on biopsy of the liver or an post-mortem examination; and not by faecal examination. In this connection, Gupta and Randhawa (1960), for example, question the role *C. hepatica* may play in diseases classified as "Tropical Eosinophilia". Regardless of the relatively small number of described human infections, hitherto, increasing attention should be directed to *C. hepatica* because the majority of proven infections ended fataly. Illnesses were accompanied by somewhat indistinct

*Supported by the German Research Association

symptoms and it was impossible to come to firm conclusions regarding pathogenesis or the cause of death. Various extra-hepatic symptoms were seen, such as in the lungs and in the intestinal tract (Calle, 1961; Ward and Dent, 1959; Cislaghi and Radice, 1970). Some cases also associated with other parasitic and organic diseases (Otto *et al.*, 1954).

Experimental investigations on capillariasis have been few, possibly because capillariasis has been considered to be of minor importance. However, reviews of the literature given by Bruckmann (1972) and Vollerthun (1972), suggest that the importance of *C. hepatica* infection as a zoonosis has been underestimated. Therefore, it seemed opportune and necessary to obtain more details on the host-parasite relationships in hepatic capillariasis.

Investigations were undertaken to establish a new animal model for the infection and to clarify the reactions of the host to the infection. The "multimammate rat" *Mastomys natalensis* (Smith, 1834) which already has been found to be naturally infected by Cochrane *et al.*, (1957) was used as experimental animal for various other helminth infections (Lämmler *et al.*, 1968a, 1968b, 1970; Zahner *et al.*, 1970, 1972; Grüner *et al.*, 1973) as well as a useful animal in which to obtain various physiological data (Schuster *et al.*, 1972; Heitmann, 1971, 1972). In the present paper, results obtained in different studies, and which are in publication or have been published elsewhere (Bruckmann, 1972; Vollerthun, 1972; Vollerthun *et al.*, 1974; Zahner *et al.*, 1974), are discussed.

DEVELOPMENT OF CAPILLARIA HEPATICA *IN THE HOST*

Infection and early development

Following ingestion of embryonated infective eggs by the host, the first stage larvae hatch in the caecum (Luttermoser, 1938; Solomon and Soulsby, 1973). The larvae penetrate into the intestinal wall and migrate via the mesenteric and portal veins to the liver (Füllenborn, 1925; Nishigori, 1925; Wright, 1961; Lee, 1964). Erratic migrating larvae have been found in various other organs of the host, including the brain (Fülleborn, 1925; Nishigori, 1925; Luttermoser, 1938). Usually the larvae migrating to the liver exhibit pronounced organo-tropic behavior, which was demonstrated when larvae, isolated 6 to 12 days after infection, were implanted in various other organs of the host (Vogel, 1930). The development of *C. hepatica* in rats to the fourth stage larva is complete within about 12 days (Wright, 1961). The worms grow very rapidly during the second and third week of infection and growth continues beyond the prepatent period (Fülleborn, 1925;

Luttermoser, 1938; Wright, 1961).

The earliest time for the appearence of eggs in the liver of animals varies; in mice it was reported to be 18 days (Luttermoser, 1938) or 21 days (Pawlow, 1955; Wright, 1961) after infection, while in rats eggs appeared 21 to 33 days after infection (Fülleborn, 1925; Nishigori, 1925; Luttermoser, 1938; Shimatani, 1960; Lee, 1964).

The findings in the multimammate rat, *M. natalensis*, generally agree with the above results. Thus hatching of the first stage larvae, which was always observed to take place in the caecum, was found to be 8 hours and 12 to 15 hours after infection in fasting and fed animals, respectively. The first appearence of eggs in the liver of *M. natalensis* occurred at 20 days post infection. Consequently the development of the parasite in *M. natalensis* is similar to that described for other animal hosts. However, massive infection of *M. natalensis* with about 50,000 eggs of *C. hepatica* per animal produced retardation of development and delayed the appearence of eggs in the liver by about two days.

Egg production

The course and duration of egg production in *C. hepatica* infection of mammals have not been fully investigated. Waddel (1969) considered the quantitative evaluation of eggs in the liver of experimentally infected rats without significance, because of the great variation in the number of eggs in different animals and in various parts of the same liver. Luttermoser (1938) claimed that the egg counting method was not applicable in the rat because many of the lesions in the liver were not egg-bearing. From the literature it appears that there is also controversy about the time of death and degeneration of the parasite in the liver (Fülleborn, 1925; Luttermoser, 1938; Wright, 1961; Lee, 1964; Waddel, 1969). The death of female parasites in mice has been reported by Pawlow (1955) to take place 26 to 28 days after infection, while Wright (1961) claimed that this does not happen prior to 60 days after infection.

In *C. hepatica* infection of *M. natalensis* a different situation was found compared to the infection in the albino rat. It has been shown that the problem of sterile lesions in the liver is of little importance, since they could be found only infrequently and then only in the case of low level infections of about 50 infective eggs or lower per animal. Hence, by the use of *M. natalensis* a quantitative evaluation of *C. hepatica* infection could be made by measuring the total egg production by egg counts of the liver. On this basis also, an estimate on the worm population could be made. As it appears difficult to fix the time of death of adult worms in the liver, the end of egg production has been used as parameter for measuring the infection.

Results have demonstred a dose dependency between infection and egg production, but host-parasite relationships may markedly influence this.

After infection of *M. natalensis* with increasing doses of 100 to 800 eggs of *C. hepatica* per animal, an increasing number of eggs per liver could be isolated 28 days after infection. Further increase of the infective dose, to 1600 eggs per animal, did not increase the egg production compared with the group infected with 800 eggs per animal. By 75 days after infection, no difference could be found in the number of eggs per liver between any of the different groups infected with increasing doses of eggs of *C. hepatica*.

On the basis of the above findings, it was concluded that there are different dynamics for egg-laying, and this promoted further studies in which infected animals were examined at shorter intervals. The results, summarized in figure 1, demonstrate the trypical course of *C. hepatica* infection and egg deposition in 6 week old *M. natalensis* after oral administration of 300 infective eggs per animal. This shows that the number of eggs retained in the liver* increased rapidly until the 50th day after infection and then remained nearly constant beyond 60 days after infection. The number of eggs deposited in the liver per day showed three phases. The first phase was an increasing phase in which the number of eggs laid per day increased rapidly. The second phase was the additive phase in which the number of eggs deposited daily remained more or less constant and the third phase, the decreasing phase, was that in which the egg output decreased gradually, until it stopped completely at the end of reproduction, about 72 days after infection.

In *C. hepatica* infection of *M. natalensis* using 50 infective eggs per animal the increasing phase showed distinct prolongation, until about 60 days after infection. The additive phase extended to the end of the experiment i.e. 85 days post infection, and no distinct decrease of egg production was observed at that time. When high doses of infective eggs (800 eggs per animal) were administered the production of eggs was found to cease as early as about 30 days after infection and only the increasing and decreasing phases could

---

*For the determination of the number of eggs per liver, livers of infected animals were grinded and digested using HCl-pepsin solution (Matsusaki, 1955), followed by egg count with the McMaster flotation technique.

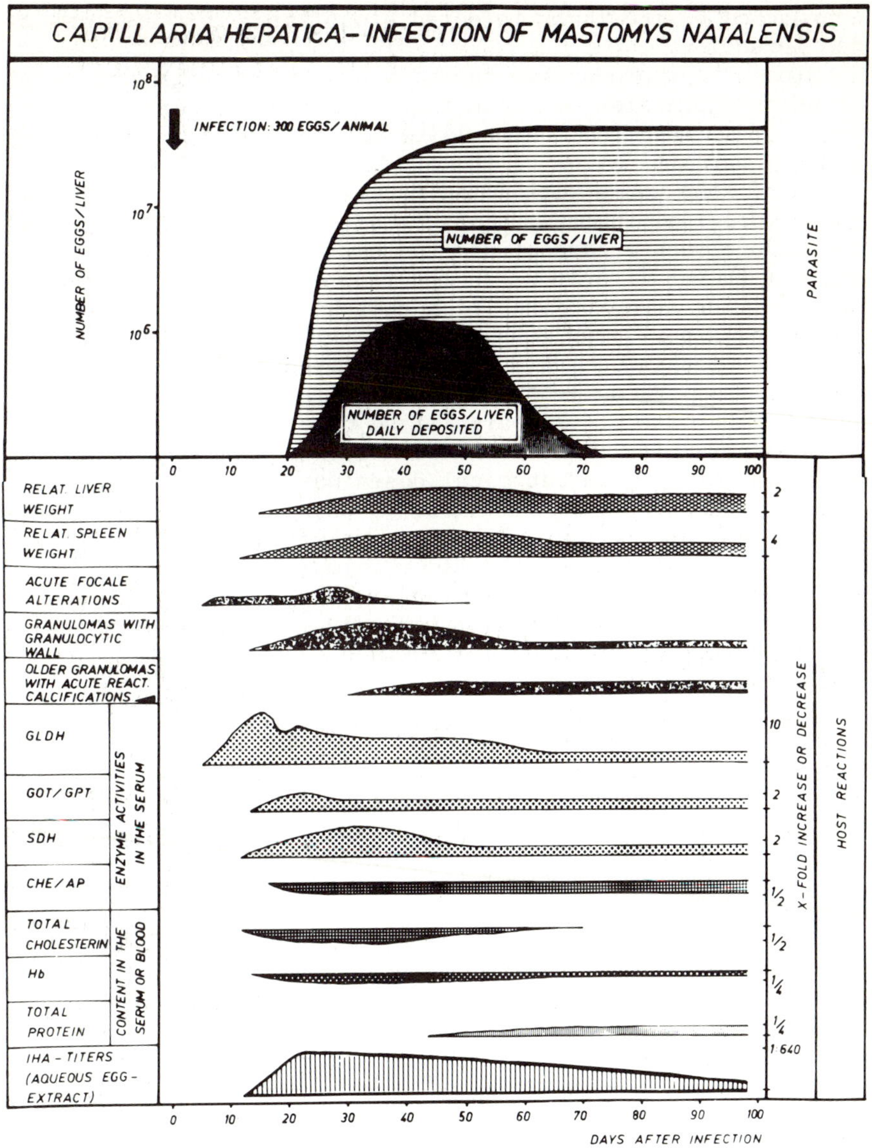

Fig. 1. Egg production and host reactions in Capillaria hepatica *infection of* Mastomys natalensis.

be observed, and the additive phase was not seen. The number of eggs per liver in the two more heavily infected groups reached the same high level after 48 days and this level was approached by the lower infected group later in the course of the infection.

Since the reproductive capacity of the worms is considered to be an expression of the bitality of the parasite, the survival of *C. hepatica* in the liver may be dependent on the degree of parasitisation of the organ. This would include early death of some worms within the prepatent period, as is seen in histological investigations. The present experimental data support such a concept and the marked differences of the reports in the literature on the time of death of *C. hepatica* in the liver are explainable on this basis.

The eggs per liver were approximately equal in the later stages of the infection regardless of the different infective doses given. This might suggest that egg production is limited by the size of the parasitized organ. It was demonstrated, for example, that the number of eggs isolated 75 days after infection with identical doses was significantly higher in four months old male *Mastomys* than in six week old animals. The latter animals at the time of infection had a liver weight half that of the older animals.

In *C. hepatica* infection of *M. natalensis* the egg production in young animals was not markedly influenced by the sex of the host. This factor did influence the later phase of infection in older animals.

HOST REACTIONS TO CAPILLARIA HEPATICA *INFECTION*

Pathological changes

The pathological changes in naturally and experimentally infected animals, including rats, mice and rabbits have been investigated by several authors. In these animals, a cirrhosis is described as the final stage of disease (Railliet, 1889; Bancroft, 1893; Kachi and Midorikawa, 1924; Fülleborn, 1925; Nishigori, 1925; Höppli, 1925; Morgan, 1932; Luttermoser, 1938; Foster and Johnson, 1939; Zajicec, 1958; Gupta and Randhawa, 1960). The mesenchymal reaction begins with a polymorphonuclear leucocytic perivascular infiltration of the tissue (Bancroft, 1893; Nishigori, 1925; Höppli, 1925; Lee, 1964). Conspicuously, there is an early onset of granuloma formation (Luttermoser, 1938) which in mice is of an immunological nature (Solomon and Soulsby, 1973). Mononuclear cells, giant cells and, predomonantly, eosinophils appear round the eggs (Höppli, 1925; Ward and Dent, 1959; Gupta and Randhawa, 1960; Smit, 1960; Calle, 1961). Parenchymal alterations are characterized by degeneration, pycnosis and karyorrhexis of liver cells and by loss of the typical structure of the liver (Bancroft, 1893; Kachi and Midorikawa, 1924; Höppli, 1925; Luttermoser, 1938; Smit, 1960; Lee, 1964).

In the opinion of most investigators resolution of the lesions does not take place but individual host variations may occur (Foster and Johnson, 1939).

In *M. natalensis*, lesions in the liver were evident macroscopically about 10 days after infection and they increased to a size to 3-6 mm by the beginning of patency. Confluence of necrotic areas occurred after various periods after infection, depending on the infecting dose of eggs. This occurred when a dose as low as 20 eggs per animal was administered. In the later phases of the infection separate foci in the liver were not descernable. These alterations were found throughout the whole liver.

With the increase of egg deposition, enlargement of the liver volume and weight occurred. These changes, expressed as the relative weight of the organ are depicted in figure 1. On one hand, this enlargement may be related to the number of eggs in the liver. Experiments with different infection doses showed that, in light infection, the liver increased in weight over a longer period of time than in the case of moderate infection. In the light infection, egg deposition continued for a longer time. Throughout the period of enlargement of the liver, the number of eggs per liver was significantly correlated with the relative weight of the liver. On the other hand, the increase in volume of the liver may be an expression of the several cellular reactions to the infection. The decrease of liver weight in the later phase of infection may be related to this.

In exceptional cases, the liver weight reached 20% of the body weight in the period between 40 and 60 days after infection. Comparison of these results with data for other hosts (Luttermoser, 1938) is not possible since there is no correlation between the body weight and the liver weight in such studies.

The relative weight of the spleen increased (Fig. 1) similarly to the liver and this increase was dependent upon the infection dose.

The histopathologic changes in the liver were characterized by initial focal necrosis, followed by granuloma formation. The acute focal changes, which diminished in the later phase of the infection may be associated with the migration of the worms. This migration is delineated by strings of eggs in the tissues in the early patency period.

As is shown in figure 1, the granulomatous changes were present as early as 10 days after infection. At first, they were a consequence of migration, intense reactions were observed at the beginning of patency and thereafter granuloma formation occurred around eggs deposited in the tissues.

It is considered that tube-like granuloma formation corresponded to the migration of the parasite and hence they showed differing stages of evolution of the granulomatous response, depending on the part of the migratory tract examined. Fig. 1 indicates that the major granulomatous response corresponded to the degree of egg deposition. The chronic granulomatous response occurs when oviposition ceases, in this phase encapsulation by connective tissue is evident, though reactive cells were still present. At a later stage, calafication occurred, with dead parasites in the center of the lesion.

The wall of the granulomas consisted mainly of polymorphonuclear cells, in which eosinophils prevailed. About 100 days post infection most of the lesions were non-reactive and were surrounded by a thin layer of connective tissue and localized without reaction within the intact liver tissue.

A conspicuous feature of the infection was the increased number of giant cells and plasma cells (the latter in Glissons capsule) at the beginning of the patent period. Later the number of these cells was decreased. In contrast to the cirrhosis described in rats, only liver fibrosis was seen in these studies. However, in some cases, mainly after infection of older female *Mastomys*, a cirrhotic response was seen.

Pathophysiological alterations

To detect hepatobilary implications of *C. hepatica* infection in *Mastomys natalensis* a spectrum of liver specific enzymes and metabolites was assayed. An increase of the indicator-enzymes in the serum indicates the loss of function and integrity of the liver cells. A decrease of activity of the so-called secretion-enzymes indicates a loss of synthesizing capacity. In contrast to the indicator-enzymes, which may show sudden changes, the concentration of some metabolites may remain constant for a considerable time despite obvious liver damages. The reason for this is that the regulatory capacity of the liver functions until the endogenous regulation breaks down.

For the examination of the influence of *C. hepatica* infection on the bilary system, the behaviour of the excreted enzymes has been evaluated. Alterations in some of the pathophysiological and haematological parameters are illustrated in Fig. 1.

An initial disorder of the liver cells was detected by "activated GLDH" in the 1st week after infection and by the other indicator-enzymes, GOT, GPT, LDH and SDH, in the 2nd and 3rd week after infection. The increase of enzyme activities, especially of GLDH, GOT, GPT as well as LDH, demonstrates marked pathophysiological changes which represent the acute phase of the *C. hepatica* infection. This was associated with the focal changes, but the mechanical effects due to the migrating juvenile parasites, and the cytotoxic effects of metabolites from growth and maturation of the parasites may also contribute to this (Fülleborn, 1925; Luttermoser, 1938; Wright, 1961).

The liver cells might be damaged by fluids produced during the process of moulting. Pathophysiologic changes occur at the end of the prepatent period and are expressed by a second peak of "activated GLDH" and by maximum values of the other enzymes. Such changes may be correlated with results obtained after infection with lethal doses of eggs. In these cases death occurred from the 20th day p.i. onwards. Similar findings were reported for the mouse by Luttermoser (1938). Therefore it is apparent that this phase of infection is associated with severe lesions of the liver parenchyma.

The maximum increase of the transaminases and dehydrogenases occurred in the 3rd week after infection and was followed by a lower but plateau-like elevation of enzyme activities. This remained until the end of the period of investigation.

Pathophysiological relationships between the decrease of ChE-activities and the increase of the indicator-enzymes were confirmed in the chronic phase of the infection. The marked decrease of the ChE-activity corresponded with a distinct increase of the SDH. Therefore, the determination of SDH-activity might be a sensitive indicator for the demonstration of parenchymal lesions of the liver in *M. natalensis*. The prolonged and constant elevation of enzyme activities points to continuing liver damage in the chronic phase.

In early patency, the liver changes can be explained on the basis of persisting migration of parasites with a high metabolic rate during egg-production. However, the enzyme changes are not directly correlated with the egg-production in the host.

In the chronic period of infection the interpretation of the results is more difficult, At this time egg-production is ceasing and acute focal changes in the liver are no longer observed. The alteration of the liver cells may be caused by disorders which cannot be seen by light microscope and could be caused by dying adult worms, though later the adult parasites become encapsulated and calcificated. The hypothesis that a direct irritation is produced by the eggs is questionable. There is no development of the eggs beyond the 6-8 cell-stage and the metabolism of the egg is unknown, but it is suggested that the high number of the eggs in the liver parenchyma and their metabolism may have pathophysiological consequences. The presence of dead eggs, as seen in histological pictures, might be an additional pathogenic factor. The immunological basis of the granuloma formation around *C. hepatica* eggs, as indicated by Solomon and Soulsby (1973), might suggest that immunological phenomen are associated with the pathophysiological phenomena.

The pronounced decrease of ChE-activity in the period beginning with the 4th week after infection corresponds with the reduction of the liver parenchyma, although in the later phase (60 days after infection with 300 eggs per animal), no further reduction of liver parenchyma can be observed by the light microscope. The decrease of the ChE is accompanied with similar decrease of the AP which might be due to an identical mechanism. According to Klein (1969), probably AP is not only excreted by the liver, but also may be produced by it. The persistent increase of "activated GLDH" suggests a persistent cytotoxic effect which could be the reason for the persistent liver damage.

A relation existed between the massive liver parenchyma lesions in the acute phase and the reduction of the capacity of esterification by the liver, i.e. the reduction of the concentration of the total-cholesterin. This along the values of the transaminases, GOT and GPT is an indication of the intensity of the pathophysiological action.

The increase of total proteins was mainly due to β-globulin fraction, whereas the values for the albumin and γ-globulin fractions remained nearly constant. The possibility of an increased turnover rate in these proteins as described by Mulligan (1971) in *Fasciola hepatica* infected rabbits, cannot be excluded, but a determination of the degradation of albumin would be necessary to evaluate this aspect.

Changes in the red blood cell picture are of interest. A slight anaemia was detected at the end of the prepatency and it persisted in moderate and severe infections. However, in lightly infected animals a normal RBC picture was seen (Vollerthun *et al.*, unpublished). The mechanism of such an anaemia requires further elucidation. Possible mechanisms for the anemia, include a toxic effect produced by the parasite and a reduced synthesizing capacity as the part of the liver.

Serologic response

In their investigations of granuloma formation in mice by *C. hepatica* eggs Solomon and Soulsby (1973) pointed out the implication of cellular immune mechanisms. Titers of humoral antibodies demonstrable by immunoprecipitation and haemagglutination (Walter *et al.*, unpublished; Soulsby, pers. comm.) respectively were found to be low in this laboratory animal. However, in comparison to these findings, in *M. natalensis* infected with *C. hepatica*, a substantial humoral antibody response was detectable.

Because isolation of larval or adult stages from the liver is difficult, a soluble antigen preparation from eggs was used for serological studies. Investigations using immunofluorescence techniques have shown that the eggs of *C. hepatica* are antigenic (Walter *et al.*, 1974) and an aqueous extract of non-embyonated eggs proved satisfactory for haemagglutination tests. This preparation was coupled to glutaraldehyd fixed and sulfosalicylic acid treated erythrocytes using difluordinitrobenzene as the coupling reagent (Ling, 1961).

Fig. 1 illustrates the antibody titers during infection. These was a peak response at the end of the prepatent period and thereafter there was a continous decline. The course corresponded to observations on precipitating antibodies which decreased in intensity in the latter phase of infection. An antigenic relationship existed between the larval stages and eggs, because, using the egg antigen, antibodies could be detected as early as 15 days after infection. Antibodies also occurred after infection with X-irradiated embryonated eggs, which did not develop to the fertile adult stages (Zahner *et al.*, unpublished).

Additional studies on the immune response in capillariasis are required. However, the present results indicate that antigens produced by the pre-adult and early adult stages of the parasite are important in the humoral immune response. The decline in antibody titers after patency may indicate decreased production or the binding of antibodies to parasite material in the liver.

The involvement of humoral antibodies in protective immunity requires further study, but initial studies by Zahner *et al.*, (unpublished) suggest that protective immunity to *C. hepatica* can be induced in *M. natalensis*. Comparison of such results with those obtained in rats and mice by Luttermoser (1938) is difficult because different criteria were used to evaluate infections, however, immunity appears to be more readily produced in *M. natalensis* than in mice.

The increase in β-globulins during the infection requires further study. This may be associated with changes in levels of specific immunoglobulins, of non-antibody components of the immune response or both. This aspect has been discussed by Lee (1964) who observed a relative increase in the β-globulin fraction of serum of rabbits infected with *C. hepatica*.

CONCLUSIONS

The results reported above represent an initial study of

the course of *C. hepatica* infection in *M. natalensis*. A relationship was demonstrated between the infection dose and the number of eggs deposited in the liver. On the basis of this relationship, it was possible to devise a practical system to quantitate the infection. Counting the number of superficial necroses, as carried out by Luttermoser (1938) in the rat, proved to be impractical in *Mastomys* because the foci in the liver became confluent in early stages of the infection. However, when the number of eggs deposited in the liver is used as a parameter of the infection, the special relationship between *C. hepatica* and its host organ must be noted. Aside from the complex cellular reactions which occur in the parasitized liver, it is probable that there is limitation on the living space available to the worm, which may be further restricted by the deposition of eggs. Such an effect would make it difficult to distinguish between immunity and crowding in superinfection experiments. Careful selection of initial and super infecting doses will be necessary to evaluate these factors.

The significance of the *C. hepatica* models extends beyond the general parasitological interest. Solomon and Soulsby (1973) have already indicated parallels with *Schistosoma* egg induced granuloma and the *C. hepatica* model may provide further knowledge of helminth granuloma in general. However, the present studies are relevant to several aspect of zoonotic infection produced by *C. hepatica*. It is clear, for example, that despite the broad spectrum of hosts for the parasite, differing host-parasite relationships occur, as is illustrated in different laboratory animals. Even strain differences can occur. For example, in C 47 black mice, the humoral antibody response is more marked than in NMRI-mice (Geyer *et al.*, unpublished).

It is anticipated that the biology of human infections with *C. hepatica* will vary according to the dose of eggs. Thus, it is not expected that patent infection will occur from a few eggs, since the large volume of the human liver may preclude the coincidence of male and female worms. Investigations relevant to this indicate that patent infections in *M. natalensis* occur only when at least 5 necrotic foci are found in the liver. In addition, we have failed to induce patent infections in pigs, even when up to 100,000 eggs were given per animal (Lämmler *et al.*, unpublished). Such results are in contrast to those of Tromba (1959).

The acute phase of the infection, which occurs before patency, is associated with a marked increase of "activated GLDH". This also occurs when infection is induced by X-irradiated embyonated eggs (Zahner *et al.*, unpublished) and hence the pathophysiological effects are also found in infections with sterile parasites.

The present investigations suggest that human infections, resulting from low doses of infective eggs, will have an extended longevity and probably greater than has been previously considered. The overcrowding effects evident in the liver of small laboratory rodents are unlikely to operate in the human liver, but the role of immunity in limiting the longevity of the parasite in man requires fuller evaluation.

These investigations also indicate that the injurious effects of *C. hepatica* infection are not limited to the phase of oviposition. The enzyme studies indicate a persisting liver damage in the chronic stage of the disease. It is possible that this is more serious than the damage which occurs in the other stages of the infection.

ACKNOWLEDGEMENT

The authors thank Dr. E. J. L. Soulsby, Chairman, Department of Pathobiology, University of Pennsylvania, Philadelphia for the supply of *Capillaria hepatica* eggs.

REFERENCES

Bancroft, T.L. (1893). *J. Proc. Roy. Soc. N. S. Wales 27,* 86.

Bruckmann, G. (1972). *Inaug.-Diss., Fachbereich Veterinärmedizin Giessen.*

Calle, S. (1961). *Pediatrics 27,* 648.

Cislaghi, F. and Radice, C. (1970). *Helvet. Paediat. Acta. 6,* 647.

Cochrane, J.C., Sagorin, L. and Wilcocks, M.G. (1957). *S. Afr. Med. J. 31,* 751.

Dive, G.H., Lafrenais, H.M. and MacArthur, W.P. (1924). *J. Roy. Arm. Med. Corps. 43,* 1.

Foster, A.C. and Johnson, C.M. (1939). *Trans. Roy. Soc. Trop. Med. Hyg. 32,* 639.

Fülleborn, F. (1925). *Arch. Schiffs. Tropenhyg. 28,* 48.

Grüner, D., Zahner, H. and Lämmler, G. (1973). *Z. Parasitenk. 42,* 221.

Gupta, I.M. and Randhawa, H.S. (1960). *Ind. J. Med. Res. 48,* 565.

Heitmann, H.H. (1971). *Blau. Hefte Tierarzt 46,* 260.

Heitmann, H.H. (1972). *Blut. 24,* 247.

Höppli, R. (1925). *Z. Infk. Hyg. Haustiere 27,* 199.

Kachi, G. and Midorikawa, B. (1924). *Trans. Jap. Path. Soc. 14,* 176.

Klein, U.E. (1961). *Dtsch. Med. Wschr. 94,* 526.

Lämmler, G., Saupe, E. and Herzog, H. (1968a). *Z. Parasitenk.* *30*, 281.
Lämmler, G., Zahner, H. and Texdorf, I. (1968b). *Z. Parasitenk.* *31*, 166.
Lämmler, G., Srivastava, V.K. and Zahner, H. (1970). *Br. Vet. J.* *26*, 467.
Lee, Ch.W. (1964). *Korean J. Parasit.* *2*, 63.
Ling, N.R. (1961). *Immunology* *4*, 49.
Luttermoser, G.W. (1938). *Am. J. Hyg.* *27*, 321.
Matsusaki, G. (1951). *Yokohama Med. Bull.* *2*, 154.
Morgan, D.O. (1930). *J. Helminth.* *10*, 65.
Mulligan, W. (1971). *In: Pathology of Parasitic Diseases.* (Ed. Gaafar, S.M.) Purdue University Studies, Lafayette, Indiana, USA.
Nishigori, M. (1925). *J. Med. Ass. Formosa* *247*, 3.
Odunjo, E.O. (1970). *Path. Microbiol.* *35*, 220.
Otto, G.F., Berthrong, M., Appleby, R.E., Rawlins, J.C. and Wilbur, O. (1954). *Bull. Johns Hopkin Hosp.* *94*, 319.
Pawlow, A.V. (1955) cited by: Skrjabin, K.I., Shikobalova, N.P. and Orlov, I.V. (1957). *In: Trichocephalidae and Capillariidae of animals and man and the diseases caused by them* Translated from Russian, Israel Program for Sci. Translation, Jerusalem (1970).
Railliet, A. (1889). *Bull. Soc. Zool.* *14*, 62.
Šlais, J. and Štěrba, J. (1972). *Folia Parasit.* *19*, 373.
Schuster, J., Lämmler, G. and Thyssen, J. (1972). *Z. Versuchstierk.* *14*, 83.
Shimatani, T. (1960). *J. Kyoto Pref. Med. Univ.* *69*, 1063.
Silvermann, N.H., Katz, J.S. and Levin, S.E. (1973). *S. Afr. Med. J.* *47*, (6) 219 (1973).
Smit, J.D. (1960). *Onderstepoort J. Vet. Res.* *28*, 473.
Solomon, G.B. and Soulsby, E.J.L. (1973). *Expt. Parasit.* *33*, 458.
Tromba, F.G. (1959). *J. Parasit.* *45*, 134.
Vogel, H. (1930). *Z. Parasitenk.* *2*, 502.
Vollerthun, R. (1972). *Inaug.-Diss., Fachbereich Veterinärmedizin Giessen.*
Vollerthun, R., Lämmler, G. and Schuster, J. (1974). *Z. Parasitenk.* (In Press).
Waddel, A.H. (1969). *Ann. Trop. Med. Parasit.* *63*, 63.
Ward, R.L. and Dent, J.H. (1959). *Bull. Tulane Univ. Med. Fac.* *19*, 27.
Wright, K.A. (1961). *Canad. J. Zool.* *39*, 167.
Zahner, H., Baudner, B. and Enders, B. (1972). *Z. Parasitenk.* *39*, 67.
Zahner, H., Herzog, H., Saupe, E. and Enders, B. (1970). *Z. Parasitenk.* *34*, 128.

Zahner, H., Lämmler, G., Bruckmann, G. and Schmidt, H. (1974). *Z. Parasitenk.* (In Press).
Zajicek, D. (1958). *Vet. medicina 31,* 211.

ALLERGIC REACTIONS IN ANIMALS CAUSED BY SOIL AND PARASITIC NEMATODES AND THE POSSIBILITY OF VACCINATION IN HELMINTH INFECTIONS

V.S. Ershov, V.K. Berezhko, A.D. Kashinsky, M.I. Naumytcheva and I.A. Nisenbaum

The All-Union K.I. Skryabin Institute of Helminthology, Moscow, USSR

INTRODUCTION

Helminthoses are diseases in which allergic reactions play a considerable role in pathogenesis. Allergic responses to helminths may persist for a long time, but in addition, their role in enhancing allergic reactions to unrelated antigens is also important.

Allergic reactions following sensitization by parasitic nematodes have been studied by several workers in various countries. It has been established that helminth antigens are complex in nature (15-25 components) and that each component may have differing immunological properties. Some produce a protective immune reaction while others produce allergic responses. Studies of the antigenic and immunogenic properties of free-living soil and plant-parasitic nematodes indicated that they were potent allergens and further studies of this aspect were necessary in connection with attempts to use these nematodes as vaccines in the prophylactical immunization of animals against helminths.

The use of free-living nematodes, such as *Rhabditis axei*, as vaccines against helminth infections such as ascariasis and dictyocaulosis have been reported by Demski (1966) and Frick (1968).

Similarly, an attempt has been made to use the free-living nematode *Caenorhabditis briggsae* as an immunogen against *Ascaris* (Guerro and Silverman, 1971). The use of free-living nematodes as immunogens is attractive since they are readily cultured and are not dangerous from the epidemiological point of view. However, little has been done to study the immunochemical and allergy inducing properties of free-living nematodes.

Consequently comparative studies on the immunogenic properties of pig ascarids, sheep lungworms and free-living nematode *Rhabditis axei* and the plant-parasitic nematode *Aphelenchus avenae*, were undertaken.

Anaphylactic shock after sensitization with Rhabditis axei *and* Aphelenchus avenae

Sensitization induced in helminth-free guinea pigs with the soil nematodes *Rhabditis axei* and the plant-parasite nematode *Aphelenchus avenae* was examined for its homologous and heterologous responses to antigens prepared from *Rh. axei, A. avenae Dictyocaulus filaria, Ascaris suum and Fasciola hepatica.* A group of animals also was sensitized to *D. filaria* and challenged with antigens from *Rh. axei* and *A. avenae.*

For sensitization of animals, 1000 living *Rh. axei* or 3000 living *A. avenae* were given orally or injected intraperitoneally. Three weeks later a challenge dose of 0.5 ml of an antigen extract of homologous or heterologous helminths was injected intracardially. Control non-sensitized animals were given a dose of 0.5 ml of the respective antigen extract intracardially.

Anaphylactic shock with a letal outcome was observed in guinea pigs sensitized with *Rh. axei* and challenged by a homologous antigen extract from *Rh. axei.* Anaphylactic shock was observed in animals sensitized by *Rh. axei* and challenged with heterologous antigens such as *D. filaria, A. suum, F. hepatica* and *A. avenae.* Anaphylactic shock was also demonstrated in animals sensitized to *D. filaria* and challenged with an antigen extract from *Rh. axei.*

In further studies anaphylaxis was marked in animals sensitized by *A. avenae* and challenged with *A. avenae* antigen or that from *Rh. axei.* The responses were less marked in animals challenged by a heterologous antigen from *A. suum.*

Thus the oral administration of free living soil nematodes (*Rh. axei*) and plant-parasitic nematodes (*A. avenae*) to guinea pigs produced anaphylactic sensitization to a challenge dose of antigen administered 3 weeks later. That indicates that *Rh. axei* and *A. avenae* have antigen components common to some of the parasitic helminths of man and animals.

Intradermal tests with extracts from Rh. axei *in ascariasis trichinellosis and cysticercosis*

Extracts of *Rh. axei* was tested intradermally in experimental trichinellosis and ascariasis in pigs and cysticercosis in calves. Extracts of living *Rh. axei* larvae or adults were used and a dose of 0.1 ml of each (60 mg and 100 mg protein respectively) was injected intradermally. Homologous antigens at a similar dose and protein content were also used.

In 6 calves infected with *Cysticercus bovis* antigen from *Rh. axei* produced a positive intradermal allergic reaction within 5 minutes after injection. In a group of *Trichinella*-infected pigs the *Rh. axei* antigen also produced a positive intradermal reaction in 5 minutes. In *Ascaris*-infected pigs the intradermal test with *Rh. axei* antigen was positive only in 50% of cases.

Since an allergen from *Rh. axei* produced positive reactions in animals infected with parasitic helminths, sensitization with free living nematodes must be considered as a factor in the immunodiagnosis of parasitic helminth infections. The results also indicate that common antigenic components exist between free-living nematodes and parasitic nematodes and cestodes.

Immunogenic properties of Rh. axei *in experimental dictyocaulosis and ascariasis*

The immunogenic properties of *Rh. axei* were evaluated in 59 guinea pigs and 17 lambs which after sensitization with *Rh. axei* were challenged with infective larvae of *D. filaria*.

The soil nematode, *Rh. axei*, was cultured on nutrient agar medium and was isolated by the Baermann method. 30,000 living *Rh. axei* were injected subcutaneously into one group of guinea pigs and this group was given 1000 infective larvae of *D. filaria* 2 weeks later. A second group of guinea pigs received 30,000 living *Rh. axei* twice at an interval of 2 weeks, and 1000 *D. filaria* larvae were given as an oral challenge 4 weeks later. A third group was injected twice, at an interval of 2 weeks, with an extract of 30,000 living *Rh. axei* prepared by ultrasonication, and challenged with 1000 infected larvae of *D. filaria* 4 weeks later. To a fourth group of guinea pigs two intraperitoneal injections, each of 50,000 living *Rh. axei* were given at an interval of 2 weeks after which 1000 infective larvae of *D. filaria* were given 3 weeks later. A fifth group were infected with *D. filaria* larvae only and a 6th group served as non-immunized, non-infected controls.

Animals were examined 2, 4, 7, 10, 14, 21 and 28 days after challenge and the mesenteric and mediastinal lymph nodes and the lung tissue was examined by the Baermann technique or the compressorium slide technique. Serum samples were examined by immunodiffusion.

In a similar trial with 5-7 months old lambs, sterilized living *Rh. axei* were injected intravenously twice at a dose rate of 300,000 or 600,000 per head (2 ml of solution) at an interval of 6 weeks, and 6-7 weeks later the lambs were challenged with 4000 infective *D. filaria* larvae. Appropriate controls were included. Lambs were slaughtered at 3 and 35-40 days after challenge and examined as above.

In a further study with 60 white mice, 20,000 *Rh. axei* were injected three times at weekly intervals to one group intraperitoneally and to a second group subcutaneously. 8 days later both groups of mice were challenged with an oral dose of *Ascaris* eggs. Larval burdens were counted 2, 4, 7 and 11 days after challenge.

Such preliminary studies showed that double immunization of animals with *Rh. axei* produced a marked resistance (up to 79.7%) to a challenge with parasitic helminths. Immunodiffusion tests with sera from guinea pigs bled 7, 12, 21 and 28 days after immunization and subsequently challenged demonstrated a common precipitation arc with antigens from *D. filaria* and *Rh. axei*. Sera from animals infected with *D. filaria* only produced two precipitation arcs with the *Rh. axei* antigen, one of which was identical to an arc produced by the *D. filaria* antigen.

DISCUSSION

It is concluded that the soil nematode *Rh. axei* and the plant-parasitic nematode *A. avenae* have antigen components common to helminths of man and animals (*Ascaris*, *Dictyocaulus*, *Trichinella*, *Cysticercus bovis* and others). Our studies have shown that *Rh. axei* and *A. avenae* can sensitize animals and produce allergic reactions in them.

These nematodes are widely distributed in nature and the number of such in the soil is enormous and reaches millions of specimens per sq.m. The soil and plant nematodes are eaten with grass and fodder and may induce sensitization in this manner. Young animals may experience their first allergic sensitization from soil and plant nematodes.

Biochemical studies over the last several years have shown that soil and plant-parasitic nematodes are closely related to nematodes parasites of man and animals in respect to amino acid and enzyme content. Such relationships may provide a basis for considering the free-living forms as immunizing agents for parasitic nematodes.

A number of vaccines have been proposed for the prophylaxis of helminth infections. Unfortunately the majority have been studied mainly from the point of view of their immunogenicity and little consideration has been to the adverse effects of vaccines, such as their influence on the quality of animal products, the fate of allergens in the body, the effect of antigen overloading, the influence of sensitization by helminths on vaccination against other infective agents and the pathology induced by helminth vaccines.

Barbaro (1972) points out the necessity to study the interrelationships between allergies and helminth infection, especially the correlation between such infections and the incidence of asthma. Since immunization of animals with vaccines will be accompanied by sensitization of the host, anaphylactic shock, autoallergy (immunopathology) and other allergic reactions might be expected in these sensitized animals after repeated exposure to helminths. For example, anaphylactic shock after the intradermal injection of pig ascarid allergen has been reported and the Cassoni test in human echinococcosis may be dangerous because of anaphylactic shock after injection of the allergen.

Sensitization by helminths may influence the immunologic response to other pathogens. For example, in children infected with helminths, prophylactic vaccination against infectious diseases may have reduced efficacy. For example, Levinas (1960) has noted that ascariasis interferes with immunization against diphtheria or paratyphoid, and Astafiev (1969) has reported that helminth antigens influence the appearance and the course of infectious diseases. In addition, Dobilas and Daniliavitchus (1973) have studied the influence of the nematode *Oesophagostomum dentatum* on immunization against paratyphoid. These authors found that piglets experimentally infected with *O. dentatum* and immunized with paratyphoid vaccine were less resistant than vaccinated helminth-free pigs. In such animals, antibody titres, total serum proteins and daily body weight gains were 4.9 times lower in helminth infected than in helminth free animals.

In 1964 Sadun pointed out that the untimely use of preliminary data with view of producing a vaccine for the control of schistosomosis without immunological knowledge of the disease may be harmful. Sadun (1964) noted that a partial protection from schistosomosis was produced in several hosts by immunizing them with inactivated cercariae, but recommended that additional studies were necessary before such methods were used for vaccination since the allergic responses in immunized animals may produce serious effects. For example, histological data in monkeys vaccinated by irradiated cercariae of schistosomes (Lin and Sadun, 1959) showed a correlation between parasitological and histological changes. Allergic reactions of the delayed type (granuloma, eosinophilia, inflammatory allergic reactions, etc.) appeared after the injection of the vaccine. Marked inflammatory reactions were noted in lung tissue, vasculitis occurred in the blood vessels of the colon and a striking reaction was noted in the liver of immunized animals.

Consequently, it is concluded that the allergies resulting from sensitization with helminth vaccines may have serious effects and may even be dangerous in certain instances. More extensive studies of the side effects of vaccination are necessary to ensure the safety of the vaccines.

REFERENCES

Astafiev, B.A. (1969). *Medits. parazit. bol. 38,* 589.
Barbaro, G.F. (1972). *In: Immunity to Animal Parasites* (E.J.L. Soulsby, Ed.) Academic Press, New York.
Berezhko, V.K. (1970). *Trudy VIGIS. 16,* 17.
Berezhko, V.K. (1973). *Bull. VIGIS. 10,* 16.
Demski, J. (1966). *Arch. Exp. Vet. Med. 20,* 599.
Dobilas, Yu. and Daniliavitchus, E. (1973). *Trudy Litovskogo NIVI,* 85.
Ershov, V.S. (1968). *Immunizatsiya selskokhozyaistvennykh zhivotnykh pri gelmintozakh,* VIGIS.
Ershov, V.S. and Naumytcheva, M.I. (1966). *Tematitch. sborn. gelmint. 12,* 175.
Frick, W. (1968). *Arch. Exp. Vet. Med. 22,* 219.
Guerrero, J. and Silvermann, P.H. (1972). *Z. Parasit. 39,* 339.
Levinas, Ya.A. (1966). Abstract of Dissertation.
Lin, S. and Sadun, E.H. (1959). *J. Parasit. 45,* 549.
Naumytcheva, M.I. (1967). *Medits. parazit. bol. 36,* 196.
Naumytcheva, M.I. and Kortchagova, A.P. (1973). *Problemy obshchei i prikladnoi gelmintologii,* VIGIS.

ARTHROPODS - OESTRIDAE, MYIASES AND ACARINES

W. N. Beesley

Department of Veterinary Parasitology, Liverpool School of Tropical Medicine, Liverpool, England

INTRODUCTION AND CLASSIFICATION OF MYIASES

Most of the species of arthropods which may affect man as zoonoses are insects and occur within the dipterous families Oestridae *s.l.*, Calliphoridae and Muscidae, or, in the acarines, mainly among the mites. Insects can cause several forms of myiasis, defined as the infestation of a living vertebrate animal with dipterous larvae, which, in at least some stage, feed on host tissues, body fluids, or ingested food (Zumpt, 1965). This broad definition incorporates myiases caused by larvae of *Hypoderma* and *Oestrus*, it includes the almost non-pathogenic *Gasterophilus*, but excludes such forms of parasitism as *Allolobophora* earthworms parasitized by *Pollenia rudis*.

The classification of myiases has been attempted by several workers, e.g. Patton (1921), James (1947) and Zumpt (1965). However, the forms of zoonotic myiasis may be examined from different standpoints such as taxonomy, degree of specificity of the insect for man, and the site of parasitisation of the tissues.

A taxonomic list of the Diptera responsible for myiasis would include at least 185 species from the Old World alone (Zumpt, 1965), ranging from the window flies (Anisopidae) and moth flies (Psychodidae) to the highly specialized oestrids. Among the more primitive species, one may find the rare example of a maggot, such as *Piophila casei* (Piophilidae), which can be ingested with food and passed live through the entire gut, having caused haemorrhagic damage to the intestinal mucosa. It is probable that several species of flies, which originally oviposited on carcasses, developed along the "saprophagous route" (Zumpt,1965), and evolved as facultative skin parasites (e.g. *Lucilia cuprina*) and then became obligatory wound parasites,(e.g. *Chrysomya bezziana*). Other species took the "sanguinivorous route", initially with a temporary and facultative (but predacious) life style (e.g. *Auchmeromyia luteola*), and gradually evolved it as a permanent habit, as in *Passeromyia longicornis* and *Cordylobia anthropophaga*. From these permanent forms of calliphorid myiasis must have come the burrowing and migrating larvae such as *Gasterophilus* spp., moving in the wall of the buccal cavity, to the more complex cycle routes followed by *Hypoderma* spp. The rather simple migration of *Oestrus ovis* larvae may have evolved originally from blood-sucking larvae that found their way to the nasal cavities, because the maggots of this species feed on both blood and mucopurulent host secretions. There is thus a tendency for the accidental myiasis-producing Diptera to include mainly the more primitive families, while those which cause specific or semi-specific human myiasis occur in the more highly evolved families.

When the myiasis-producing Diptera are considered in detail, it is convenient to divide the myiases biologically into obligatory and facultative parasitisms. Very few Diptera are *obligatory* parasites of mammals in the larval stage. Examples of such include most species in the 12 genera, *Wohlfahrtia, Callitroga, Chrysomya, Auchmeromyia, Cordylobia,* (including *Stasisia*), *Hypoderma, Gasterophilus, Oestrus, Rhinoestrus, Dermatobia, Cuterebra* and *Cephenemyia*. The *facultative* species have larvae which normally are free-living and develop in decaying organic matter, such as carcasses, sewage and decomposing plant material. Such forms may be subdivided further into the "semi-specific myiasis" group (mainly Sarcophaginae and Calliphorinae) and the heterogeneous "accidental myiasis" group. The non-specific producers of myiasis ideally should be widely-distributed flies which live in close association with man, and possessing larvae which have very plastic feeding habits and requirements able to adapt to the rather unusual conditions of a parasite way of life (James, 1964).

Therefore, in man, the following forms may be encountered; (a) larvae which seem specific to him, (b) larvae which normally parasitize animals, and (c) larvae which are there quite by accident. The final classification would include these features as well as the site and the form of myiasis:- thus skin blood-feeders, skin tissue-feeders, larvae which occur in the head cavities, those which invade the urinogenital tract, and those which occasionally, and at random, occur in the alimentary canal, usually in the lower end.

FORMS OF HUMAN MYIASIS

HAEMATOPHAGOUS LARVAE

Haematophagy among dipterous larvae is exceptional and seems possible only at the expense of rather sedentary hosts which have a slightly hairy skin.

The only blood-sucking larvae which attack man are those of the Congo Floor-maggot, *Auchmeromyia luteola*, which at night sucks the blood of people asleep on the earth floors of huts. It is commonly and erroneously stated that *A. luteola* is specific to man, but its usual hosts are wild animals, probably wild pigs and ant bears, although Zumpt (1965) believes that the original true animal host has still to be identified. *A. luteola* is thus zoonotic, rather than a completely specific human parasite. The other species, *A. bequaerti, A. reidi, A. choerophaga* and *A. boueti,* all live in the burrows of warthogs, although they can take human blood. This latter form of association is similar to that seen with the calliphorid *Choeromyia*, larvae of which attack warthogs. The blood-sucking larvae of *Protocalliphora* (Calliphoridae), *Passeromyia* (Muscidae) and *Neottiophilum* (Dryomyzidae) all attack young birds in their nests, which could be regarded as a 'domesticated' parasitic association. Large numbers of larvae of *N. praeustum* in one nest can kill the fledglings, and the female flies dispose their eggs accordingly so as not to overwhelm their hosts. It is perhaps surprising that none of these species has been found to transmit disease, although *A. luteola* was suspected formerly of being a vector of human trypanosomiasis.

CUTANEOUS MYIASES

This large group includes mainly saprophytic species which on the whole rarely attack animals (e.g. *Sarcophaga* and *Lucilia*) although some are obligatory parasites. Man may become infested because of his close contact with domestic live stock. Development of the larvae to the third stage may occur in man with insects with non-migratory life-cycles, but in those species with migratory larvae, (e.g. *Hypoderma bovis*), the larvae rarely develop beyond first stage in man.

Non-migratory life-cycles

The commonest sarcophaginid species which attack human skin include *Sarcophaga lambens, S. carnaria, S. ruficornis* and *Wohlfahrtia magnifica*. In addition to the skin, the larvipositing females also attack the ears and eyes. Indeed Wohlfahrt originally described *W. magnifica* from the eye of a patient in Halle, Germany, in 1770 (cited by Zumpt, 1965). In the warmer parts of the Palaearctic Region, humans are frequently attacked by *W. magnifica* while the species *W. vigil* and *W. opaca* can cause a furuncular myiasis in the New World (James, 1947; Stabler *et al.*, 1962). It seems likely that *W. magnifica* is an obligatory myiasis fly, while the other species of *Sarcophaga* and *W. nuba* - which is a minor myiasis species of Africa and India, are facultative parasites.

The New World Screw-worm, *Callitroga hominivorax = (Coch-*

liomyia americana) is an obligatory and primary myiasis-producing arthropod while *C. macellaria (= Chrysomya macellaria)* is a secondary myiasis fly. In man *C. hominivorax* lays its eggs mainly in existing wounds on the body and head, but in animals it can produce very severe lesions rapidly in previously unbroken skin. Human infestations are usually furunculous, but there are several reports of myiasis of the navel, eyes, ears, turbinal mucous membranes, frontal sinuses and mouth.

Chrysomya bezziana, the Old World Screw-worm, is a green blowfly which lays its eggs in the wounds and body orifices of man and his domestic stock; this contrasts with the carrion-feeding behaviour of the other species of *Chrysomya*. Of animal hosts, the larvae develop most readily in agricultural live stock, which tend to have lost the grooming habits still found in their wilder relations. The most severe lesions are found on sheep, goats, cattle and buffalo. Human infestations are much less common in Africa than in India, for example, probably reflecting the differences in the environmental conditions and the way of life in certain parts of these continents.

Perhaps the most notorious species causing dermal myiasis in man is the calliphorid *Cordylobia anthropophaga*, the African Tumbu Fly. This obligatory parasite occupies a similar niche to *Auchmeromyia luteola*, in that it is often assumed to be a parasite specific to man, whereas it is probably a parasite mainly of burrowing animals (Zumpt, 1965). Dogs, rabbits and many other species of warm-blooded animals can be infested, and human myiasis is quite common in central and southern Africa. The eggs are laid on dry sand which has been contaminated with urine or faeces, or on contaminated clothing such as babies' napkins even when these have been washed. The larvae penetrate the intact skin in 25 seconds to 30 minutes, eventually produce severe boils from which the mature maggots emerge about one week after penetration. A child recently developed an infestation in Bristol, England, following a visit to Nigeria (Chaddah and Warin, 1966).

A second species of *Cordylobia* which may cause human myiasis is *C. rodhaini*, sometimes referred to as *Stasisia rodhaini*; the larvae, which are 23 mm. in length, are larger than those of *C. anthropophaga*, and cause more painful lesions (Lavoipierre and Beesley, 1957). The most important wild reservoirs are thought to be the African Giant Rat (*Cricetomys gambianus*) and certain antelopes (Zumpt, 1965).

Dermatobia hominis is an oestrid forest fly, which, despite its specific name, is common on cattle in South America. Deep running lesions are produced along the sides and back of animals, these may be confluent, so that large sores containing many larvae appear. A most unusual feature is that the *Dermatobia* eggs are carried (phoresy) by mosquitoes, (e.g. *Psorophora, Janthinsoma*), by stableflies or by ticks. Eggs are then left behind on the skin of the vertebrate host. Though many oestrid flies have a migratory larval stage, *D. hominis* infestation resembles more the blowfly "strike" type of lesion seen in sheep or cattle. The purulent lesions may encourage oviposition by screw-worms, so that a very heavy final infestation with dipterous larvae is possible. In man, boils follow infection of the body and scalp, and Dao (1963) listed 156 cases seen in Venezuela; more recently Flew and Grundy (1967) discussed infestation by this species of five soldiers in Guyana. There is one record of an infection of the brain (Dunn, 1934), but this may have been a misidentification for *Callitroga hominivorax*.

Another oestrid fly which rarely causes human skin myiasis is *Cuterebra*. This normally affects small rodents, but occasionally the fly lays its eggs on the skin of man. The larvae bore into the skin and produce small boils (Rice and Douglas, 1972). With this species there is only minor larval migration. Skin myiasis of man is also rarely caused by larvae of *Lucilia*, the green-bottle fly.

There have been few studies of human skin reaction to calliphorid or oestrid larvae (Zumpt, 1965). Some individuals may experience a pricking sensation as larvae bore in, others may feel nothing.

Larvae of the sarcophagid fly *Wohlfahrtia nuba* have been used deliberately for the treatment of slow-healing wounds, e.g. osteomyelitis, by Grantham-Hill (1933), in the same way that Baer (1931) first employed *Lucilia sericata* larvae for this purpose. It could be considered that such maggots were feeding on a carcass within the living body of the animal.

The severity of natural infestations with blowfly and fleshfly larvae probably is considerably modified by the secretion of inorganic and organic bacteriostatic substances. Such have been demonstrated for *Lucilia sericata* (Baer, 1931), *Gasterophilus* (Landi, 1960) and *Hypoderma* (Beesley, 1968).

MIGRATORY LIFE-CYCLES

Migrations either short and simple, or long and two-stage, are a necessary part of the development of several species of the Oestridae *s.l.*, including the Oestrinae, Hypodermatinae and Gasterophilinae.

Many of the human infestations so far considered occur because of chance exposure to flies primarily attracted to decaying refuse and offal. Few of them are obligatory myiasis species. Oestrids on the other hand are all obligatory parasites, and the four of most importance medically are *Oestrus*, *Gasterophilus*, *Hypoderma* and *Dermatobia*, the last of which can be considered to have a non-migratory dermal myiasis larva. *Oestrus* has a very short migration, in natural hosts hardly more than up the nostril and down again. This genus will be discussed in more detail in the section on myiases of the head cavities. Both *Gasterophilus* and *Hypoderma* can cause myiases of the eye, but since they also cause true skin myiases, they are discussed at this point.

Gasterophilus normally parasitises equines; it usually oviposits on the hairs of the host, but *G. pecorum* lays its eggs on pasture plants which are eaten together with the embryonated eggs. The eggs laid on hairs may (*G. haemorrhoidalis*, *intestinalis*) or may not (*G. nasalis*) need the stimulation of licking before they will hatch. The first instar larvae burrow into the gum, cheek or tongue, and migrate to the stomach or duodenum. Second instar larvae of *G. haemorrhoidalis* detach from the mucosa of the stomach or small intestine and pass through the gut. They re-attach to the rectum and here develop to the final instar. The only external signs of infestation in horses, apart from the presence of eggs on the hairs, may be occasional "summer dermatitis" (Dinulescu, 1929), usually due to *G. intestinalis*. In addition, this latter species can also occasionally infect non-equines. It was recently reported from New York State that 11 of 17 cattle pastured with or near horses had *G. intestinalis* eggs laid on them (Mock, 1969); one steer had more eggs than were laid on a pony in the same pasture. However, it is not known whether *Gasterophilus* will oviposit on cattle if these alone are presented to the fly. These recent findings have a bearing on the likelihood of the flies laying their eggs on humans.

Newly hatched larvae quickly penetrate human skin, as has been shown for *G. nigricornis*, *G. pecorum* and *G. haemorrhoidalis* in self infections by Chereshnev (1954). There are several instances of natural human infections. For example in New Zealand a 32-year old farrier complained of chronic irritation and lesions in his right axilla and upper forearm. Early first stage 1 mm. larvae of *G. intestinalis* were recovered from the pustules (Heath *et al.*, 1968) and it was considered that infection was associated with the close contact between man and horses while shoeing.

Many of the recorded cases of human myiasis by oestrids have been due to *Hypoderma*, normally a parasite of cattle (*H. bovis*, *H. lineatum*) or deer (*H. diana*, *H. capreola*, *H. actaeon*, *H. moschiferi*). *Hypoderma* from cattle can also affect other animals, and larvae have been recovered even from the surface of the brain of horses. Human infestations are often correlated with some form of agricultural work, and these can be manifest variously as, larva migrans, furunculosis, abscesses and pain and oedema (O'Rourke, 1968). Doby and Beaucornu (1965) found that in Brittany there are about two cases annually, the condition being particularly common in the Département of Morbihan.

The migrations of larvae of the ox warble flies (cattle grubs) are still not fully understood. It is known that the larvae of *Hypoderma lineatum* burrow into the skin from eggs laid on the hairs of the cow, and some weeks later they are found in the wall of the oesophagus. Larvae remain at this site for 5-6 months (Beesley, 1966) and they reach a length of 15-17 mm. By some unknown mechanism they are stimulated to resume their migration, and soon they appear under the skin of the back, which they penetrate, hence doing this for a second time while they are first instar larvae. Larvae of *H. bovis* behave in a similar manner, but they migrate to the epidural fat which surrounds the spinal cord (Haberman *et al.*, 1949; Beesley, 1962). Here they may cause severe lesions, especially if the larvae are killed by systemic organophosphorus insecticides.

MYIASES OF THE HEAD CAVITIES

Medically, the most important myiasis fly consistently affecting the head cavities is *Oestrus ovis*, the sheep nasal bot. Ill effects in sheep from parasitism by the larvae are variable, often amounting to no more than irritation caused by the third stage larvae as these crawl down the nasal passages. There may be a mucopurulent discharge and a few immature larvae may be sneezed out, but most hold on with their mouth hooks and cuticular spines to the folds of skin around the turbinates. There appears to be no protective immunity against *Oestrus* nasal maggots in sheep, goats, or antelopes, and older animals are usually more heavily infested than the younger.

Of considerable practical importance, however, are the effects of infestation with *O. ovis* on abnormal hosts, especially men and dogs. There is a tendency for the adult females to flick or drop their larvae into the eye, ear or mouth. Shepherds in Italy and North Africa seem prone to this infection as they become heavily contaminated by the odour of their sheep or goats, and often eat goat cheese (Zumpt, 1965). Ocular myiasis, or ophthalmomyiasis may be diagnosed clinically as an acute catarrhal conjunctivitis; as with the other oestrids, the larvae do not develop beyond the first instar, and the condition usually clears up within a few days although 50 larvae have been removed from the conjunctival sac of a single patient. The course of the eye infection is nearly always benign, and the eyeball itself is never invaded, but the larvae may also invade the nasal cavities, causing considerable pain and swelling.

In the same way that man suffers from the effects of *O. ovis*, so another nasal fly, *Gedoelstia*, normally a symptomless parasite of antelopes in Southern Africa, can cause serious trouble in domestic stock. The epidemiology of a severe ophthalmomyiasis known as "uitpeuloogsiekte", or Bulging Eye disease, was unknown until Basson (1962) showed that both *G. hässleri* and *G. cristata* (and probably also a hybrid of the two species) were responsible. The disease takes the form of a severe ophthalmic lesion, leading to an encephalitis five days later. Explosive outbreaks of the condition appear to be associated with migration of hartebeest, and up to 75% of groups of sheep, goats, cattle or horses can be severely affected, with as much as 75% mortality (Wetzel, 1969). Fortunately, there are few records of human infestations with *Gedoelstia* (Zumpt, 1963).

More unusual forms of human nasal myiasis have been reported following infestation with larvae of the rodent bot fly, *Cuterebra* (possibly *emasculator* or *grisae*: Beachley and Bishopp, 1942) and by the psychodid *Telmatoscopus albipunctatus* (Neville *et al.* 1969). The latter are also known as moth flies, and breed in drains, sinks, water closets, rain barrels and wet mud.

Human myiasis of the eye region may be caused by first instar larvae of *Hypoderma*, and these parasites have also been extracted from the gums. Glaser (1912) recovered a larva from the back of his throat after allowing a first instar larvae to penetrate the skin of his leg. It is probably valid to suggest that *Hypoderma* represents the current final evolutionary stage in the development of migratory dipterous larvae within the body of the host, and just as ascarid larvae migrate to ectopic sites if they gain access to unusual hosts, so *Hypoderma* larvae move, possibly in response to gravity, toward such parts of the human body as the scalp, eyes and shoulders. It is, of course, possible that some of these larvae had the advantage of starting life as eggs on the hairs of the eye-brows or eyelids (Zumpt, 1963).

INTESTINAL AND URINOGENITAL MYIASES

In intestinal myiasis, the eggs or larvae are ingested with the food, or larvae may even enter the anus. Myiasis of this type is often recorded in error, the original eggs having been laid on passed faeces - an easy mistake in the tropics with the great abundance of blowflies and flesh flies. Genera which have been incriminated in intestinal myiasis include *Musca, Muscina, Fannia, Calliphora, Sarcophaga, Stomoxys, Lucilia, Teichomyza, Tipula* and *Anisopus*.

First stage larvae of the *Eristalis tenax* are common along the edges of pools, and so can be taken into the mouth. When eventually passed with the faeces some days later these larvae may be alive (Canese, 1970) and their long respiratory siphons may suggest to the non-entomologist a nematode infestation. In rather the same way, eristalid larvae may be found in standing human excreta; when the corresponding event occurs in farm manure heaps the brown larvae and pupa cases can easily give the impression of masses of spikey worms.

Leclerq (1969) cites an extraoridinary case in which larvae of *Fannia scalaris* and *Teichomyza fusca* (a latrine fly) apparently produced a chronic diarrhoeal infection over a period of several years. After very careful investigation it was suggested that this might have been an example of "paedogenesis", in which the larvae were able to produce mature eggs without development of the pupal and adult stages.

There are also genuine instances of the passage in the faeces of larvae of leaf-miners (the leaf-miner *Pegomyia hyoscanii*; Laarman and van Thiel, 1967) and of termites (Reynolds, 1963). Certain Phorid dung flies (*Megaselia rufipes, M. scalaris*) have occasionally been incriminated in intestinal myiasis and may be commoner than generally realized.

Urinogenital myiasis is usually caused by calliphorine or muscid larvae invading a genital or urinary opening which is already the site of a lesion and perhaps discharging pus or serous material. The larvae may then ascend the tract and may survive for considerable periods, but rarely attain larval maturity. Recent cases have also involved larvae of *Anisopus* and *Scenopinus*, the latter producing symptoms which closely resembled those of cystitis (Thompson *et al.*, 1970).

INFESTATIONS BY NON-DIPTEROUS INSECTS

FLEAS

Fleas are unlike most ectoparasites in that they pass their entire pre-adult life off the host, their larvae feed on organic dust and the semi-digested blood excreted by the adult fleas. The larvae, pupae and adults need virtually no contact with the host for long periods, and it is useful to their survival that the adults can often cross-infect other hosts, as the cat flea (*Ctenocephalides felis*) and dog flea

(C. canis) can attack dogs and cats, respectively, while the hen flea *(Ceratophyllus gallinae)* attacks various birds, as well as man. Narrow specificity has been attained by several species of fleas, but the practical ecological conditions within the nest of the host mammal or bird are often at least as important as the species of the host. Thus, several species of bird fleas can each cross-infest the nests of various species of birds as long as these have a suitable humidity, regardless of the final host which will be used as a source of blood meals. Again, *Pulex irritans*, the human flea, is often abundant in pig sties and is probably a true parasite of the badger or related animal.

Primates and carnivores, which generally do not make permanent lairs or burrows, have less chance of coming into contact with fleas than do rodents and birds, and their populations of fleas tend to be small and to consist of few species. A possibly compensating mechanism allows these fleas of the larger mammals to lay more eggs than are produced by the rodent fleas.

LICE

All developmental stages of lice are spent on the host, and transfer between animals is by direct contact, in the flock or herd, or during suckling. Lice tend to be host-specific or to occur on a few closely related species of hosts and chewing lice tend to be more host-specific than sucking lice. There is no particular problem of survival arising from louse host-specificity, as plenty of hosts are usually available.

Man appears to genuinely have his own species of lice, in the genera *Pediculus* and *Phthirus*, and these genera also occur on the higher apes, but not on monkeys.

MOTHS

Larvae of several species of Lepidoptera cause urticarial lesions on man and animals (erucism), and the adults of at least two genera of moths can sting: the saturniid *Hylesia* and the zygaenid *Zygaena*. Recently, adult noctuid, pyralid and geometrid moths, which normally feed on fruit juices, have been incriminated in persistent attacks on the eyes of people and stock (Guilbride, *et al.*, 1959; Büttiker, 1969). The probosces of the moths are equipped with strong barbs and serrated edges, and the oscillation of the mouthparts while feeding on the lachrymal secretions causes considerable irration and pain, even keratitis. Man seems less attractive than cattle and water buffaloes, but he may be attacked while asleep or doing night work on farms. Büttiker (1969) suggests that this peculiar form of parasitism is recent, and it is likely that certain species of moths will develop increasingly close associations with man and animals. Bänziger (1971) considers that the evolution of piercing-feeding in moths has taken place along two main lines: one from fruit-sucking to fruit-piercing, the other from feeding on animal dung or skin secretions (perspiration, wound exudates, etc.) to lachrymal secretions or even extravasated blood, as in the noctuid *Calpe eustrigata*.

ACARINES

Most of the acarine infestations of animals transmissible to man occur among the mites, but ticks, and some pentastomids, may also pass to humans.

MITES

Man has his own species of mange mites in *Sarcoptes scabiei* and the virtually non-pathogenic *Demodex folliculorum*, but several animal mites can also infect him, either from his pets or domestic stock. Mites are generally not so precisely host-specific as, for example, lice, and recently there has been a tendency to aggregate many of the "species" of mange mites more realistically into units founded on true affinity rather than on the assumption that each host must automatically have its own species or subspecies of a genus of mites.

We can refer to mites of the families Sarcoptidae, Psoroptidae, Demodicidae, Dermanyssidae, Tyroglyphidae and Cheyletidae. Of the Sarcoptidae, the best known is *Sarcoptes scabiei*, formerly split off into many subspecies, as *S. scabiei* var. *bovis*, but now best upgraded, here to *S. bovis*. Human scabies becomes very common in times of national diaster, as after the Chilean earthquake (Schenone *et al.*, 1972), and the disease probably exists in every country. *S. scabiei* appears to be transmissible either way between man and the great apes of the Pongidae, but *S. canis*, *S. bovis*, *S. ovis* and *S. rupicaprae* are separate species, each of which can infect several related host species, as *S. canis* on dogs, foxes and wolves (Kutzer, 1966). One problem in these studies on the specificity of mites is that the general health and nutritional status of the host must be taken carefully into account; mange develops best if the host is predisposed to it by such factors as a deficiency of vitamin A, protein or phosphorus, also perhaps by an excess of calcium or the presence of concomitant helminth infection.

Sarcoptes canis causes a transient infestation in man, unpleasant but fortunately easy to cure with modern acaricides.

S. cuniculi occurs in pet rabbits, and *S. equi* in horses, the latter being a very serious and notifiable condition in many countries. Sarcoptic mange often passes from farm animals to man, resulting in "dairyman's itch", "cavalryman's itch", etc., but these temporary infestations never produce typical scabies like that caused by *S. scabiei*, and they usually quickly resolve, often without treatment. The two other sarcoptid genera, *Notoedres* and *Cnemidocoptes (Knemidokoptes)* have never been known to infect man (Yunker, 1973).

Of the psoroptids, neither *Psoroptes bovis* (which causes both cattle scab and sheep scab: Sweatman, 1958) nor *Chorioptes* of stock have been recorded from man (Yunker, 1973). The third psoroptid, *Otodectes*, represented by *O. cynotis*, normally in the ears of dogs and cats, can cause *Sarcoptes* type lesions on the skin of man (Hewitt *et al.*, 1971).

Continuing investigations on *Demodex* are showing an increasing number of new morphological types, and it has been assumed that man is affected solely by *D. folliculorum*. However, Hewitt *et al.*, (1971) reported a case of apparent demodectic mange in a dog owner, causing a fine papular reaction, but which cleared following successful treatment of the pet.

Larvae of the harvest mite or Herbstgrasmilbe, *Trombicula (Neotrombicula) autumnalis* may be a serious pest during the late summer and autumn months, causing irritating wheals; the nymphs and adults are not parasitic. Rabbits, dogs and various rodents are commonly infested with the larvae, and it is difficult to link this parasite with any one species of host. *Neotrombicula americana, Eutrombicula batatas* and *E. alfreddugèsi* are closely related trombiculids which commonly attack man (Yunker, 1973).

Dermanyssus gallinae, the chicken red mite, can be a serious pest in chicken houses, particularly when these are organised on a back-yard scale. The nymphs and adults feed on blood and transfer very easily to man from poultry and from wild birds, including the vacated nests of birds which have lived under the eaves of houses. *D. gallinae* can feed on human blood (Williams, 1958), although this is unusual. Infestations in man can result in a severe erythematous pruritus or papular response, mainly over the trunk and face; the lesions often resemble those produced by fleas (Hewitt *et al.*, 1971). The northern fowl mite, *Liponyssus (Ornithonyssus) sylviarum* seems generally more frequent on birds than the red mite, but is uncommon on man. *L. bacoti*, the tropical rat mite, and *L. bursa*, the tropical fowl mite, will readily attack people and can transmit several species of micro-organisms. The family Parasitidae is closely related to the Dermanyssidae, and includes *Echinolaelaps echidninus*, a blood-sucking mite which normally infests rats but which may attack man, and *Haemolaelaps casalis* which can apparently feed on poultry and rodents but often occurs among broiler house litter, when it may attack farm workers. Cases are on record in which the itching and general irritability in already hot and humid conditions has made work almost impossible.

Cheyletiella parasitivorax, which occurs on rabbits, cats and dogs, was once thought to be hyperparasitic on another fur mite, *Listrophorus gibbus*; it is now realised that this mode of life, like its occasional phoretic attachment to fleas and hippoboscids, is unusual, and it has been shown to be a completely independent parasite in all its developmental stages. Smiley (1965) has described morphological features (Table I) which distinguish *C. yasguri* from *C. parasitivorax*, and a total of five species have now been recognised. It is apparent that many of the earlier records of *parasitivorax* must have been *yasguri*, and current studies that *C. parasitivorax* may be a true parasite of rabbits and cats, while *C. yasguri* infests canids. Work on the two species has recently been carried out in Liverpool (Gething, 1973), and the results can conveniently be considered with those of a survey of zoonotic ectoparasites which covered south-west England (Hewitt *et al.*, 1971).

Table I

Species Differentiation of Cheyletiella parasitovorax *and* C. yasguri *(after Smiley, 1965).*

Feature	*C. parasitivorax*	*C. yasguri*
Sensory organ on genu I	spade-shaped	heart-shaped
female: hysterosome	entire surface striated	striated save for pair of dorsal platelets
Body setae	fine	coarse

C. parasitivorax in cats and rabbits usually causes little trouble, perhaps a light scurfiness, while in dogs there is excessive exfoliation, heavy scurfiness, alopecia and scale formation - most severe in 2-8 week old puppies, this possibly indicating an acquired immunity. The lesions produced in human skin after contact with infected pets do not follow the pattern seen in animals, often occurring more as irritating and hyperaemic spots which progress to yellow crusted lesions; the general pattern of lesions in man is similar with both *C. parasitivorax* and *C. yasguri*. Some two thirds of the people seen in the English survey developed only mild reactions with *Cheyletiella* there consisting of general irritation, papules and wheals. It was also observed that not all members of a household showed a reaction, possibly indicating an allergic mechanism or a difference in attractivity on the part of different people. On the question of attractiveness, it may be relevant to add that several species of ectparasites are attracted to their hosts by "odour", including carbon dioxide and amino acids excreted in association with the perspiration. Worth (1950) examined the attraction of various ectoparasites to rats in the Florida Everglades, and showed that cotton rats had five times the total number (but fewer actual species) of mites and other parasites than rice rats, despite the common environmental niche shared by the two hosts. Worth suggested that the overall differences between the two hosts must have included their blood components, hair and skin texture, microclimate of the skin, and perhaps, chiefly, their different grooming behaviours.

A final group of mites which may cause some distress to man and animals are the tyroglyphids. These are normally free-living on foodstuffs, but on man can cause "grocer's itch", "copra itch", "miller's itch", etc. In the survey carried out by Hewitt *et al.*, (1971) several human patients suffered increased skin sensitivity, urticaria, papular rashes and even bullous eruptions, and there were sometimes infestations with forage mites on pets in the same households as the human patients. The incidence of human infestations with mites from pets has hardly been investigated, and much more work should be done on this large and complex field of comparative dermatology. In Hewitt's survey it was estimated that at least 5% of the patients who entered dermatological clinics suffered from lesions directly attributable to animal ectoparasites.

The analysis of the antigenic components of related "subspecies" of mange mites and of the host reactions to mite invasion are linked problems. Fisher (1972) recently employed the gel-diffusion technique to demonstrate common antigens between *Ps. bovis* (= *Ps. ovis*) and the accepted separate species *Ps. cuniculi* of the rabbit; no reaction was obtained when extracts of sheep *Psoroptes* were tested against sera from sheep which harboured the ked, *Melophagus ovinus*. These results are interesting in view of the successful - if fatal-infestation of a rabbit with *Ps. bovis*. Further investigations could be carried out on the relations between animal and human species of *Sarcoptes* and *Demodex*, for example. In the *Cheyletiella* work, Hewitt used standard skin test techniques on human patients, and extended studies would profit, as did his, by the cooperation of specilists in parasitology, veterinary science and human medicine.

TICKS

Ticks are obligatory parasites of vertebrates, often transmitting micro-organisms, and sometimes responsible for paralysis. Their bite-lesions may become secondarily infected with bacteria or the larvae of screw-worm flies.

One tends to think of ticks as taking blood from man or animals, man thus furnishing either a specific or alternative (zoonotic) food supply. This state of affairs is due largely to our long association of such species pairs as *Ornithodorus moubata* and *Borrelia duttoni* (relapsing fever spirochaete). It seems more likely, however, that *O. moubata* is primarily a parasite of warthogs, porcupines and ant bears. This and similar eyeless species of ticks may have originally lived in the lairs and burrows of wild animals, from which it would be a short step to the darkness of a mud hut or pigsty (Geigy and Mooser, 1955). It is interesting that the hairless parts of warthog skin resemble human skin, and that these hairless areas are preferred by *O. moubata* (El Ziady, 1958). It is also well known that different stages of one species of tick prefer to feed on different parts of the same host, as in the occurrence of larvae and nymphs of *Rhipicephalus evertsi* in the ears of hares and rabbits, while the adults infest the peri-anal area (Arthur, 1973). In this case the feeding larvae begin to stimulate a strong waxy host reaction, which then makes feeding increasingly difficult for the nymphs. A further stage of differentiation occurs in the Karoo tick, *Ixodes rubicundus*, the immatures of which occur largely on shrews and hares, while the adults infest domestic stock. Experiments with *O. moubata* have shown that the blood of snakes and lizards is quite acceptable to the adults, while nymphs placed on this diet suffer a high mortality but the precise reasons for some species of ticks having different sites of predilection or different hosts in their different stages, remain to be investigated.

Many surveys have been carried out, which indicate how certain species of ticks, "so called animal ticks", can attack man. Sandosham and Keeling (1967), working in Malaysia, for example, showed that men were parasitised by larvae of *Dermacentor auratus* and *Amblyomma testudinarium*, normally parasitic on pigs and tapirs, and by species of *Haemaphysalis* from various carnivores. It is quite common for man to be attacked by dog ticks, such as *Rh. sanguineus* and even by bat species, such as *Argas pusillus* and *O. batuensis*. In Europe, man is occasionally infected by louping ill virus or the bovine piroplasms following contact with the sheep/cattle tick, *Ix. ricinus* (Garnham, *et al.*, 1969). It is becoming very obvious that as people move into the countryside more and more in search of recreation, they must be in contact with ticks more often, so that diseases such as tick-borne encephalitis have become a very real hazard in central Europe and North America (Hoogstraal, 1972).

Tick paralysis is also a condition to be reckoned with. The problem occurs mainly in North America (*Dermacentor andersoni, D. variabilis*), South Africa (*Rh. sinus, H. truncatum, Ix. rubicundus*) and Australia (*Ix. holocyclus*). Most human cases involve children, and in Canada and the United States reported deaths have been of persons aged up to 16; 30 children have died in North America during the past 60 years due to this condition (Schmitt, *et al.*, 1969). Paralysis may be particularly dangerous if the parasites attach in the head or neck regions, and Jellison and Gregson (1950) pointed out that long hair tends to hide ticks which may have begun feeding on the nape of the neck, where they may then remain for several days. Paralysis can be very damaging in herds of cattle, and Rich (1971) reported a very acute outbreak in British Colombia, Canada, where 320 out of 700 cattle were paralysed, 30 dying before they could be treated.

The tropical fowl tick, *Argas (Persicargas) persicus* may attack man, and Gothe (1971) has studied the onset of paralysis in chickens bitten by this tick. It was shown that a weak protective immunity slowly develops against both engorgement and against inoculated toxin.

PENTASTOMIDA

Larvae of the linguatulids (tongue worms) are found in the viscera of several species of mammals, while the adult stage parasitises the respiratory passages of reptiles and mammals. Encysted larvae of *Armillifer armillatus* in Africa, and of *A. moniliformis* in Africa, Asia and Australia are sometimes recovered at human autopsies, the subjects probably having been infected by eating the flesh of snakes which harboured adult worms. The dog tongue worm, *Linguatula serrata*, also occurs in man, perhaps following the ingestion of vegetables or other material contaminated by dog excreta. In one case in the United States, *L. serrata* was taken from the eye of an 8-year old child (Rendtorff *et al.*, 1962).

CONCLUSIONS

During the course of evolution, and partly because of the unfavourable action of host tissues against pathogens, potential ectoparasites must have slowly passed from wholly free-living to a stage which included facultative parasitism. Well-balanced parasitic relationships probably came about as a result of long-evolved immunological reactions, and severe pathological conditions occur when this balance is upset, as in the transfer of *Gedoelstia* from the native antelope to domestic stock. Most ectoparasites have a reasonably balanced relationship with their host, and pathological signs range from the virtually non-existent or very mild, as in human infections with *Demodex* or *Linguatula*, and in most equine infections with *Gasterophilus*, to the severity of human *Cordylobia* and animal *Callitroga* infestations.

In order to examine the host-ectoparasite relationship in detail, we may attempt to identify the immune reactions associated with the infestation. Previously there have been considerable practical difficulties, but modern techniques of immunoelectrophoresis, haemagglutination, immune lysis, immunofluorescence and complement fixation are now used to demonstrate antigen-antibody reactions only vaguely suggested by older analytical methods. As an example, Doby *et al.*, (1970) used immunoelectrophoresis to indicate the presence in human serum of antibody against a current or recent infestation with *Hypoderma*, distinguishing ten precipitin lines. A difficulty here has been that host antibodies are produced mainly in response to the actively migrating first instar larvae rather than to the quiescent second and third instar larvae (Beesley and Breyev, 1969). Using passive haemagglutination and electrophoresis, Boulard and Weintraub (1973) have further demonstrated a rapid rise in antibody titre during the first two months of artifical infestations of rabbits with *Hypoderma*, persisting for seven further months. Larval collagenase seems to be responsible for the main immune stimulus, and interesting finding in view of Lienert and Thorsell's (1955) earlier suggestion that if the collagenase of *Hypoderma* larvae could be inhibited by a suitable chemical agent, then the parasites would become immobilised and soon die from the strong host reaction that would then result.

The immune response which develops after exposure of the tissues to the secretions and excretions of oestrid larvae appears to be weaker than that produced against calliphorid larvae, first demonstrated by Blacklock and Gordon (1927): guineapigs were shown to develop a skin immunity after they had been inoculated with extracts of larvae of the African

Tumbu Fly, *Cordylobia anthropophaga*. Subsequent attempted infestations with entire larvae failed because of the skin reactions. In the same way, repeated attacks on sheep by the ked, *Melophagus ovinus*, become progressively less effective in older animals following the increasing development of a histamine-mediated "sealing-off" reaction by the sheep, which prevents the parasites from extracting blood from the dermal capillaries (Nelson and Bainborough, 1963). It seems quite possible that sheep are also capable of a skin reaction against certain blowflies, *Lucilia* spp., and we are currently investigating this aspect of parasitism in Liverpool.

Parasitism does not affect either "animals" or "man", and we have seen in this review that man, himself an animal, may or may not be affected by various ectoparasites of "animals". Careful consideration of, for example, *Cordylobia anthropophaga*, indicates that many "human" parasites are probably more at home in the lairs and burrows of various wild animals than on ourselves. It has been suggested here that it may be wrong to think that there are a large number of truly human ectoparasites, and perhaps we are limited to such species as *Pediculus humanus* and *Sarcoptes scabiei*. There are, however, many insects, ticks and mites which, given the opportunity, will attack us in one or more of their developmental stages, and which can do this so expertly that we may appear to adopt them well before they have evolved as strictly hominoid parasites.

REFERENCES

Arthur, D.R. (1973). *J. Wildl. Dis.*, *9*, 74.
Baer, W.S. (1931). *J. Bone Jt. Surg.*, *13*, 438.
Bänziger, H. (1971). *Fauna*, *1*, 3.
Basson, P.A. (1962). *Onderstepoort J. vet. Res.*, *29*, 211.
Beachley, R.G. and Bishopp, E.C. (1942). *Virginia Med. Mthly.*, *69*, 41.
Beesley, W.N. (1962). *Res. vet. Sci.*, *3*, 203.
Beesley, W.N. (1966). *Brit. vet. J.*, *122*, 91.
Beesley, W.N. (1968). *Ann. trop. Med. Parasit.*, *62*, 8.
Beesley, W.N. and Breyev, K.A. (1969). *Parazitologiya*, *3*, 472.
Blacklock, D.B. and Gordon, R.M. (1927). *Ann. trop. Med. Parasit.*, *21*, 181.
Boulard, C. and Weintraub, J. (1973). *Int. J. Parasit.*, *3*, 379.
Büttiker, W. (1969). *Mitt. schweiz. ent. Ges.*, *42*, 305.
Canese, A. (1970). *Rev. Paraguay Microbiol.*, *5*, 26 (cited in *Rev. appl. Ent. ser. B. 59*, 122).
Chaddah, V. and Warin, R. (1966). *Br. J. clin. Tract.*, *20*, 215.

Chereschnev, N.A. (1954). *Dokl. Acad. Nauk SSSR (N.S.)., 99,* 661.
Dao, L. (1963). *Derm. trop., 2,* 158.
Dinulescu, G. (1929). *Ann. Parasit. hum. comp., 7,* 419.
Doby, J.M. and Beaucornu, J.C. (1965). *Bull. Soc. Path. Exot., 58,* 520.
Doby, J.M., Rosin, G. and Rault, B. (1970). *Bull. Soc. Path. Exot., 63,* 716.
Dunn, L.H. (1934). *J. Parasit., 20,* 219.
El Ziady, S. (1958). *Ann. ent. Soc. Amer., 51,* 317.
Flew, G.P. and Grundy, J.H. (1967). *J.R. Army med. Cps., 113,* 148.
Fisher, W.F. (1972). *J. Parasit., 58,* 1218.
Garnham, P.C.C., Donnelly, J., Hoogstraal, H., Kennedy, C.C. and Walton, C.A. (1969). *Brit. med. J., 4,* 768.
Geigy, R. and Mooser, H. (1955). *J. trop. Med. Hyg., 58,* 199.
Gething, M.A. (1973). *Vet. Bull., 43,* 63.
Glaser, A. (1912), cited by Zumpt, F. (1965).
Gothe, R. (1971). *Z. Parasitenk., 35,* 308.
Grantham-Hill, C. (1933). *Trans. Roy. Soc. trop. Med. Hyg., 27,* 93.
Guilbride, P.D.L., Barber, L. and Kalikwani, A.M.G. (1959). *Bull. epiz. Dis. Africa., 7,* 149.
Haberman, W.O., Morgan, B.B. and Dicke, R.J. (1949). *J. agric. Res., 78,* 637.
Heath, A.C.G., Elliott, D.C. and Dreadon, R.G. (1968). *N.Z. med. J., 68,* 31.
Hewitt, M., Walton, G.S. and Waterhouse, M. (1971). *Br. J. Derm., 85,* 215.
Hoogstraal, H. (1972). *Wiad. Parazyt., 18,* 501.
James, M.T. (1947). "The Flies that cause Myiasis in Man." *U.S. Dept. Agric. Misc. Pub.,* no. *631,* 175pp.
James, M.T. (1964). *Proc. 1st Int. Congr. Parasit. (Rome)., 2,* 955.
Jellison, W.L. And Gregson, J.D. (1950). *Rocky Mt. Med. J., 47,* 28.
Kutzer, E. (1966). *Z. Parasitenk., 28,* 60.
Laarman, J.J. and van Thiel, P.H. (1967). *Trop. Geog. Med., 19,* 187.
Landi, S. (1960). *Can. J. Microbiol., 6,* 115.
Lavoipierre, M.M.J. and Beesley, W.N. (1957). *Trans. Roy. Soc. trop. Med. Hyg., 51,* 295.
Leclerq, M. (1969). "Entomological Parasitology". pp. 158. Pergamon Press, Oxford, London and New York.
Lienert, E. and Thorsell, W. (1955). *Expt. Parasit., 4,* 117.
Meleney, W.P. (1967). *Amer. J. vet. Res., 28,* 892.
Mock, D.E. (1969). *J. Med. Ent., 10,* 34.

Neville, E.M., Basson, P.A., Schroonraad, J.H. and Swanepoel, K.A. (1969). *S. Afr. med. J.*, *43*, 512.

Nelson, W.A. and Bainborough, A.R. (1963). *Expt. Parasit.*, *13*, 118.

O'Rourke, F.J. (1968). *J. Irish Med. Ass.*, *61*, 19.

Patton, W.S. (1921). *Bull. ent. Res.*, *12*, 239.

Rendtorff, R.C., Deweese, M.W. and Murrah, W. (1962). *Amer. J. trop. Med. Hyg.*, *11*, 762.

Reynolds, W.B. (1963). *J. Amer. Med. Ass.*, *186*, 210.

Rice, P.L. and Douglas, G.W. (1972). *Ann. ent. Soc. Amer.*, *65*, 514.

Sandosham, A.A. and Keeling, M.N. (1967). *Med. J. Malaya*, *22*, 16.

Schenone, M., Falaha, F., Villarroel, F., Rojas, A., Szekely, R., Rojo, M. and Palamino, H. (1972). *Bol. Chil. Parasit.*, *27*, 2.

Schmitt, N., Bowmer, E.J. and Gregson, J.D. (1969). *Canad. med. Ass. J.*, *100*, 417.

Smiley, R.L. (1965). *Proc. ent. Soc. Wash.*, *67*, 75.

Stabler, R.M., Nelson, M.C., Lewis, B.L. and Berthiong, M. (1962). *J. Parasit.*, *48*, 209.

Sweatman, G.K. (1958). *Can. J. Zool.*, *36*, 905.

Thompson, J.H., Knutson, L.V. and Culp, O.S. (1970). *Mayo Clinic Proc.*, *45*, 597.

Wetzel, H. (1969). *Berl. Münch. tierärztl. Wschr.*, *82*, 330.

Wohlfahrt, J.A. (1770). *Novae Acta phys. med. Acad. Caes. Leop. Car.*, *4*, 277. (cited in Zumpt, 1965).

Williams, R.W. (1958). *Amer. J. trop. Med.*, *7*, 627.

Yunker, C.E. (1973). "Mites" in "Parasites of laboratory animals" (R.J. Flynn, ed.), pp. 425-492. Iowa St. Univ. Press, U.S.A.

Zumpt, F. (1963). *S. Afr. med. J.*, *37*, 425.

Zumpt, F. (1965). "Myiasis in Man and Animals in the Old World". Buterworths, London., 267 pp.

NEUROPHARMACOLOGICAL INVESTIGATIONS ON TICK PARALYSIS OF CHICKENS INDUCED BY LARVAE OF *ARGAS (PERSICARGAS) WALKERAE*

Rainer Gothe and Klaus Kunze

Institute of Parasitology and Parasitic Diseases of Animals and Department of Clinical Neurophysiology, Centre of Neurology, Justus Liebig University Giessen, Federal Republic of Germany

INTRODUCTION

Tick paralysis induced by larvae of *Argas (Persicargas) walkerae* can be defined as a toxicosis (Gothe, 1971) which shows the typical signs of a generalized affection of the peripheral nervous system (Gothe and Kunze, 1970; Gothe *et al.*, 1970; Gothe *et al.*, 1971b; Kunze and Gothe, 1971; Kunze *et al.*, 1970). It can be demonstrated that efferent fibres as well as afferent ones are involved (Gothe and Kunze, 1971a) and of the fibre types affected, the fast conducting motor fibres are affected markedly (Gothe and Kunze, 1971a; Kunze and Gothe, 1971). This affect on peripheral nerves by the tick larvae is not associated with morphological changes; there is, for example, no lesion in the parenchyma of the nerve fibre (Gothe *et al.*, 1971a). The clinical affect on the peripheral nervous system is reversible if the tick larvae are removed early enough. Electrophysiological investigations show an almost complete reversability following removal of the ticks (Kunze and Gothe, 1971).

Not only are the peripheral nerves affected, as has been shown by neurophysiological studies, but also there is a functional lesion in neuromuscular transmission, in tick paralysis. Thus if the distal parts of the nerves are stimulated supramaximally at a frequency of 30/sec, the muscle response show a response which is 65% of the initial values (Gothe and Kunze, 1970, 1971b; Gothe *et al.*, 1970; Kunze and Gothe, 1971; Kunze *et al.*, 1970). If stimulation of the distal parts of the nerves is performed at frequencies under 10/sec. then the response was reduced in amplitude by only 10% from the initial values.

Such neurophysiological studies indicate that the neuromuscular endplate is concerned in the pathogenesis of this type of tick paralysis. Naturally, the question arises as to the role of acetylcholine in the process.

This report deals with investigations performed to assess whether the assumed toxin in tick paralysis has an action on the acetylcholine system and whether such action has a role in the pathogenesis of tick paralysis.

MATERIAL AND METHODS

For the electrophysiological investigations chickens (HNL-Leghorn), 4 weeks of age, and bred tick-free in batteries, were used. Larvae of *Argas (Persicargas) walkerae* were used in numbers that would produce a complete paresis. The chickens were infested beneath one of the wings and housed separately in plastic cages. The cages were placed in tubs filled with water to control the larvae. The infestation rate was assessed by counting the number of the engorged larvae daily and, finally, by counting the number of larvae which were removed from the animal after death.

A selected population of a South African (Onderstepoort) strain of *A. walkerae* was used. The larvae were bred in an incubator at 26-28°C and a relative humidity of 92-95%.

Infested chickens were investigated neurophysiologically at the time of the most marked clinical signs. Anaesthesia was produced with Jetrium(R) (25 mg/kg body weight) and body temperature of the bird was maintained by the use of a warming lamp.

Electrophysiological investigations were performed on the sciatic nerve. This nerve was stimulated as proximally as possible and distally at the tarsal joint. The stimulations were performed supramaximally using needle electrodes and the duration of the stimulus was 0,2 sec. Muscle responses were assessed by the belly tendon technique using the interdigital muscle of the foot.

The neuromuscular endplate reactions were tested by applying supramaximal stimuli to the distal parts of the nerve at a frequency of 30/sec. using pulses with a duration of 1 sec. and at time intervals of 30 seconds. Pharmacological tests were performed with acetylcholine (20 mg/kg body weight), neostigmine (0,05 mg/kg body weight) and with "Tensilon" (Edrophoniumchloride, 0,4 or 2 x 0,4 mg/kg body weight) administrated intravenously. For the quantitative evaluation of the function of neuromuscular transmission the first amplitude and the amplitude of the thirtieth pulse was determined. The thirtieth amplitude was related to the first amplitude which was considered as 100% responsiveness.

Control measurements were performed on paralysed animals not subject to the pharmacological tests and on non-paralysed animals subject to the pharmacological tests.

The DISA-3-channel-EMG-apparatus and the DISA-Multistim-stimulator were used for the electrophysiological measurements. Evaluations of the responses were done from film records.

RESULTS

Measurements on non-infected and non-paralysed chickens.

Maximum conduction velocity of the sciatic nerve of healthy animals ranged between 40,1 - 44,3 m/sec. with an amplitude of the muscle response of the interdigital muscles of more than one mV. On repetative stimulation of the distal parts of the nerve at a frequency of 30 sec. using pulses with a time interval of 30 sec., the amplitude of the 30th potential showed a decline to a minimum of 90% of the initial amplitude.

The influence of acetylcholine (20 mg/kg body weight) (Fig. 1.) on neuromuscular transmission was seen in two phases. Initially, a marked depression of the first as well as the thirtieth potential was evident. This depression reached about 20% of the initial value. One minute later this depression became less, and by two minutes after injection of the acetylcholine, the initial amplitudes during the pulses were in the range of 80% of normal values before drug administration. There was no marked dissociation in the amplitude values for the first and the thirtieth potential (with the exception of a small time delay in the recovery of the thirtieth potential). Five minutes after the application of acetylcholine (i.e. at the 15th and 16th pulses), a second phase of depression of the amplitudes of the potentials takes place.

Under the same conditions, the administration of neostigmine (0,05 mg/kg body weight) to healthy animals, produced a slowly developing and progressive depression of amplitudes of the first and the thirtieth potential (Figs. 2, 3). At 9 minutes after injection of the drug, (28.-30. pulse) minimum values of approximately 20% of the initial values were reached.

Under the influence of the short acting cholinesteraseinhibitor edrophoniumchloride, a depression of the first and the thirtieth potential was seen, but this did not amount to more than 50% of the normal values and was reached only after 2 minutes (i.e. at the 6-7th pulse). The depression lasted approximately one minute, and by 3½ minutes (12-13th pulse) the responses reached a steady state of approximately 70% of the normal values. It is of note that, during these investigations with "Tensilon", the thirtieth potential during each pulse, showed only a small alteration and maintained a value of about 60% of the initial amplitude values during the whole period.

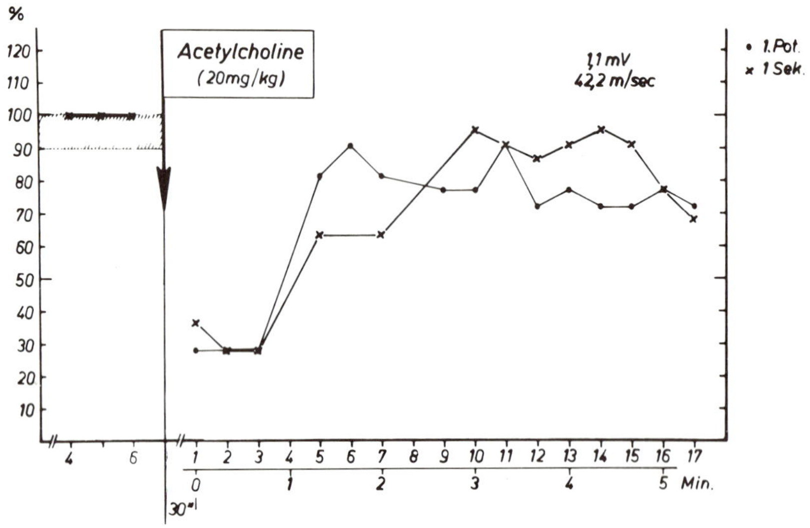

Fig. 1. Neuromuscular transmission studies in chicken. Plot of the amplitudes of the 1st and 30th potential from interdigital muscles after supramaximal stimulation of the nerve. Stimulation series 1 sec duration at 30 stimulations/sec. Ordinate: Percentage of initial amplitude. Abscissa: Number of stimulations and (below) time scale in minutes. Solid circles: 1st potential Crosses: 30th potention.

Normal animal, before and after administration of acetylcholine.

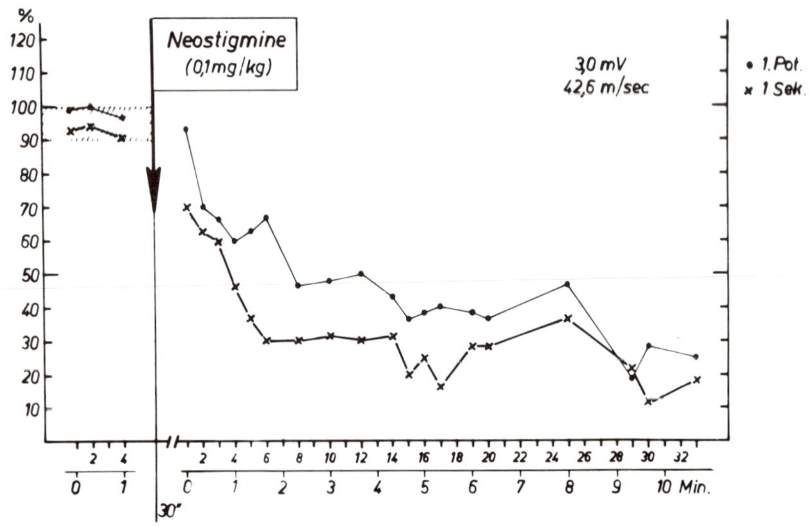

Fig. 2. Normal animal, before and after administration of neostigmine. (See Fig. 1. for caption details).

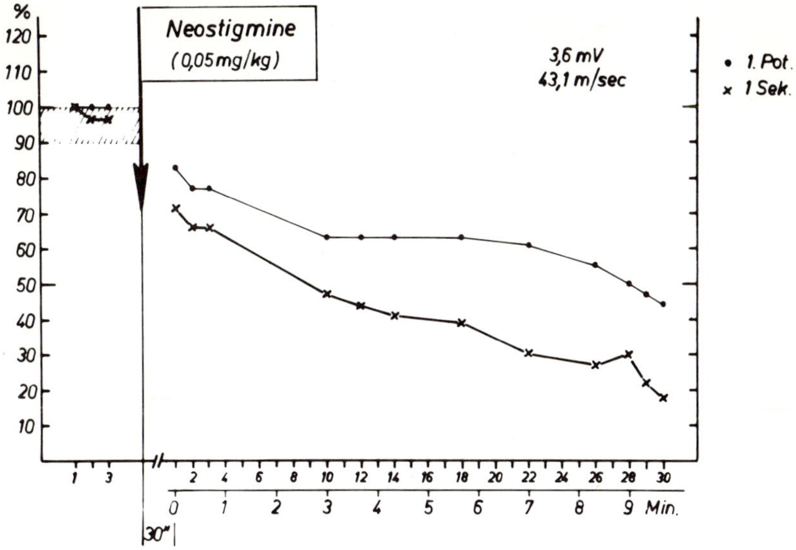

Fig. 3. Normal animal, before and after administration of neostigmine. (0.05 mg/kg). (See Fig. 1. for caption details).

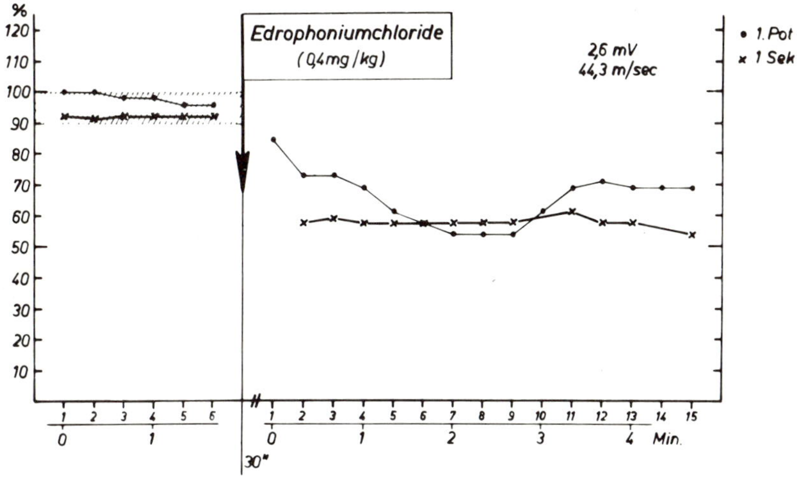

Fig. 4. Normal animal, before and after administration of edrophoniumchloride. (See Fig. 1 for caption details).

Measurements in paralyzed animals

The action of the pharmacological test-substances in animals differed according to the grade of paresis and of the degree of the effect on the peripheral nerves, respectively, caused by the ticks. This was especially evident with acetylcholine in animals with slight paralysis and those with pronounced paralysis. Thus, at a maximum conduction velocity of 23,8 m/sec. and at an initial amplitude of 0,6 mV (Fig. 5) for the muscle response, there was only a slight initial depression for the first potential, but a marked secondary depression occurred starting after about 1 minute and which lead to nearly complete blocking of neuromuscular transmission. Before the administration of acetylcholine, there was a marked difference between the first and the thirtieth potential which showed a decrease of about 40%. After acetylcholine this difference was smaller (Fig. 5).

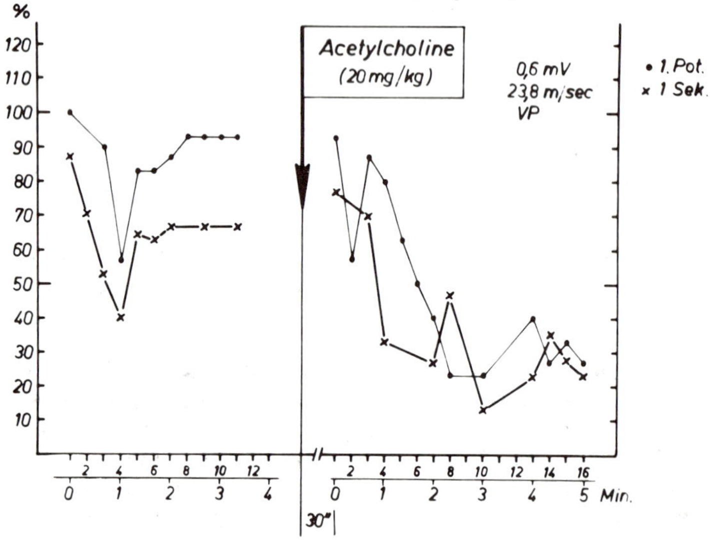

Fig. 5. Paralyzed animal (slightest case). Before and after administration of acetylcholine. (See Fig. 1. for caption details).

In a more pronounced case of paralysis showing a maximum motor nerve conduction velocity of 24,5 m/sec. and a potential of 0,3 mV (Fig. 6), the difference between the first and the thirtieth potential before acetylcholine was initially about 40% and during the first 9 pulse series the 30th potential decreased to about 40% of the amplitude of the first potential. After acetylcholine injection in a case of pronounced paralysis the difference between the first and the thirtieth potential was between 20 and 30% over 11 pulse series. An initial slight depression of the first and thirtieth potential was evident, and thereafter, there was a progressive decrease of the amplitude of the two potentials until the 9-10 pulses, after which a slight increase occurred.

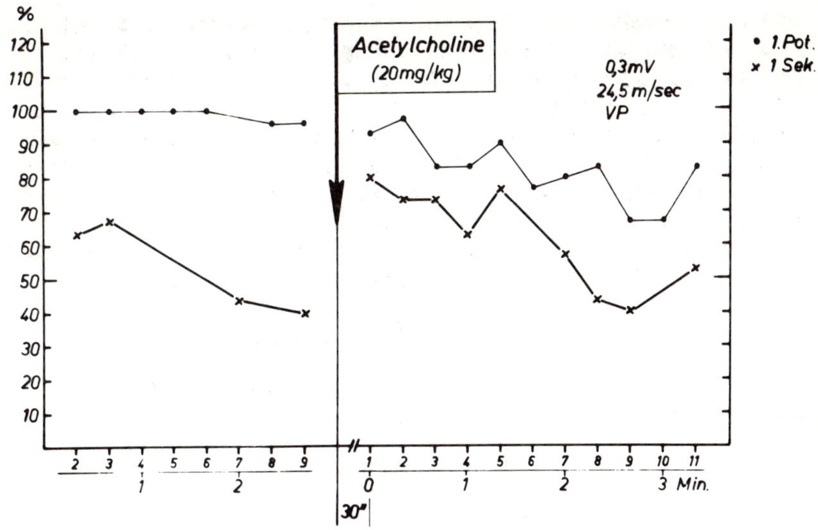

Fig. 6. Paralyzed animal (pronounced case). Before and after administration of acetylcholine. (See Fig. 1. for caption details).

In cases of very pronounced paralysis in which animals had a complete paresis, the neurophysiological parameters showed a maximum conduction velocity of 19,5 m/sec. and an amplitude of 0,075 mV (Fig. 7). A progressive decrease of the amplitude of the first and the thirtieth potential was observed during the series of pulses and both potentials reached a level of about 50% of the initial values, with little difference between the first and the thirtieth potential. After injection of 20 mg/kg body weight acetylcholine both potentials increased. The first potential showed a maximum during the 7th pulse (2½ minutes after acetylcholine administration) after which it showed a slight decrease, but it remained higher than it was before acetylcholine administration. The thirtieth potential showed a linear course over the 12 pulses after acetylcholine injection (Fig. 7).

In the most pronounced case of tick paralysis we have investigated the amplitude of the muscle response after a single stimulus was only 0,027 mV at a maximum conduction velocity for the sciatic nerve of 20,0 m/sec. (Fig. 8). This animal showed clinical signs of complete paresis but was essentially similar, clinically, to the other cases of complete paresis. In this animal, there was, initially, essentially, no difference between the first and the thirtieth potential during stimulation. After the administration of acethycholine the first and the thirtieth potential showed a rapid increase in amplitude. At the fourth pulse the first and thirtieth potential increased to 160%, and at the 5th pulse to approximately 200% of the initial values.

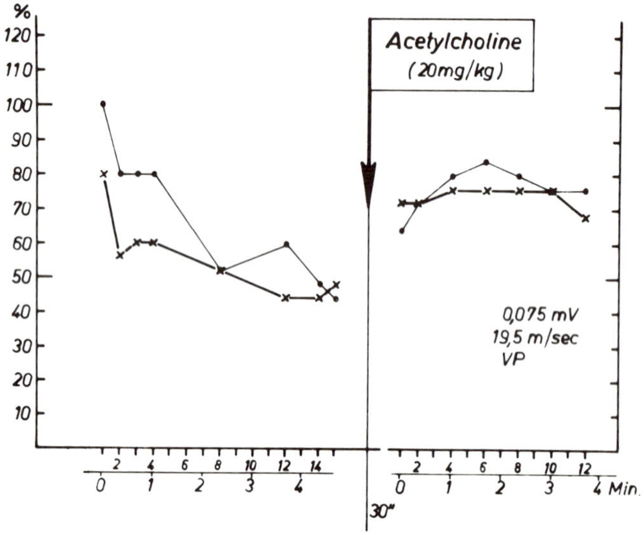

Fig. 7. Paralyzed animal (more pronounced case). Before and after administration of acetylcholine. (See Fig. 1. for caption details).

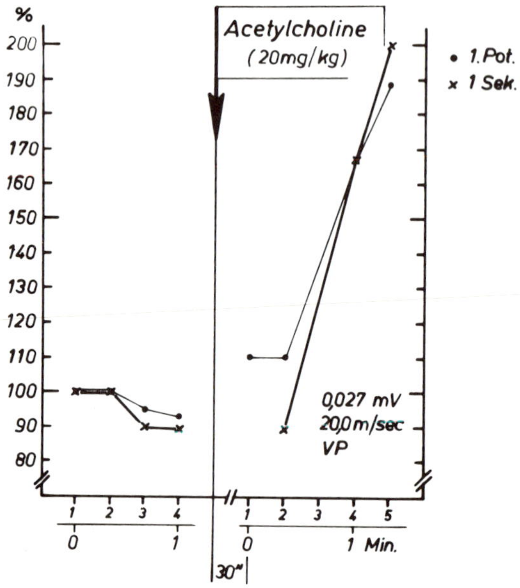

←Fig. 8. Paralyzed animal (most pronounced case) Before and after administration of acetylcholine. (See Fig. 1. for caption details).

In the case of administration of neostigmine (0,05 mg/kg B.W.), completely paralyzed animals, at initial values of 0,44 mV amplitude and 31,4 m/sec. (Fig. 9) and 0,44 mV and 33,2 m/sec. (Fig. 10) respectively, a distinct increase of the amplitudes for the first and the thirtieth potential was seen initially. This increase persisted from the second to the ninth pulse (Fig. 9). A second neostigmine injection resulted in an increase of the amplitude of the first potential only, though the second peak response did not reach that of the first peak (Fig. 10).

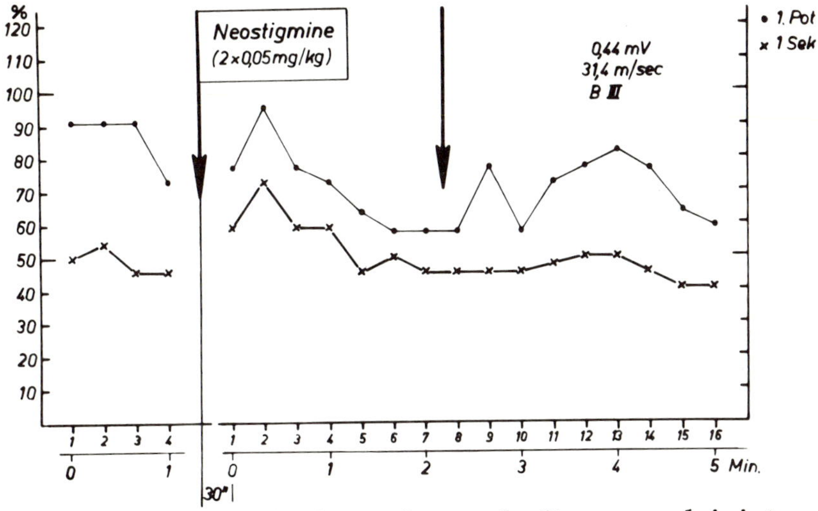

Fig. 9. Paralyzed animal. Before and after one administration of neostigmine. (See Fig. 1. for caption details).

When edrophoniumchloride (0,4 mg/kg body weight) was administered to an animal with a complete paresis, showing a maximum conduction velocity of 25,0 m/sec. and an amplitude of the muscle response to a single nerve stimulus of 0,36 mV, a rapid increase of the first as well as of the thirtieth potential amplitude was seen (Fig. 11). This increase was about 50% of the initial value. The increase took place within 1 minute after injection of edrophoniumchloride and thereafter, the amplitudes showed a linear course over the subsequent 20 pulses. Only a very slight and slow decrease of amplitudes occurred. The amplitudes for first potential during the first series of pulses were higher than the initial value and then ranged at normal levels. This is in distinction to the responses prior to edrophoniumchloride injection, where the amplitude of the first potential showed a marked decrease from 100 to 70% at the 7th pulse.

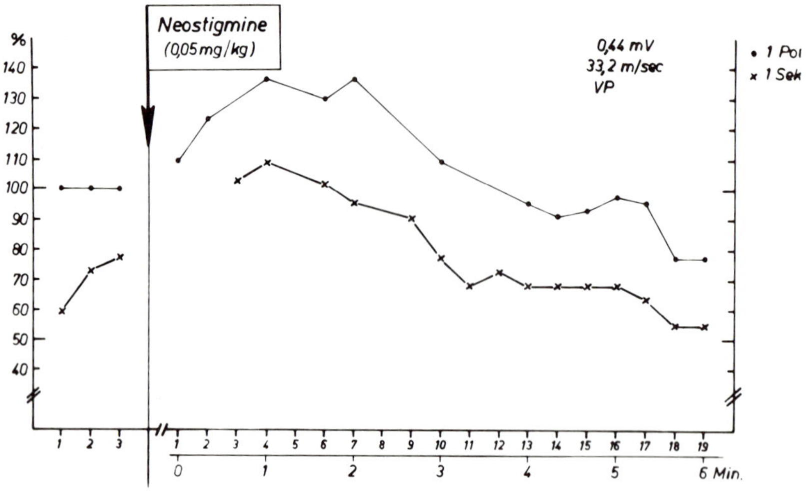

Fig. 10. Paralyzed animal, before and after twofold administration of neostigmine (arrow indicates the second administration). (See Fig. 1. for caption details).

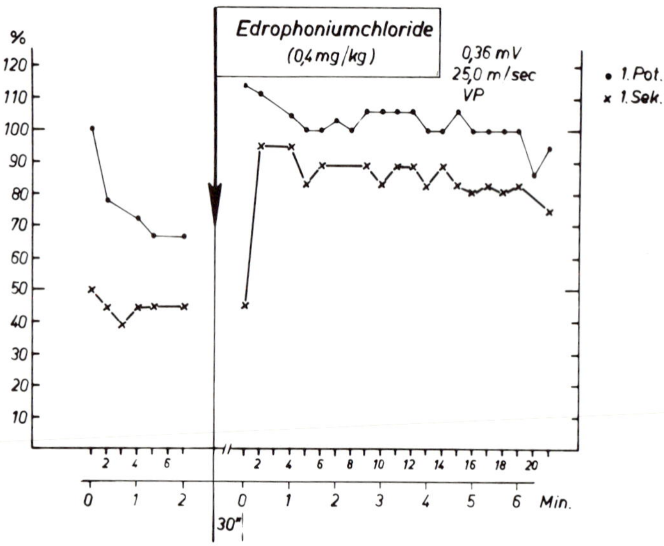

Fig. 11. Paralyzed animal, before and after administration of edrophoniumchloride. (See Fig. 1. for caption details).

DISCUSSION

Animals, infested with larvae of *Argas (Persicargas) wal-*

kerae and developing a more and more completing paresis of cross striated muscles, show a disturbance in neuromuscular transmission. Following supramaximal stimulation of the distal parts of the motor nerve, an increasing decrement of the amplitude of the muscle response is evident with stimulation frequencies of 30/sec. The use of lower stimulation frequencies (e.g. under 10/sec.) did not result in any appreciable amplitude decrement. This type of neuromuscular transmission defect shows no facilitatory effect but is manifest by an alternating blocking effect on individual responses during the series of pulses, and becomes more apparent as paresis increases. When acetylcholine and the cholineesteraseinhibitors, neostigmine and edrophoniumchloride, were administrated to healthy animals the neuromuscular junctions behaved as expected. Thus after acetylcholine, a short and a late depression phase of the responses was observed. Neostigmine and edrophoniumchloride led to a more increased depression due to the increased depolarization block caused by these drugs.

The opposite occurred in infested and paretic animals. In these investigations, all animals had developed a complete paresis of all cross-striated muscles, with the exception of the respiration muscles. Though the animals showed nearly the same clinical features, there were differences in the severity the paresis from the electrophysiological standpoint. This resulted in a different behaviour to the drugs tested.

Thus, the more the nerve derangement had progressed, the more acetylcholine improved the neuromuscular transmission. This was especially so in a case which was practically dead from paralysis, though, this improvement was of a temporary nature.

The two cholineesterase inhibitors similarly influenced neuromuscular transmission in paretic animals, but the effect was more pronounced than with acetylcholine. After neostigmine, the improvement lasted only a short time, whereas, with edrophoniumchloride, a longer lasting effect occurred, resulting in facilitation of neuromuscular transmission. This occurred with both the first and the 30th potential responses.

While measurements of the circulating acetylcholine esterase levels in blood proved to be very difficult, an influence on the pseudo-choline-esterases, possibly caused by disturbance of liver function, has been shown by Gothe and Kraft (1972).

The literature on the pathogenic mechanisms in tick paralysis has been reviewed by Kunze and Gothe (1971) and Gregson (1973). Extensive work has been done on the influence of tick toxin on neuromuscular transmission and on the action of different drugs on this. Compounds such as succinylcholine, tubocurarine, syncurine, atropine, eserine, epedrine, potassium chloride or calcium chloride etc. (Murnagham, 1960; Yarborough, 1955; Nelson and Weintraub, 1962; Webb and Earnest, 1963; Gregson, 1973) have been used to influence or alleviate paralysis in animals. No consistent success has been achieved.

In fact, it is difficult to compare the various results because differing techniques have been applied. Investigations by Rose and Gregson (1956), Emmons and McLennan (1959, 1960) and, especially, Murnaghan (1958) showed a disburbance of neuromuscular transmission. This was shown by the fact that there was no muscle response if motor nerves were stimulated but there was a muscle response if the muscle itself was stimulated. Emmons and McLennan (1959) and Murnaghan (1960) claimed a presynaptic blockade of the neuromuscular junction, because they could show that during nerve stimulation the acetylcholine release was diminished in their nerve muscle preparations from paralyzed animals. On the other hand, these findings can be explained by the fact, proved by Emmons and McLennan (1959, 1960), Murhaghan (1958, 1960) and Kunze and Gothe (1971), that during the development of paresis by tick infested animals, more and more motor fibres become blocked. Hence the acetylcholine release must be lower because the exitable motor axon pool is smaller. Kunze and Gothe (1971) demonstrated this effect by stimulating and recording simultaneous from mixed nerves and from muscle responses. McLennan and Oikawa (1972) raised the question whether there is a neuromuscular transmission disturbance in paralysed animals. Basing their work on earlier studies by Emmons and McLemman (1959, 1960) and Murnaghan (1958, 1960) McLennan and Oikawa conducted microelectrode studies in neuromuscular endplates in phrenic nerve-diaphragm preparations. Their very extensive investigations did not permit an answer to their initial question, and in the discussion of their results, these authors conceded that their measurements neither confirmed nor excluded an additional action of the toxin on the processes of mobilization and/or release of transmitter at the neuromuscular junction.

With this background of doubt in the action of the tick toxin on neuromuscular transmission, it is difficult to evaluate the different results which have been obtained by the use of pharmacological agents at the site of neuromuscular transmission disturbance in tick paralized animals.

The investigations of Murnaghan (1958) are of special interest. He investigated, among other drugs, acetylcholine and neostigmine. With acetylcholine he confirmed the sensitizing effect of acetylcholine on muscle. He found that paralyzed muscle behaved like a denevated muscle to intra-arterial injection of acetylcholine. With neostigmine he could not see any effect on muscular transmission. These investigations serve as an example of the difficulty of comparing results of different authors. Thus Murnaghan (1958) only reported the action of different substances, without mentioning the technique he had used for the special cases. It is considered that reports of changes of physiological parameter following pharmacological maniputation of tick paralysis must also give exact data on the grade of paresis which has developed up to the point of the investigation.

Generally, it is accepted that tick paralysis is caused by a toxin which originates from, or in connection with the secretion of the saliva. The investigations of several authors (Murnaghan, 1958, 1960), Emmons and McLennan (1959, 1960), Kunze and Gothe (1971), Gothe and Kunze (1971a) have shown, without any doubt, that this toxin produces a generalized effect on the peripheral nerves, and both the larger as well as the smaller motor and sensory nerve fibres are affected. The evidence would suggest that the larger motor fibres are affected earlier and much more severely than the smaller motor fibres.

The results reported in this paper suggest the hypothesis that the effect on the peripheral nerves is caused by the toxin blocking the impulse propagation along these nerves. In addition to this action on the nerves, there is doubtless an interaction with the processes which take place at the neuromuscular junction of motor nerves. Whether this interaction is on the presynaptic or postsynaptic side of the neuromuscular junction has yet to be determined. No evidence is available to determine whether the toxin acts specifically on acetylcholine, its synthesis or its turn over rate. The electro physiological studies would suggest a post-synaptic defect, perhaps through an altered sensitivity of the post-synaptic receptor.

Such results provide information on the secondary, or effect or, manifestations of the toxin, which are responsible for the clinical signs of tick paralysis.

There is no information about the nature of the toxin itself. It can be assumed that it has much affinity to peripheral nerve tissue but only a slight affinity to spinal and cerebral tissue. It has never been described that cerebral seizures take place under the influence of a tick toxin. This toxin must have a very short half-life since the typical features of paralysis disappear when the tick is removed early enough. This must be done before the animal is moribund.

The following conclusion may serve as a possible working hypothesis for tick paralysis: The paralysis activating substance, liberated by various species of ticks, acts on motor and sensory nerves and on neuromuscular transmission. By its action on motor nerves, the liberation of acetylcholine is dimished and by its action on neuromuscular transmission, the receptor site is changed in its sensitivity. An increasing number of blocked motor fibres is evident, and the neuromuscular block produced at frequencies of 30/sec or higher is acelycholine and cholinesterase sensitive.

REFERENCES

Emmons, P., and McLennan, H. (1959). *Nature 183*, 474.

Emmons, P., and McLennan, H. (1960). *J. Exp. Biol. 37*, 355.

Gothe, R. (1971). *Z. Parasitenk. 35*, 298.

Gothe, R., Hager, H., Jehn, E., Kunze, K., and Thoenes, W. (1971a). *Z. Tropenmed. Parasit. 22*, 285.

Gothe, R., and Kraft, W. (1972). *Vet. Med. (B.), 19*, 213.

Gothe, R., and Kunze, K. (1970). *J. Parasit. 56*, 123.

Gothe, R., and Kunze, K. (1971a). *Z. Tropenmed. Parasit. 22*, 292.

Gothe, R., and Kunze, K. (1971b). Abstracts of papers, V. Tagung der Deutschen Tropenmedizinischen Gesellschaft, Tübingen.

Gothe, R., Kunze, K., and Alt, H. (1970). *Z. Parasitenk. 34*, 31.

Gothe, R., Kunze, K., and Mechow, O. (1971b). *Z. Tropenmed. Parasit. 22*, 430.

Gregson, J.D. (1973). Monograph No. 9, Canada Department of Agriculture.

Kunze, K., and Gothe, R. (1971). *Z. Parasitenk. 36*, 251.

Kunze, K., Gothe, R., and Muskat, E. (1970). *Pflügers Arch. 319*, 105.

McLennan, H., and Oikawa, I. (1972). *Can. J. Physiol. Pharm. 50*, 53.

Murnaghan, M.F. (1958). *Nature 181*, 131.

Murnaghan, M.F. (1960). *Can. J. Biochem. Physiol. 38*, 287.

Nelson, W.A., and Weintraub, J. (1962). *Can. Insect Pest Rev. 40*, 54. (In: Gregson, J.D. (1973). Monograph No. 9, Canada Department of Agriculture.)

Rose, I., and Gregson, J.D. (1956). *Nature 178*, 95.

Webb, I.H., and Earnest, F. (1963). *Ohio State Med. J. 59*, 395.

Yarborough: Personal communication. (In: Gregson, J.D. (1973). Monograph No. 9, Canada Department of Agriculture.)

THE FLEAS *CTENOCEPHALIDES FELIS FELIS* (BOUCHÉ, 1833), *CTENOCEPHALIDES CANIS* (CURTIS, 1826), AND THE MITE *CHEYLETIELLA* (CANESTRINI, 1886) IN THE DOG AND CAT: THEIR TRANSMISSIBILITY TO HUMANS.

W. P. Beresford-Jones

Royal Veterinary College, London, England

INTRODUCTION

Reports on the incidence of fleas on cats and dogs and of the transmission of the cat and dog flea to humans are not numberous. No figures of the incidence of the cat flea *Ctenocephalides felis felis* and the dog flea *Ctenocephalides canis* have previously been recorded for the Beaumont Animal Hospital Clinic at the Royal Veterinary College, London.

The incidence of fleas on the dog has recently been reported by Baker and Hatch (1972). Fleas were collected from 50 dogs; 43 carried *C. canis*, 2 carried *C. felis*, 12 carried *Pulex irritans*, 6 had concurrent *C. canis* and *P. irritans* and one had *C. canis* and *C. felis*. Ressl (1963) who found *P. irritans* on one dog and Haas and Wilson (1967) who found *P. irritans* and *P. simulans* on 186 dogs in Hawaii. The only other report from Britain is that of Edwards (1969), who examined 135 fleas from dogs and 27 from cats. No *P. irritans* was found. Of the fleas from dogs, 113 were *C. canis* and 22 were *C. felis* and of the fleas from cats all were *C. felis*.

The effect of cat and dog flea bites on humans by natural contact have been reported by Hewitt, Walton and Waterhouse (1971) in patients entering dermatological clinics serving a scattered rural population living in Cornwall, in the South West of England. In the same survey cutaneous reactions were also noted to a mite of the *Cheyletiella* spp. and to other mites. Such clinical records are derived from medical and veterinary clinicians. Experimental data relating to cat and dog flea sensitization have been concerned either with hyposensitisation in dogs and cats to flea bites (Michaeli and Goldfarb 1968) or with the evolution of flea bite sensitivity in humans (Hudson, Feingold and Kartman 1960). The induction of flea-bite sensitivity to the cat flea (*C. felis*) has been studied in the guinea pig (Hudson, Feingold and Kartman 1960). More recently Feingold, Benjamini and Michaeli, (1968) have reviewed the allergic responses to insect bites and refer to a sequence of events following exposure of the guinea pig to cat-flea bites.

The first part of this paper refers to the incidence of fleas and mites *Cheyletiella* spp.) found on cats and dogs from two different sources. The second part reports the skin reaction of humans to the bite of cat fleas.

MATERIALS AND METHODS

Fleas were collected from dogs and cats admitted to The Beaumont Animal Hospital, Royal Veterinary College, London, or to the Field Station of the Royal Veterinary College. The Field Station material included samples submitted by veterinary surgeons in private practice and medical dermatologists. Some of the dogs and cats in the Beaumont Animal Hospital were examined *post-mortem* for fleas and mites, but the remaining material was obtained from living animals.

The fur was examined on either the same day *post-mortem* or the following day after the cadavers had been kept at +2°C overnight. Fleas were collected live by means of lightly sprung forceps, placed in glass specimen tubes 50 x 19 m.m. sealed with polythene closures and either killed, cleared in 5% potassium hydroxide and mounted in Canada Balsam or maintained alive in the specimen tubes for feeding experiments. *Cheyletiella spp.* were obtained by brushing the hair along the back of the cat and dog on to sheets of brown paper which was examined with a dissecting microscope for mites or eggs attached to the hairs. Hair was further treated with 5% potassium hydroxide and the mites isolated by this procedure and those obtained by brushing were mounted in Farrants Medium after staining in Lignin Pink. The identification of the cat and dog flea was based on the features of the hind tibia (Lapage 1968) and identification was verified by Dr. F.G.A.M. Smit, British Museum (Natural History) London, England.

Figures 1 and 2 illustrate specimens which were designated as *Ctenocephalides felis felis* and *Ctenocephalides canis*, respectively.

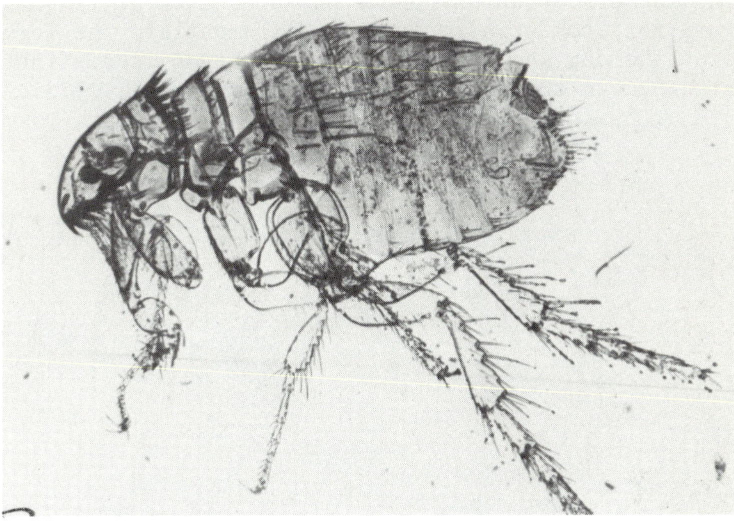

Fig. 1. Ctenocephalides felis felis x 35

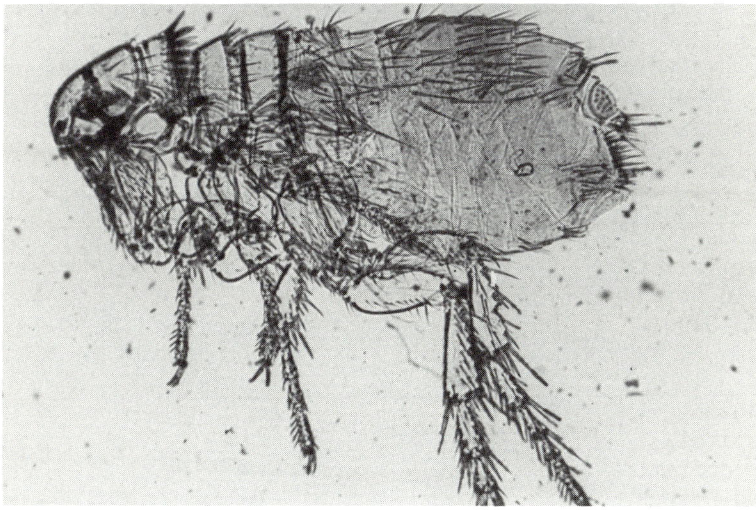

Fig. 2. Ctenocephalides canis x 35

The sensory organ on genu 1 was used as a distinguishing feature for *Cheyletiella* spp. to differentiate the form of mite on the dog and cat. The sensory organ is distinctly heartshaped in the dog (Smiley, 1965, Pfeiffer, 1973).

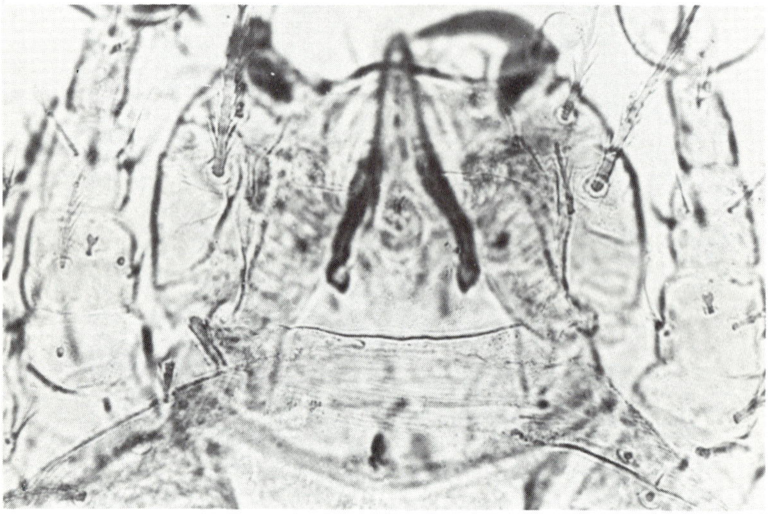

Fig. 3. Cheyletiella yasguri x 550.

RESULTS

The incidence of *C. felis* and *C. canis* on dogs and cats at the Beaumont Hospital and the Field Station is presented in Table 1.

Table 1

LOCATION	NUMBER EXAMINED	POSITIVE	CTENOCEPHALIDIS *felis*	CTENOCEPHALIDIS *canis*
DOG				
Beaumont Hospital	65 (51)	14	10	4
Field Station *and Others	71	9	8	1
CAT				
Beaumont Hospital	95 (75)	64	64	nil
Field Station *and Others	32	10	10	nil

*"Others" - Material supplied by veterinary surgeons and medical dermatologists.

Parentheses - Number of animals examined at *post-mortem*.

In addition to the fleas reported in Table 1, four specimens of *Archeopsylla erinacei* were obtained from dogs and 2 specimens of *Spilopsyllus cuniculi* were obtained from cats.

The ratio of fleas to the sex of the dog or cat is presented in Table 2. In the case of the cat, "male" and "female" include neutered males and females respectively.

Table 2.

The Ratio of fleas to the sex of the dog and cat

	MALE	FEMALE
Dog	14	9
Cat	36	38

The incidence of *Cheyletiella* spp. on dogs and cats at the Field Station and from other sources is presented in Table 3. Of 65 dogs and 95 cats examined at the Beaumont Animal Hospital none were infected with these mites.

Table 3.

HOST	FIELD STATION AND OTHERS NUMBER EXAMINED	*CHEYLETIELLA* *PARASITIVORAX*	*YASGURI*
DOG	71	nil	4
CAT	32	3	nil

Though recorded as *C. parasitivorax* the speciation of the *Cheyletiella* mites from the cat requires further study. Information obtained from Dr. Schillhorn van Veen and from the work of Smiley (1970), suggests that the commest species in the cat is *Cheyletiella blakei*.

Skin sensitivity due to the bite of Ctenocephalides felis felis.

The sequence of skin reactivity has been described by Benjamin *et al.*, (1961) following exposure of guinea pigs to the bite of the cat flea *C. felis*. Five stages of reactivity occur: No observable skin reactions; delayed skin reactions; immediate and delayed skin reaction; immediate reactions only and finally, no reactivity.

Most of the human experiments on flea bite sensitivity have used multiple exposure to fleas. The present results record the reaction to a single flea bite on the left inner surface of the forearm of subjects with no previous history of flea bites. A single *C. felis* female was removed from a cat and was fed on the human subject. The flea was allowed to feed for 13 minutes and then was removed. Within 8 minutes erythema was evident. This reached a maximum size of 4 - 5 mm. in diameter, it began to fade in approximately 30 minutes, and had disappeared 30 minutes later. The same flea was allowed to feed daily on a different area of the same arm for 12 days.

After 3 days of successive bites, the area of the first bite reacted with a raised papule which increased in size progressively as application of the flea continued, so that the lesion reached a size of 3 - 4 mm. in diameter by the 6th to 7th day of exposure. During the last 6 days of exposure the papular lesion at the area of the first bite resolved. This type of response was evident with the areas of individual bites subsequent to the first bite. Thus on any day, it was possible to detect the erythema of the initial bite in a new area of skin along with papular formation on areas of the skin subject to a flea bite on previous days.

Skin sensitivity due to Cheyletiella *spp.*

In two cases of *Cheyletiella yasguri* infection in the dog, there was obvious allergic dermatitis on a human living in the same house.

A single experimental attempt was made to study the effects of this mite on a human subject. This was unsuccessful and because of lack of material was not repeated.

DISCUSSION AND SUMMARY

Although further study is required, *Cheyletiella* spp. infection was not detected on dogs or cats entering the Beaumont Animal Hospital in London. In many of the cases, excessive scurf was present along the back, which was suggestive of clinical evidence of *Cheyletiella* infection, and further work is needed with such cases to evaluate the relationship between scurfiness and *Cheyletiella*.

The *Cheyletiella* genus has been reviewed by Smiley (1970) who states it consists of five species, namely *Cheyletiella yasguri* (Smiley) on dogs, *Cheyletiella blakei*, n. sp. on cats, *Cheyletiella strandt manni* n. sp. on hares and *Cheyletiella parasitivorax* (Mégnin) and *Cheyletiella furmani*, n. sp. on rabbits.

Over 50% of the cats entering the Beaumont Animals Hospital carried *C. felis*. The incidence in dogs was much lower.

Studies of the skin reaction to the bite of a single flea simulated the relationship between the cat and its human environment. The area of the initial bite of the flea always reacted in the same manner by showing erythema, and was adjudged to be an immediate type reaction. Previous opinions of the five stages of flea bite reactivity have stated that in Stage 1 no observable skin reaction takes place. The erythema observed in the present studies could be a sensitising reaction of a haptenic nature.

The second type of reaction kind could be classified as Stage 2 or a delayed skin reaction. Whether stage 3, consisting of immediate and delayed reactions, would occur if the flea bites were continued beyond the 12th day remains to be determined.

The skin reactions of the human to flea bites require further study. The present work has shown that a single flea is able to sensitize the skin and this indicates that it is not necessary to use a large number of fleas to produce skin reactions.

ACKNOWLEDGMENTS

I am grateful to Dr. F.G.A.M. Smit, British Museum (Natural History), Cromwell Road, London S.W.7. for verification of the identity of fleas. For technical assistance I am grateful to Miss E.J. Pegg and Mr. F.A. Shephard. I wish to offer my thanks to Dr. Schillhorn van Veen who drew my attention to the species differentiation of *Cheyletiella* in the cat.

REFERENCES

Baker, K.P. and Hatch, C. (1972). *Vet. Rec. 91*, 151.

Benjamini, E., Feingold, B.F. and Kartman, L. (1961). *Proc. Soc. Exp. Biol. Med., 108*, 700.

Edwards, F.B. (1969). *Vet. Rec. 85*, 665.

Feingold, B.F., Benjamini, E. and Michaeli, D. (1968). *Ann. Rev. Ent., 13*, 137.

Haas, G.E. and Wilson, N. (1967). *J. Med. Ent. 4*, 25.

Hewitt, M., Walton, G.S. and Waterhouse, M. (1971). *Br. J. Dermatol., 85*, 215.

Hudson, B.W., Feingold, B.F. and Kartman, L. (1960). *Exp. Parasit., 9*, 18.

Lapage, G. (1968). "Veterinary Parasitology" 2nd edit.

Oliver and Boyd Edinburgh and London.
Michaeli, D. and Goldfarb, S. (1968). *Aust. Vet. J.*, *44*, 161.
Pfeiffer H. (1973). *Wien tierärztl Mschr 6/7*, 201.
Ressl, F. (1963). *Z. Parasitk.*, *23*, 470.
Smiley, R.L. (1965). *Proc. Ent. Soc. Wash.*, *67*, 75.
Smiley, R.L. (1970). *Ann. Entomol. Soc. Amer.*, *63*, 1056.

Subject Index

D

E

F

M

N

O

P

R

S

T

V

A 4
B 5
C 6
D 7
E 8
F 9
G 0
H 1
I 2
J 3